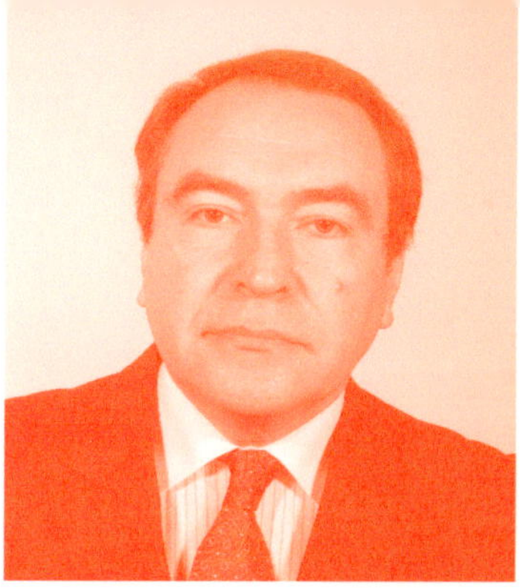

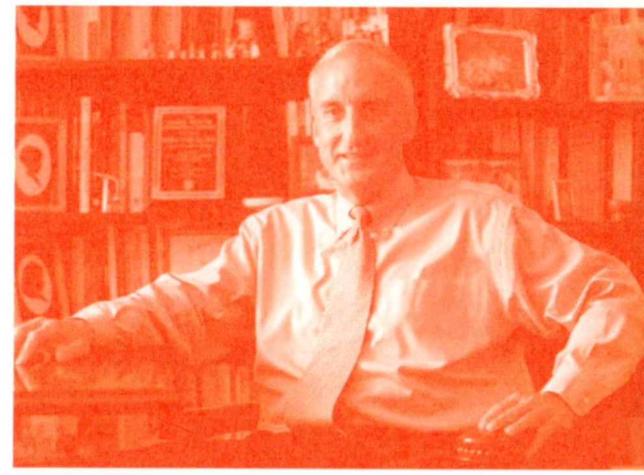

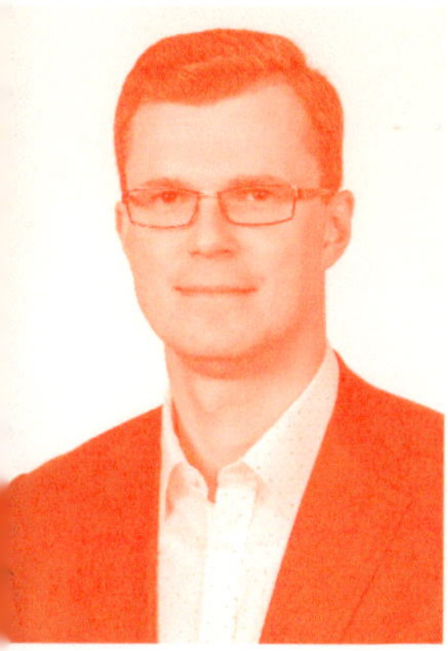

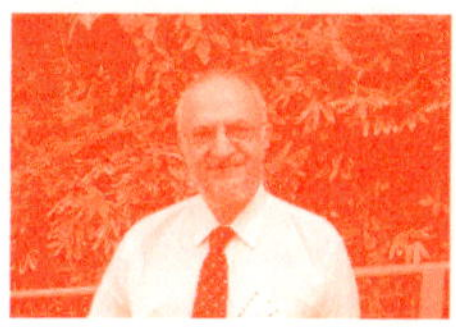

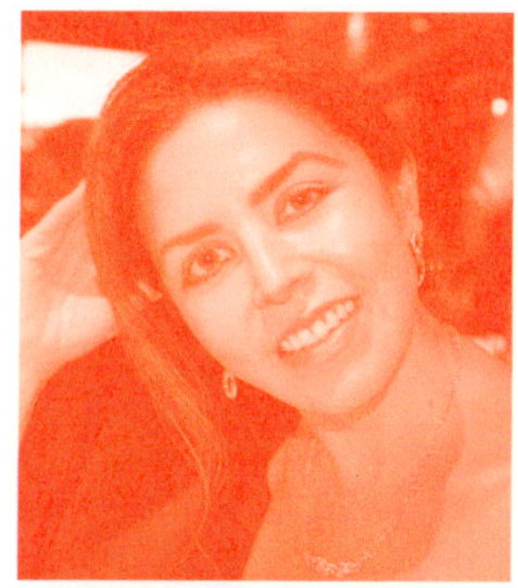

Supporting open minds since 2005

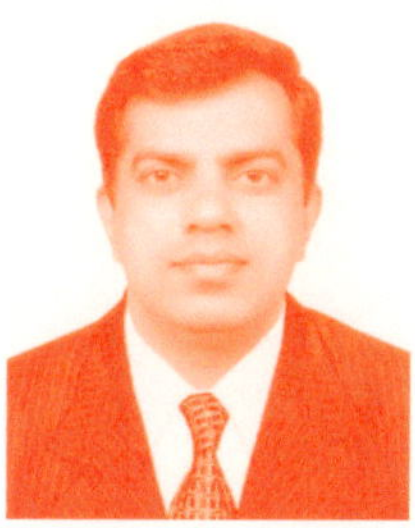

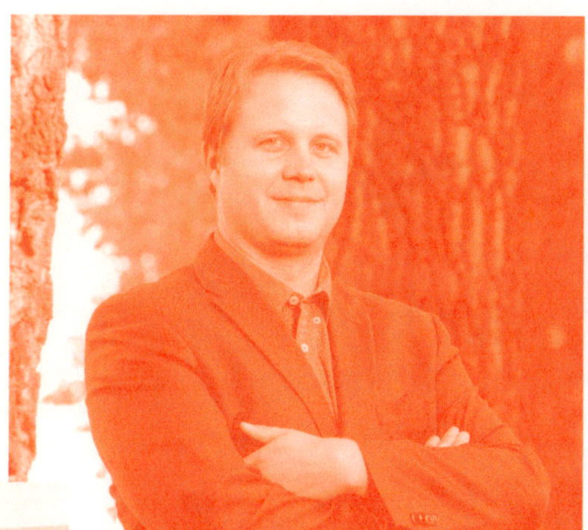

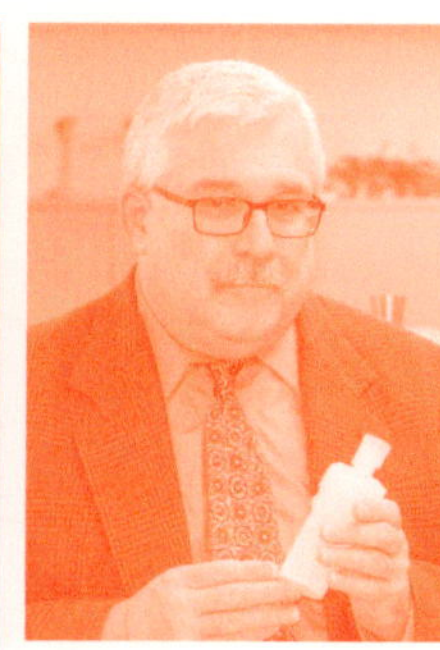

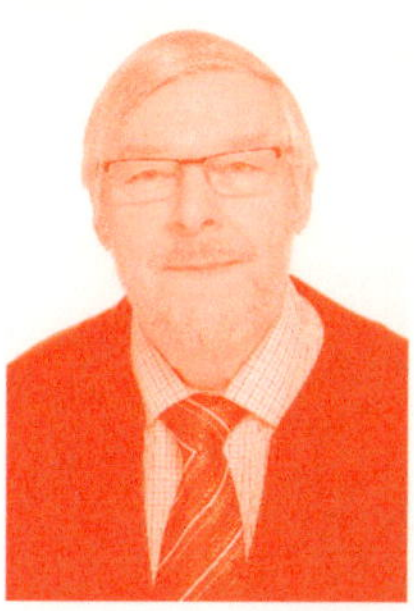

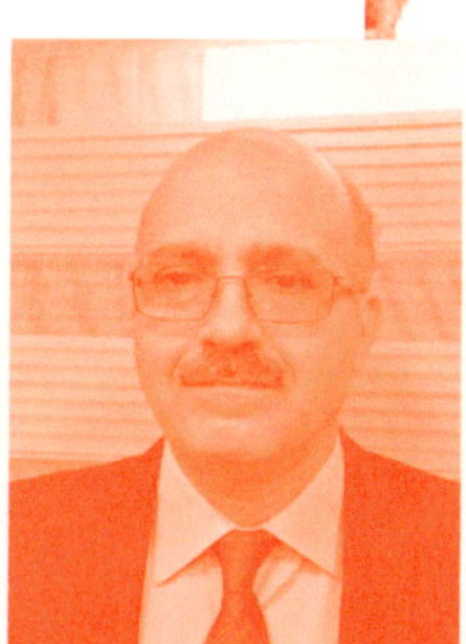

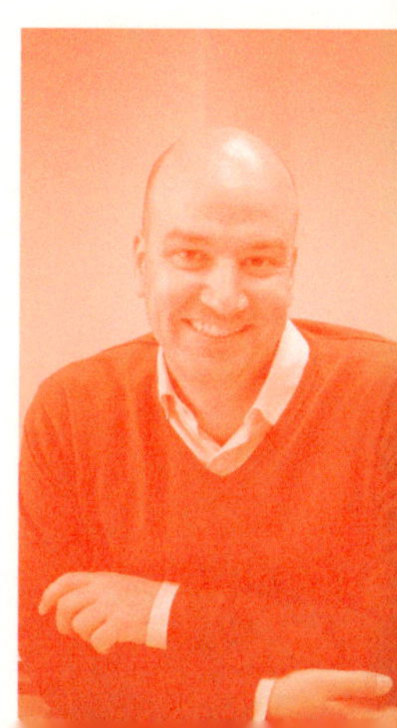

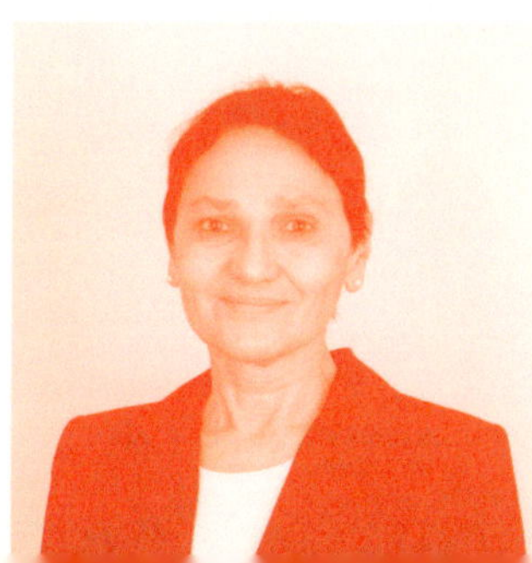

Translational Research in Cancer
http://dx.doi.org/10.5772/intechopen.73772
Edited by Sivapatham Sundaresan and Yeun-Hwa Gu

Contributors

Yeun-Hwa Gu, Mirko Salomón Alva-Sánchez, Thatiane Alves Pianoschi, Erik Bey, Edward Motea, Naveen Singh, Xiumei Huang, S. Louise Pay, Colton Starcher, Jayne Silver, I-Ju Yeh, Xiaolin Su, Kristen A. Russ, Thomas J. Fitzgerald, Elena Lastraioli, Jessica Iorio, Claudia Duranti, Petru Teodor Dragos Iancu, Tao Lu, Aishat A. Motolani, Annie Sun, Matthew Martin, Steven Sun, Adam McCluskey, Cecilia Russell, Maria Teresa Gonzalez Garza, Joaquín M. Campos, Ana Conejo-García, Olga Cruz-López, Mehmet Sait Bakır, Sivapatham Sundaresan, Palanirasu Rajapriya, Delia Elva Cruz-Vega, Carmen Maldonado-Bernal, David A. Boothman, Maryann Bishop-Jodoin, Fran Laurie, Richard Hanusik, Matthew Iandoli, Kathryn Karolczuk, Sandra Kessel, Fred Prior, Joel Saltz, Ashish Sharma, Michael Knopp, Mark Rosen, Ying Xiao, David Followill, Jeff Michalski, Ameer Elaimy, James Shen, Peter Lee, Maria Giulia Cicchetti, Janaki Moni, Camil Ciprian Mirestean, Călin Gheorghe Buzea, Roxana Irina Iancu

Notice

Statements and opinions expressed in the chapters are these of the individual contributors and not necessarily those of the editors or publisher. No responsibility is accepted for the accuracy of information contained in the published chapters. The publisher assumes no responsibility for any damage or injury to persons or property arising out of the use of any materials, instructions, methods or ideas contained in the book.

First published in London, United Kingdom, 2021 by IntechOpen
IntechOpen is the global imprint of INTECHOPEN LIMITED, registered in England and Wales, registration number: 11086078, 5 Princes Gate Court, London, SW7 2QJ, United Kingdom
Printed in Croatia

British Library Cataloguing-in-Publication Data
A catalogue record for this book is available from the British Library

Additional hard and PDF copies can be obtained from orders@intechopen.com

Translational Research in Cancer
Edited by Sivapatham Sundaresan and Yeun-Hwa Gu
p. cm.
Print ISBN 978-1-83880-534-0
Online ISBN 978-1-83880-535-7
eBook (PDF) ISBN 978-1-78984-837-3

For EU product safety concerns:
IN TECH d.o.o., Prolaz Marije Krucifikse Kozulić 3, 51000 Rijeka, Croatia, info@intechopen.com or visit our website at intechopen.com.

Meet the editors

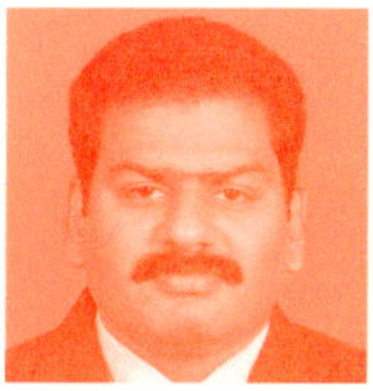

Dr. S. Sundaresan has been working in the field of cancer chemoprevention, cancer immunotherapy, and tumor marker detection. Translational research (TR) has been described as translating research into medical practice and translating science into better healthcare. Translational research on tumor biomarkers has successfully promoted the development of tumor treatment and has brought new hope for cancer patients. It is important to direct cancer research on diagnosis and treatment toward applying fundamental research findings to the clinic as soon as possible, and applying novel tumor molecular markers to early diagnosis, targeted therapy, and individualized treatment. Focused medical treatment should be given through the analysis of new tumor biomarkers and appropriate treatments. Dr. S. Sundaresan has been working with oral cancer and cancer biomarkers. There are newer molecular markers that are of clinical significance and they need to be studied in various populations. The administration of indoles and triterpenes for preventive and curative effects was studied in laboratory animals. Dr. S. Sundaresan's research study also demonstrates interferon beta synergistically works with chemotherapeutic drug cisplatin for liver, breast, and cervix cancer cells.

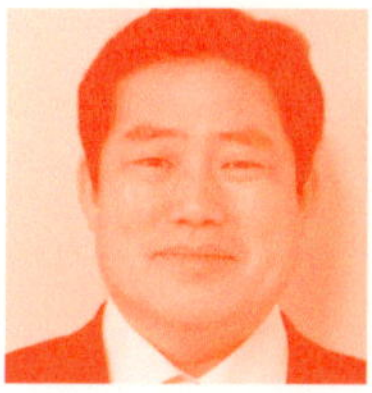

Dr. Yeun-Hwa Gu is working as a Professor for the Department of Radiation Oncology, Graduate School of Health Science, Junshin Gakuen University, Japan. He has worked as a Professor for the Department of Health and Medicine, Suzuka Medical Science University for 15 years. He graduated from the University of Tokyo with his Master's and Ph.D. degrees. He is currently working as an academic advisory committee member of the Korea Society of Health Sciences and academic director of the Korean Ultrasound Cancer Therapy (HIFU) Society and co-researcher of the Russia Space Radiation Chemistry Protection Study Group. He is a board member and editor of the International Journal of Food Science, Editor-in-Chief of Clinical Microbiology and Infectious Diseases and Current Traditional Medicine. He has published more than 250 papers in various peer-reviewed journals.

Contents

Preface

This book is intended primarily for researchers in translational oncology research, clinical oncology, and members of other professions such as medical researchers and radiography. It focuses on translational research in oncology, which has led to improvements in molecular diagnosis, tumor heterogeneity, and newer systematic therapies. This has brought challenges to the clinic in terms of patient education, toxicity management, workflow, and prognostication for palliative care.

Normally, the immune system is responsible for monitoring and getting rid of molecules or cells outside the body that can be potentially malignant. The immune system works to eliminate malignant cells; however, for reasons not well established yet, at some point, the immune system fails, and the malignant cells survive and establish. Importantly, IL-10 can exert the antitumor effect by mechanisms such as the activation of natural killer cells (NK), lymphocytes T, macrophages, and nitric oxide. The authors have presented the importance of IL 10 in cancer diagnosis and prognosis.

The book includes a chapter on ion channels and transporters (ICTs), emerging as potential cancer biomarkers. ICTs are aberrantly expressed in several types of human cancers, and exert a relevant role in mediating interactions between tumor cells and the tumor microenvironment. Such interactions drive different functions that in turn regulate neoplastic progressions, such as cell proliferation and survival, cell invasiveness, and pro-angiogenetic programs. Hence targeting ion channels and transporters for cancer diagnosis with antibodies becomes the need for cancer research to throw light on the discovery of many novel methods.

The book highlights that the epigenetic enzyme activity has been altered in cancer and contributes to the genomic instability in cancer cells. It is crucial to develop targeted therapeutic treatments to restore their normal function. Targeted therapy involves the use of drugs that target a specific biological molecule/pathway or drug treatment that requires genome profiling of an individual before it can be administered. Further it brought about the current update on epigenetics in the cancer treatment paradigm.

An effort has been made to give a synopsis of each different aspect of translational research in clinical oncology at the present time, which we hope will be of interest and benefit to all future researchers in clinical oncology.

Sivapatham Sundaresan
SRM Institute of Science and Technology,
India

Yeunhwa Gu
Junshin Gakuen University,
Japan

Chapter 1

Discovery of Small Molecule Inhibitors for Histone Methyltransferases in Cancer

Aishat A. Motolani, Mengyao Sun, Matthew Martin, Steven Sun and Tao Lu

Abstract

Cancer is the second leading cause of mortality in the United States. There are several therapeutic regimens employed to mitigate the mortality rate of cancer. This includes the use of chemotherapy, radiation, immunotherapy, and precision medicine/targeted therapy. Targeted therapy involves the use of drugs that target a specific pathway or biomolecule compromised in cancer for cancer treatment. Aberrant expression of epigenetic enzymes has been well documented for their contribution in driving tumorigenesis and other cancer hallmarks. Hence, there is an urgent need for novel drug discovery and development in epigenetics to help combat various cancer morbidities. Herein, we review the roles and consequences of dysregulated function of several epigenetic enzymes, with a focus on histone methyltransferases (HMTs). Additionally, we discussed the current efforts made in the development of small molecule inhibitors for a few representative HMTs implicated in different cancers. Furthermore, the common screening assays used in discovering potent small molecule inhibitors were also detailed in this chapter. Overall, this book chapter highlights the significance of targeting HMTs in different cancers and the clinical application potentials/limitations faced by the developed or emerging small molecule inhibitors of HMTs for the purpose of cancer therapy.

Keywords: cancer, drug discovery, epigenetics, histone methyltransferases, small molecule inhibitors

1. Introduction

Since the conception of the term “epigenetic landscape” by Conrad Waddington in 1940, the field of epigenetics has rapidly evolved with technological advances. In the study of embryonic development, it was observed that a single gene has the ability to produce different phenotypes, so epigenetics was used to describe the mechanisms through which that happens [1]. Today, epigenetics is defined as the study of changes in organisms caused by modification of gene expression through addition and removal of chemical groups to nucleotides and proteins rather than the alteration of the genetic code itself [2]. The human genome contains approximately 3 billion bases of nucleotides and they are compacted into chromosomes in the nucleus via histone proteins. About 146 base pairs of nucleotides are wound around core histone octamers and are sealed with the linker histone (H1) to form a nucleosome.

The linker histone connects multiple nucleosomes in the chromatin. The core histone octamers consist of two dimers of H2A-H2B and a tetramer of H3-H4 proteins [3]. These core histones contain two regions namely: the histone fold and the histone tails. The C-termini of H2A and N-termini of other core histones protrude out of the fold to form histone tails and are commonly subjected to epigenetic modifications [4]. DNA and RNA also undergo epigenetic modifications, and these modifications control gene expression and maintain genomic integrity. Epigenetic enzymes can be broadly categorized into three components: the writers, the erasers, and the readers. Writers are enzymes responsible for adding the modifications, erasers remove it, and readers recognize it. These modifications include but are not limited to methylation, acetylation, phosphorylation, ubiquitination, GlcNAcylation, and SUMOylation [5].

DNA mainly undergoes methylation, and this occurs through the action of a family of DNA methyltransferases (DNMT1, DNMT2, DNMT3a, and DNMT3b). DNMTs covalently modify DNA by catalyzing the transfer of methyl group from S-adenosylmethionine (SAM) to the C5 position on a cytosine ring. DNA methylation mostly occurs in CpG islands, a region of the DNA rich in cytosine and guanine base repeats [6]. This modification to the DNA functions to repress transcription when it occurs in gene promoters and regulates splicing when it occurs in gene bodies [7]. DNA methylation is a reversible mechanism, which can be either passive through reduced DNMT1 activity during DNA replication or active through activity of its erasers, DNA demethylases. For instance, the ten-eleven translocation proteins (TET 1/2/3) are human demethylases that catalyze the oxidation of 5-methyl-cytosine to 5-hydroxymethylcytosine [8]. Following DNA methylation, often readers such as the family of methyl binding domain proteins recognize the methylation marks to drive transcriptional repression [9].

RNA is also methylated on C5 position of cytosine (m^5C) and N6 position of adenosine ring(m^6A) by family of RNA methyltransferases such as Dnmt2, NOP2/Sun, Mettl3, and Mettl14. RNA methylation can be reversed by these RNA demethylases: fat mass and obesity associated protein (Fto) and α-ketoglutarate-dependent dioxygenase alkB homolog 5 (AlkBH5) [10]. Methylation modification on RNA is interpreted by readers such as the YTH domain family, and they mediate RNA splicing, export, stability, maturation, decay, secondary structure switch, and translation [11]. There have also been reports of RNA acetylation by NAT10 acetyltransferase, which functions to promote mRNA stability and efficiency in translation [12].

Moving up the central dogma, lysine and arginine residues on histone proteins are mostly subjected to various post-translational modifications by their respective epigenetic enzymes to either activate or repress transcription. Although the focus of this chapter is histone methylation, histone acetylation will be briefly discussed. Histone methyltransferases (HMTs) and histone acetylases (HATs) are the writers of histone methylation and acetylation, respectively. HMTs can be further subdivided into lysine methyltransferase (KMT) and protein arginine methyltransferase (PRMT) [13]. The families and functions of HMTs will be further explored in this chapter. On the other hand, several HATs have been discovered, with the major ones being the GNATs (Gcn5-N-acyltransferases), the MYST families, and p300/CBP [5]. These enzymes catalyze the transfer of acetyl group from acetyl Co A to the side chain amino group on histone lysine residues, inducing transcriptionally active chromatin [13]. Histone deacetylases and histone demethylases are involved in reversing the histone modifications discussed above. The families of lysine-specific histone demethylase 1 (LSD1) and Jumonji histone demethylases (JMJD) mediate the removal of methyl groups from histone through respective mechanisms [13, 14]. Readers of histone methylation include protein containing the MBT, PHD, chromo, Tudor, double/tandem Tudor, Ankyrin Repeats, zf-CW, WD40, and PWWP domains [15].

Given this array of epigenetic enzymes and their broad spectrum of function in regulating several gene expression in humans, the roles of epigenetic enzymes have been implicated in tumorigenesis. The epigenome of cancerous cells has widespread changes in DNA methylation and histone modification patterns [16]. For instance, hypermethylation of CpG islands in the promoter of chromodomain helicase DNA-binding protein 5 (CHD5), a chromatin remodeler, was observed in colon, breast, hepatocarcinoma, cervix, and glioma cell lines [17]. This results in the downregulation of CHD5, which plays a tumor suppressive role in cells. Similarly, hypomethylation of DNA at promoters of oncogenes such as insulin-like growth factor 2 (IGF2) has been observed in breast and colon cancers. The differential methylation patterns on promoters of tumor suppressors and oncogenes mediated by increased/reduced activity of DNMTs and TETs enzymes have been used as biomarkers to predict the predisposition of individuals to cancer [18]. Also, aberrant expression of histone acetyl transferases (HATs) and histone deacetylases (HDACs) has been linked to tumor development. Studies have shown that that p300/CBP acts as a coactivator with c-Myb to activate the transformation of fusion oncoproteins in myeloid leukemia [19]. Increased expression of HDACs was reported in gastric, prostate, colon, and breast carcinomas, and this results in repression of tumor suppressor genes like cyclin-dependent kinase inhibitor, see p21 [20]. Of all the histone modifications, histone methylation dysregulation is mostly attributed to poor prognosis in several cancers, which we will further elaborate in detail in *Section II* "Histone Methyltransferases in Cancer."

As these epigenetic enzymes' activity has been altered in cancer and contributes to the genomic instability in cancer cells, it is crucial to develop targeted therapeutic treatments to restore their normal function. Aside from surgery, some common treatment options for cancer patients can be broadly categorized as thus: chemotherapy, immunotherapy, radiotherapy, and precision medicine/targeted therapy [21]. These classes of treatments are not mutually exclusive and can be used in concert for treating cancer patients. Among these different therapeutic approaches, targeted therapy is the future for cancer treatment. Targeted therapy involves the use of drugs that target a specific biological molecule/pathway or drug treatment that requires genome profiling of an individual before it can be administered [22]. For optimal development of drugs for targeted therapies, it is important to identify a well-defined biological target whose activity contributes to one to several hallmarks of cancer including propagating growth signals, evading immunosurveillance, cell death resistance, activating metastatic programs, suppressing antigrowth signals, inducing angiogenesis, and enabling immortal replication of cells [23, 24]. For example, cancer patients whose tumors are driven by high activity of epidermal growth factor receptor (EGFR) signaling can be treated with specific monoclonal antibodies or small molecule kinase inhibitors antagonizing the aberrant signaling, and thereby reducing tumor proliferation [25]. Similarly, targeting an epigenetic enzyme, PRMT5, which is highly expressed in gastrointestinal cancers, with small molecule inhibitor, PR5-LL-CM01, was shown to slow down cancer cell growth and invasion *in vitro* [26]. The limitations of targeted therapies include cancer cell resistance to drug treatment by activating a parallel pathway or sometimes targets can undergo mutation, making drug accessibility to target difficult [27].

Given the myriad of biological targets that have been discovered to mediate cancer progression, there has been increasing interest in the development of small molecule inhibitors capable of decreasing the activity of those targets. Small molecules are intracellular targeting compounds with low molecular weight of less than 900Da. They can modulate their target activity as an agonist or antagonist [23]. The growing interest in the use of small molecules for drug development is not only due to their small size, which enables easy permeability into the cell, but also their desirable pharmacokinetics, pharmacodynamics, longer shelf life, and easy synthesis [28]. Several small molecule modulators have been developed into drugs to treat various types of cancers. The range of small molecule inhibitors developed to enable tumor regression can be broadly categorized into small molecule kinase inhibitors, proteasome inhibitors, metalloproteinases and heat shock protein inhibitors, and apoptosis targeting inhibitors [29]. The most common small molecule inhibitors, kinase inhibitors, have been used to inhibit the several protein kinases whose activity is dysregulated in cancers. The first tyrosine kinase inhibitor drug, Imatinib, is a small molecule ATP analog that competitively inhibits Bcr-Abl fusion protein kinase activity in chronic myeloid leukemia patients [30]. Similarly, a number of small molecule inhibitors targeting epigenetic enzymes implicated in tumorigenesis are in development or have been FDA approved for cancer treatment. For instance, drugs like belinostat and romidepsin are HDAC inhibitors that are FDA approved for the treatment of lymphoma [31]. After the first clinical trial in 2014, tazemetostat, an EZH2 small molecule inhibitor, moved to phase 2 clinical trial and was fast tracked by FDA in 2017 for the treatment of follicular lymphoma [32]. The use of tazemetostat for treatment of epithelioid sarcoma in adults 16 years and above was also granted accelerated approval by the FDA. These examples, among many others, show the potentials of epigenetic modifiers as a druggable target for cancer treatment. More of these small molecule inhibitors for histone methyltransferases will be explored later on in this chapter. However, challenges in the clinical application of certain small molecule inhibitors as drugs remain due to their off-target effects or development of resistance by cancer cells [29].

2. Histone methyltransferases in cancer

As we mentioned above, epigenetic enzymes, including histone methyltransferases, are novel targets for cancer therapy. In this section, we will review the role of histone methyltransferases in cancer.

2.1 Lysine methyltransferases

Lysine methylation of histones was first characterized in the 1960s [33, 34] and was initially described as an "irreversible" post-translation modification. This dogma was challenged by the discovery of histone demethylases by Shi et al. indicating a dynamic function of methylation allowing the addition and removal of methyl groups [35]. The proteins responsible for the addition of methyl groups to histones are known as lysine methyltransferases (KMTs). KMTs are broadly defined as SET [Su(var)3-9, Enhancer of Zeste, Trithorax] domain-containing proteins and non-SET domain-containing proteins [36]. The only non-SET domain-containing KMTs identified so far are DOT1 (disrupter of telomeric silencing 1) family members, which methylate K79 of histone H3 and which also do not share structural similarities with SET-containing proteins [37–39]. KMTs act by catalyzing the transfer of 1~3 methyl groups to lysine residues of histone and non-histone proteins through the addition of the cofactor S-adenosyl methionine (SAM), which acts as a methyl donor group [40]. In the case of SET domain-containing proteins, SAM interacts and orients with a lysine residue of the substrate histone tail within the catalytic pocket of the SET domain. Then, a tyrosine residue acts to deprotonate the ε-amino group of the lysine residue, which allows the lysine chain to nucleophilically attack the methyl group of the SAM molecule, transferring the methyl group to the lysine side chain [41]. In the case of non-SET domain-containing KMTs, the enzyme DOT1 acts to methylate a lysine residue in the histone core [40]. As we described above, histone methylation is a critical epigenetic modification of chromatin that can impact genomic stability, alter expression of different genes, determine cell lineage, alter DNA methylation, as well as control cell mitosis [42].

SET-containing proteins have been characterized in greater detail than non-SET-containing proteins. SET domain proteins are characterized as seven families of the superfamily of KMTs: SUV39, SET1, SET2, EZ, RIZ, SMYD, and SUV4-20 [36]. There are also several SET domain proteins that do not fall into these groups including SET7/9 and SET8 [36]. The SUV39 family has been characterized the most out of these groups of KMTs. Specifically, *Schizosaccharomyces pombe* Cryptic loci regulator 4 (CLR4), human SUV39H1, and murine SUV39H2 were among the first identified SET domain protein lysine methyltransferases characterized when their sequence homology between their SET domains was discovered. These proteins methylate lysine 9 of histone H3 (H3K9) [43]. SET1 and SET2 complexes are involved in the RNA polymerase II holoenzyme [44, 45]. TSET1 acts to tri-methylate H3K4 and is associated with early gene transcription as opposed to SET2-mediated methylation of H3K36, which is associated with later transcriptional elongation of downstream genes. The mammalian nuclear-receptor-binding SET domain-containing protein (NSD1, a member of the SET2 family) has an important function in methylation of H3K36 and H4K20 in development [46]. Lu et al. in our research group also reported that NSD1 could methylate non-histone protein, NF-κB, at K218/221 of its p65 subunit, leading to the activation of NF-κB and its downstream target gene expression [47–50]. Another example is SETDB1, a H3K9 methyltransferase, which is amplified in primary tumors of lung cancer patients and contributes to the invasive phenotype of tumor cells [51]. Additionally, SETDB1 methylates H3K9 in euchromatin, and is also required for development [52]. Human SET7/9 acts to mono-methylate H3K4 [53]. Furthermore, SET domain enzymes' functions are not specifically tied to histone methylation. Human SET7/9 methylates K189 on transcription factor TAF10, which increases RNA polymerase II affinity and transcriptional activity, thereby expression of TAF10-dependent genes [54]. SET7/9 is also involved in p53 methylation, which increases its stability [55]. These examples described are only a few of the many SET-containing proteins of which over 50 different proteins have been discovered [56]. While SET domain proteins are typically referred to as histone lysine methyltransferases, it may be more accurate to refer to them as protein lysine methyltransferases due to their identification of non-histone targets for these KMTs.

These examples of SET and non-SET domain-containing proteins exhibit the importance of KMTs in the regulation of histone and non-histone proteins. Therefore, it is not surprising that dysregulation of KMT function can result in dysregulation of cellular functions. Specifically several KMTs have been associated with tumorigenesis of several different cancers.

H3K9 methyltransferases SETDB1 and G9a are both known to have roles in gene silencing and embryo development [57]. G9a regulates cancer metabolism in several types of cancer [58]. Overexpression of G9a is associated with worse prognosis in patients with prostate cancer. Intriguingly, G9a knockdown in breast and lung cancer has been shown to promote E-cadherin expression and thus tumor metastasis [59, 60]. Moreover, G9a's higher expression predicts higher mortality of ovarian cancer patients [61] and is reported to be associated with cell growth and proliferation in neuroblastoma [57]. Furthermore, G9a has been shown to have a critical role in the development of pancreatic carcinoma and acute myeloid squamous cell carcinoma. G9a-dependent repression of genes is also associated with development of leukemia as well as squamous cell carcinomas [57]. SETDB1 is another H3K9 methyltransferase reported to play a role in numerous types of human cancer.

SETDB1 is involved in regulation of several cellular processes, including apoptosis, DNA damage repair, and regulation of transcription factors [62]. SETB1 is associated with oncogenic activity and is upregulated in several cancers including lung cancers, gliomas, and prostate cancer [63–66]. For instance, in lung cancer, overexpression of SETDB1 promotes invasiveness and knockdown reduced lung cancer cell growth. In gliomas, cell proliferation was reduced by suppression of SETDB1. In prostate cancer, downregulation of SETDB1 led to reduced cellular proliferation, migratory ability, and invasive ability.

EZH2 (Enhancer of zeste homolog 2), a H3K27 methyltransferase, plays an important role in transcriptional repression [36]. EZH2 plays a critical regulatory role in as many as 46 types of human cancer [57, 67]. Typically, EZH2 is overexpressed in cancers, and its high expression has been linked to worse patient survival. For instance, EZH2 downregulation in breast cancer can block cell growth and survival [68]. Moreover, EZH2 knockdown inhibits invasive ability and cellular proliferation in prostate cancer [69]. Additionally, EZH2 has also been shown to have roles in gliomas and renal cell carcinoma, wherein decreased EZH2 expression reduces cellular proliferative ability and promotes apoptosis [70].

Another example is SMYD3 (SET and MYND domain-containing 3). It is a KMT that methylates H3K4 and is extremely important for initiation of transcription. High SMYD3 activity is indicative of an epigenetic signature of active enhancers [71]. SMYD3 knockdown in colorectal cancer can impair cellular proliferation [72]. In breast cancer, knockdown of SMYD3 also inhibits cell growth, and overexpression can promote carcinogenesis by regulation of the Wnt signaling pathways [73]. Additionally, reduction of SMYD3 expression in prostate cancer inhibits cellular proliferation, migration, and colony formation [74].

H3K36 methylation is critical for transcriptional elongation, and H3K36 methyltransferases have been identified to play important regulatory roles in several types of cancer. NSD1, a H3K36 KMT, is involved in prostate cancer androgen receptor transactivation, which results in prostate tumorigenesis [75]. Overexpression of NSD1 in neuroblastoma reduces cellular growth ability and colony formation [76]. NSD1 has also been reported to play a role in myelomas and lung cancers [57]. As we described above, our lab also found that NSD1 activates NF-κB to induce its target gene expression. The function of these genes is frequently involved in oncogenic phenotype, or cytokine, chemokine secretion [47]. Another example is H4K20 methylation, which is reported to be important for gene transcription. For example, overexpression of methyltransferases of H4K20 SUV420H1 and SUV420H2 is associated with decreased cell invasiveness in breast cancer, and knockdown increases epithelial to mesenchymal transition [77].

DOT1, the only known H3K79 methyltransferase and non-SET containing KMT, also plays an important role in cancer development. DOT1 is involved in cell survival and colony formation in several forms of leukemia [78]. The activity of human DOT1L (hDOT1 like) methyltransferase is compromised in mixed lineage leukemia (MLL) and is required for maintaining proliferative state of transformed cells [79]. Also, downregulation of DOT1 in lung cancer can cause cell cycle arrest and reduce cellular proliferation [80].

Together, these examples show several of the pathways regulated by KMTs and also highlight the critical importance of tight regulation of these pathways wherein dysregulation of KMTs can result in promotion of tumorigenesis.

2.2 Protein arginine methyltransferases

In contrast to KTMs, there is another important family of protein methyltransferases, namely, protein arginine methyltransferases (PRMTs). It is a family of nine members (PRMT1-9) and specifically catalyzes the methyl transfer from SAM to the guanidine nitrogen (ω-NG) of the arginine residues of protein substrates [81]. After the donation of methyl groups, SAM forms S-adenosyl-L-homocysteine (AdoHcy, SAH) and methylarginine is produced [81]. There are three forms of methylarginine recognized in mammalian cells: ω-NG-monomethylarginine (MMA), ω-NG, NG-asymmetric dimethylarginine (ADMA), and ω-NG, N'G-symmetric dimethylarginine (SDMA) [82]. The family of PRMTs is categorized into three major types: type I, II, and III. Type I and II PRMTs first catalyze the formation of MMA, and then type I PRMTs (PRMT1, 2, 3, 4, 6, and 8) further catalyze the formation of ADMA, while type II (PRMT5 and 9) would instead catalyze the production of SDMA. For type III PRMTs (PRMT7), they only catalyze the formation of MMA [83]. These three types of PRMTs methylated similar substrates, such as histone, but they also can catalyze different non-histone substrate proteins. Additionally, although the majority of PRMTs methylate glycine-arginine-rich (GAR) motifs in their substrates [84, 85], some of them display a preference of methylation on the proline-glycine-methionine rich (PGM) motifs in substrate proteins such as PRMT4 [86, 87], while PRMT5 is characterized with the methylation of both types of motifs in proteins [86, 88].

PRMTs are widely expressed in mammalian cells and regulate primary cellular processes, including cell proliferation and differentiation. The abnormal expression of some types of PRMTs such as PRMT1, 4, 5 and 6 frequently leads to tumorigenesis and malignancy.

PRMT1 was the first protein arginine transferase recognized in mammals and assumes the large fraction of arginine transferases activity in mammalian cells [89, 90]. It has been reported that PRMT1 is related to various kinds of cancer. Le Romancer et al. suggested that PRMT1 governed the interaction of estrogen receptor α (ERα) with steroid receptor coactivator proteins (Src), the p85 subunit of phosphatidylinositide 3-kinases (PI3K) and focal adhesion kinase (FAK) [91]. PRMT1-mediated ERα methylation is integral for the activation of the Src-PI3K-FAK signaling pathway [91]. In their subsequent report, the authors further demonstrated arginine methylation of ERα by PRMT1 might remarkably activate protein kinase B (PKB, also known as AKT) [92]. Another example is methylation of Axin by PRMT1. Cha et al. showed that arginine methylation of Axin by PRMT1 may activate the WNT pathway by destabilizing Axin and promote tumorigenesis [93, 94]. Importantly, it is reported that methylation of meiotic recombination 11 (MRE11, also known as MRE11A) and p53 binding protein 1 (53BP1) by PRMT1 can block the DNA repair pathway, contributing to cancer progression [95, 96]. MRE11 combines with DNA repair protein RAD50 and Nijmegen breakage syndrome 1 (NBS1) to form MRE11-RAD50-NBS1 complex (MRN complex). The mammalian MRN complex plays significant role in repairing DNA double-strand breaks (DSBs). Yu et al. reported that the deficiency of arginine methylation of MRE11 in its GAR motif resulted in exonuclease and DNA-binding defects and finally failing to repair DNA damage [96]. Interestingly, Boisvert et al. found that 53BP1 could not relocalize to DNA damage sites and γ-H2AX formation was decreased in fibroblasts treated with methylase inhibitors [95, 97]. Moreover, Mitchell et al. discovered that depletion of PRMT1 affected the length and stability of telomere [98]. Since dysfunction of both DNA repair pathway and telomere maintenance is known to be the cause of cancer, deregulation of PRMT1 may lead to tumorigenesis by these pathways.

In addition to PRMT1, another PRMT member, PRMT4 (also known as CARM1), is reported to be tightly associated with estrogen-mediated oncogenesis of breast cancer through the upregulation of transcription factor E2F1 expression [99]. Moreover, CARM1 is suggested to be overexpressed in human colon cancer and exert a crucial role in Wnt signaling through mediating the action of β-catenin on Wnt target genes as a transcriptional coactivator [100]. Moreover, c-fos is a proto-oncogene and overexpressed in a set of cancers. Some groups reveal that PRMT4 regulates transcriptional activation of c-fos, and that matrix metalloproteinases (MMPs), c-fos target genes, are significantly downregulated in CARM1-deficient cells [101]. Therefore, arginine methylation by PRMT4 is related to multiple oncogenic signaling pathways.

An important PRMT member that plays a critical role in cancer is PRMT5. As a primary type II PRMT, PRMT5 functions in the presence of other binding partners, such as MEP50. Hou et al. discovered that E-cadherin expression was remarkably repressed by SNAIL and PRMT5 recruited by bridge molecule AJUBA, which was favorable for tumor metastasis [102]. It was also reported that p53 can be methylated on multiple arginine sites by PRMT5 in response to DNA damage [103]. Scoumanne et al. proposed that PRMT5 inhibition may promote cancer cells to progress toward apoptosis under chemotherapy/radiotherapy [104]. Moreover, Cho et al. found methylation of E2F1 by PRMT5 weakened its ability to promote apoptosis and repress proliferation, indicating PRMT5 overexpression may enhance cancer cells' growth and survival [105]. It is well known that continuous NF-κB activation exists in most cancers. Our group uncovered that PRMT5 dimethylated the p65 subunit of NF-κB at arginine 30 (R30) to activate NF-κB pathway [106], an important transcription factor that is involved in the progression of many cancers. Also, PRMT5 is reported to promote its own overexpression in several cancers through a feedback loop involving NF-κB signaling [107].

Besides the PRMTs we discussed above, PRMT6 is widely taken as a transcriptional repressor. Neault et al. reported that embryonic fibroblast cells from the PRMT6 knockout mouse were subjected to a premature senescence, while the cellular senescence can be rescued in PRMT6 and p53 double knockout mouse embryonic fibroblast (MEF) cells [108], affirming growth suppression effect of excess p53 due to PRMT6 deficiency. Thus, PRMT6 actively suppresses p53 cascade to promote tumorigenesis in cancer.

Taken together, many members in the PRMT family have shown essential role in cancer development and progression. Thus, it is unsurprising that these PRMTs have become the rising targets in cancer therapeutics in recent years.

3. Discovery of small molecule inhibitors for histone methyltransferases in cancer treatment

3.1 Screening assays for epigenetic drug discovery

The timeline of drug development from conception of the idea to a feasible drug available in the market for treatment of diseases takes between 12 and 15 years and can cost up to $1billion [109]. Drug discovery process begins with identifying a druggable biological target that contributes to a disease progression. These targets can be identified through text mining from online databases, microarray data mining using bioinformatic tools, proteomic data mining from proteomic databases, and chemogenomic data mining, which involves simultaneous exploration of multiple cell phenotypes by screening small molecules from chemical libraries to a number of biological targets [110]. Then, promising or known targets can be validated *in vitro* and *in vivo* to confirm that their activity influences phenotype associated with a disease. This step is followed by screening or high throughput screening (HTS), which describes the process of sifting through compound libraries for molecules with high affinity for a target of interest [111]. The two approaches of developing assays for compound library screening are the biochemical target-based approach and the cell-based approach. Biochemical target-based approach is often employed as the primary screening assay in epigenetic compound screen because it allows the direct monitoring of ability of a target activity as opposed to cell-based assays wherein changes in cell phenotypes are measured [112]. Listed below are some of screening assays used in the preclinical development of drugs for epigenetic enzymes.

3.2 AlphaLISA screen (amplified luminescent proximity homogeneous assay-linked assay)

AlphaLISA is a high throughput screening approach used to analyze and measure post-translational modifications, protein-protein interactions, and concentrations of analytes. The robust, highly sensitive, reproducible, miniaturized, scalable, and automated nature of AlphaLISA assays earned them their widespread application in research and drug discovery. The principle behind AlphaLISA technology is based on the mechanism of another methodology, Luminescent oxygen channeling immunoassay (LOCI). LOCI involves chemiluminescent reaction of a singlet oxygen transfer and was developed in 1994 by Ullman et al. to quantify latex particle binding [113]. Similarly, AlphaLISA assays employ biotinylated antibody bound to streptavidin donor beads and an acceptor bead bound to a second antibody. These antibodies are specific to different epitope on a protein (could also be product of a bimolecular interaction or a modified protein). The binding of these antibodies to the proteins brings the donor and the acceptor bead into proximity of at most 200nm. Upon excitation of donor beads at 680nm, a singlet oxygen is excited from the donor bead and this triggers singlet oxygen reaction with the chemical dyes (thioxene and europium) on the acceptor bead, which results in chemiluminescent emission at 615nm [114, 115]. Multiplate readers equipped with AlphaLISA screen detections can be used to record signals. A systematic method used to validate the quality of HTS assay output like AlphaLISA is called the Z-factor. The Z-factor is calculated by accounting for the positive and negative controls' mean signal-to-mean background ratio. Hence, in the design of AlphaLISA assay, to ensure quality control, wells containing maximum signal and no signal solution mix must be included [116]. This assay is widely optimized to screen for small molecule modulators for different epigenetic enzymes. For example, in our lab, Prabhu et al. used an optimized AlphaLISA screen protocol to identify a lead compound capable of targeting PRMT5, and subsequently, the compound was shown to be more potent in reducing pancreatic and colon cancer cells' proliferation compared to another commercially available compound EPZ015666 [26]. Not only is this assay used to screen for compounds for epigenetic targeted therapy, but also they uncover new roles of different epigenetic enzymes in cancer. Consequently, together with other assays, it was uncovered using AlphaLISA HTS assay that an inhibitor of G9a lysine methyltransferase, A-366, limits cell growth and differentiation in leukemic cells [117]. Potent small molecule inhibitors for EZH2, a methyltransferase known to silence tumor suppressor genes, are also being identified using this particular HTS assay [118]. AlphaLISA kits specific for histone methyltransferase modifications, among many other epigenetic enzymes, are commercially available for research and drug development purposes [119].

3.3 FRET (Förster/fluorescent resonance energy transfer) assay

Discovered in 1946 by Theodor Förster, FRET is cell-based assay that enables real-time observance of molecular interactions within cells [120]. This phenomenon depends on the proximal interaction (1-10nm) of a donor fluorophore and an acceptor fluorophore, whereby upon excitation, the donor fluorophore transfers energy to the acceptor, increasing its emission wavelength [121] (**Figure 1**). The measure of FRET is taken as the ratio of the intensities of the donor/acceptor fluorophore. Although highly sensitive in distance, FRET assay does not permit the level of sensitivity and high throughput as AlphaLISA [122]. A type of FRET, FLIM-FRET (fluorescence lifetime imaging FRET) was used to conduct epigenetic biomarker screening in ER-positive breast cancer cell line and patients. The utilization of FRET in this study was based on the presence of certain histone modifications around ERα in the nucleus. Consequently, the assay revealed H3K27ac and H4K12ac interaction with ERα, making HATs a potential therapeutic target in compound screening [123]. Another study optimized TR-FRET (time-resolved FRET) for high throughput screening, following the treatment with HDAC inhibitors, to detect the methylation levels of histone 3(H3) in U-2 OS cells using terbium-tagged antibodies specific to a particular H3 modification and green fluorescent protein (GFP)-tagged H3 [124].

3.4 In silico screen

In silico screening or virtual screening is a common method used in drug discovery as a pre-filtering method for identifying promising compounds that can be used for experimental studies. Drug development using this method of screening is estimated to save approximately $130 million and 0.8 years per drug [125]. The approach to virtual screening can be broadly divided into structure-based methods

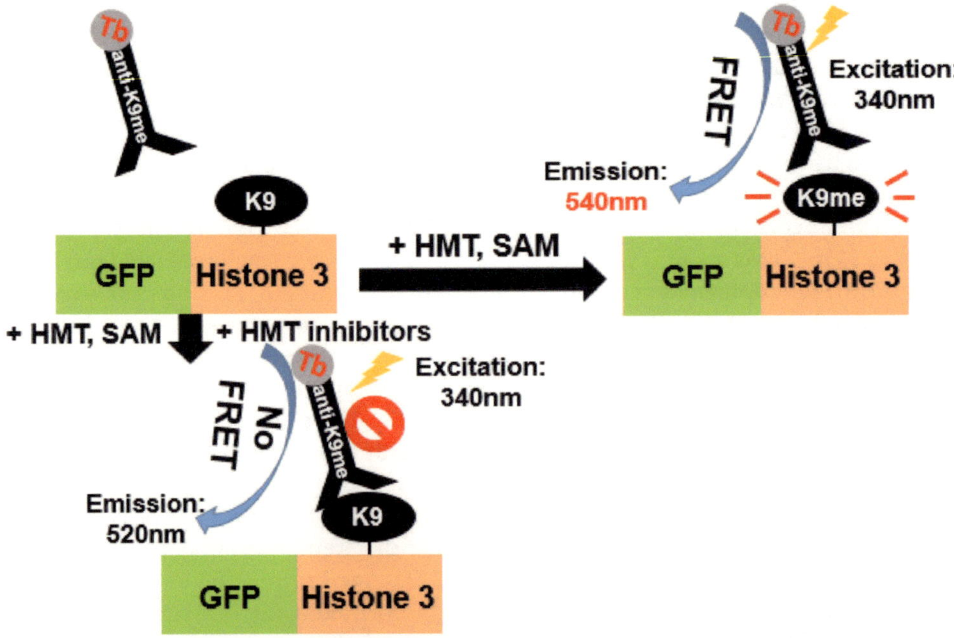

Figure 1.
*Schematic demonstrating the use of FRET for epigenetic screen. In the presence of histone methyltransferase and its methyl donor, SAM, a GFP-tagged Histone 3 becomes methylated on lysine-9 (K9) and undergoes FRET as terbium (Tb) conjugated antibody binds to the monomethylated K9 (K9me). This leads to increased GFP emission at 540nm wavelength (*Right arm of the diagram*), demonstrating the occurrence of K9 methylation. In contrast, when in the absence of K9 methylation mediated by HMTs, due to the addition of potent HMT inhibitors (*Lower arm of the diagram*), FRET does not occur as K9 cannot be methylated and thereby the antibody cannot bind to its epitope. As a result, the wavelength of GFP will be at lower end of the emission spectra, 520 nm.*

and ligand-based methods. Structure-based approach encompasses docking candidate molecules against available 3D structure of the target protein. When there is no crystal structure of the target protein, ligand-based approach is more useful because it relies on the screening of bioactive ligands of a similar chemical structure [126]. This approach is similar to pharmacophore-directed homology modeling: a process that involves superposing known active ligands for structurally similar targets and then extracting matching chemical properties of the ligand that are required for their bioactivity. Pharmacophore from different bioactive molecules can be generated using commercially available software such as HipHop, PHASE, DISCO, HypoGen, among others [127].

In computer-aided design of epigenetic drugs, there are a plethora of databases like ZINC containing over 35 million compounds available for screening. Other databases like *SPECS, Chembridge,* and *Enamine* have been used to identify inhibitors for most subsets of histone methyltransferases [128]. Molecular dynamics simulation also aids in drug discovery as they are employed to understand the conformational changes in the different domains of a target protein [129]. For instance, a study developed analogs of eosin, a template molecule known for having anti-methyltransferase activity, using pharmacophore methods. These molecules were docked on to PRMT1, SET7, and CARM1, and the AutoDock analysis revealed that compounds that target SAM substrate-binding site were more active in PRMT1 and CARM1 while those that target lysine and co-factor binding site were more promising in SET7 [126].

4. Current small molecule inhibitors of histone methyltransferases

Development of small molecule inhibitors for histone methyltransferases has garnered remarkable attention over the past years due to their combined efficacy and potency in various cancer treatments. In this section, we will discuss small molecule inhibitors of a few HMTs that have either shown promising results in preclinical development, clinical trial stage, or that have been FDA approved.

4.1 Small molecule inhibitors of EZH2

As aforementioned, EZH2 is a lysine methyltransferase that is overexpressed and found to contribute to many cancer progressions including but not limited to breast, prostate, colon, ovarian, liver, bladder, lymphoma, skin, and lung cancer. The overabundance of EZH2 causes hypersilencing of genes that restrain proliferation and promotes differentiation [67]. As a result, several studies have been conducted to understand the mechanism of action and structure of the enzyme so that appropriate drugs can be developed to inhibit its aberrant activity. For example, FDA has approved the use of tazemetostat (EPZ6438) (**Table 1**), an EZH2 small molecule inhibitor, for the treatment of epithelioid sarcoma (not qualified for resection) in 16 years and above patients. Tazemetostat has an inhibition constant (Ki) of 2.5nM and works by competitively inhibiting SAM binding site on EZH2 [32]. Another small molecule inhibitor, CPI-1205 (**Table 1**), completed phase 1 clinical trial for B-cell lymphoma and solid advanced tumor and is in phase 1b/2 clinical trial for metastatic castration-resistant prostate cancer (mCRPC) [130, 131]. Furthermore, another potent small molecule inhibitor, GSK2816126 (**Table 1**), which showed remarkable preclinical potential entered phase 1 clinical trial for the treatment of lymphoma and solid cancers but proved to be unsuitable target for inhibiting EZH2 due to its unfavorable pharmacokinetic profile [132]. More than 50 small molecule inhibitors for EZH2 are in preclinical development [133]. A few are highlighted in **Table 1**.

Epigenetic enzyme	Small molecule inhibitors	Stage of development	Cancer treatment	Reference
Lysine methyltransferases				
EZH2	EPZ6438 (Tazemostat)	FDA approved	Epithelioid sarcoma	[32]
		Phase 1 clinical trial	Various lymphomas and advanced solid tumors	[ClinicalTrials.gov] Identifier: NCT03010982
	GSK2816126	Phase 1 clinical trial	Lymphoma and advanced solid tumors	[132]
	CP1-1205	Phase 1b/2 clinical trial	B-cell lymphoma, advanced solid tumors metastatic castration-resistant prostate cancer (mCRPC)	[130, 131]
	EI1	Preclinical stage	B-cell lymphoma with Y641 mutation	[134]
	EPZ011989	Preclinical stage	Lymphoma	[135]
	UNC 1999	Preclinical stage	Diffused B-cell lymphoma with Y641N mutation and MLL rearranged leukemia	[136, 137]
hDOT1L	EPZ5676 (Pinometostat)	Phase 1 clinical trial	Acute myeloid leukemia (AML)/ acute lymphoblastic leukemia (ALL)	[138] [ClinicalTrials.gov] Identifier: NCT03724084
	EPZ 004777	Preclinical stage	MLL rearranged leukemia	[139]
	SGC0946	Preclinical application	MLL rearranged leukemia	[140]
Protein Arginine Methyltransferases				
PRMT5	GSK3326595(formerly EPZ015938)	Phase 1 clinical trial	Solid tumor and non-Hodgkin's lymphoma	[ClinicalTrials.gov] Identifier: NCT02783300
	JNJ-64619178	Phase 1 clinical trial		[Clinical Trial identifier: NCT03573310]
	EPZ015666	Preclinical stage	Mantle cell Lymphoma	[141]
	PR5-LL-CM01	Preclinical stage	Colon and Pancreatic cancer	[114]
	LLY-283	Preclinical	Ovarian, lung, breast, gastric, skin, and hematological cancers	[142]

Table 1.
List of representative small molecule inhibitors for EZH2, hDOT1L, and PRMT5.

4.2 Small molecule inhibitors of hDOT1L

There are over 20 hDOT1L small molecule inhibitors and can be categorized into four groups based on their mode of action: (i) SAH(S-adenosyl-L-homocysteine)-mimicking compounds; (ii) benzimidazole or (iii) urea group-containing compounds; and (iv) carbamate-containing compounds [143]. The activity of human homolog of yeast DOT1L or hDOT1L is mostly dysregulated in a subset of acute myeloid leukemia that has MLL gene translocation. This results in an onco-MLL protein which aberrantly recruits hDOT1L to the promoter of MLL target genes. Together with other transcription factors, hDOT1L drives the overexpression of HoxA9 and HoxA7 which leads to leukemia [141]. Hence, the need for inhibitors of hDOT1L. The first potent inhibitor of this HMT was EPZ004777 (**Table 1**), but it failed to progress through clinical development due to poor pharmacokinetics [139]. Another small molecule inhibitor, EPZ5676 (pinometostat) (**Table 1**) with Ki of less than 0.08nM, was shown to have improved pharmacokinetics and has now completed phase 1 clinical trial [138].

4.3 Small molecule inhibitors of PRMT5

PRMT5 is overexpressed in a several types of cancers. There are currently over 50 PRMT5 small molecule inhibitors, and PRMT5 is emerging as a hotspot for cancer targeted therapy [144]. Some small molecule inhibitors of PRMT5 are currently undergoing assessment in phase 1 clinical trial for non-Hodgkin lymphomas and solid cancers include GSK3326595 and JNJ-64619178 (**Table 1**). PRMT5 has also been implicated in the progression and metastasis of pancreatic and colon cancer. As a result, a lead compound, PR5-LL-CM01 (**Table 1**), has been discovered by our group to have more potent inhibitory properties compared to EPZ015666 in pancreatic and colon cancer cells [114]. However, EPZ015666 showed high potency *in vitro* and in mantle lymphoma cells with an IC50 of 22nM (**Table 1**) [145]. Another potent inhibitor of PRMT5, LLY-283 (IC50 = 20 nM) (**Table 1**) showed an outstanding inhibition of breast, lung, skin, ovarian, and hematological cancer cells' proliferation [142].

5. Conclusion, perspective, and future directions

Taken together, in this chapter, we discussed the important roles that epigenetic enzymes play in a variety of cancers. We also summarized several popular methods currently used for screening small molecule inhibitors of epigenetic enzymes. As shown in **Table 1**, we provided a list of representative small molecule inhibitors of HMT that are either FDA approved, or at preclinical or different stages of clinical trials. Notably, compared to the well-developed HDAC small molecule inhibitors, the development of small molecule inhibitors for HMTs is a rising and cutting-edge drug development area. We can envision that in the next 5~10 years, intense attention will continuously be drawn to the discovery of HMTs small molecule inhibitors. We have no doubt that many HMTs small molecule inhibitors will be shifted into clinical trials, more will be approved by FDA, and most likely, more members of HMTs will be targeted for cancer treatment. Additionally, it is very possible that novel HTS methods will emerge, which will further accelerate the discovery of anti-HMTs drugs. Moreover, it is viable that the clinical indications of HMTs small molecule inhibitors could be further expanded to other diseases beyond cancer. In summary, the development of new classes of anti-HMTs drugs will offer brand new and exciting opportunities for diseases treatment.

Acknowledgements

This publication is made possible, in part, with support from NIH-NIGMS Grant (#1R01GM120156-01A1) (to TL), and NIH-NCI Grant (#1R03CA223906-01) (to TL).

Conflict of interest

The authors declare no potential conflicts of interest.

Author details

Aishat A. Motolani[1], Mengyao Sun[1], Matthew Martin[1], Steven Sun[1] and Tao Lu[1,2,3]*

1 Department of Pharmacology and Toxicology, Indiana University School of Medicine, Indianapolis, IN, USA

2 Department of Biochemistry and Molecular Biology, Indiana University School of Medicine, Indianapolis, IN, USA

3 Department of Medical and Molecular Genetics, Indiana University School of Medicine, Indianapolis, IN, USA

*Address all correspondence to: lut@iu.edu

References

[1] Waddington CH. The epigenotype. Endeavour. 1942;**1**:18-20

[2] Kanwal R, Gupta S. Epigenetic modifications in cancer. Clinical Genetics. 2012;**81**(4):303-311

[3] Stefanelli G, Walters BJ, Ramzan F, Narkaj K, Tao C, Zovkic IB. Epigenetic mechanisms of learning and memory. In: Molecular-Genetic and Statistical Techniques for Behavioral and Neural Research. Cambridge, Massachusetts: Academic Press; 2018. pp. 345-382

[4] Iwasaki W, Miya Y, Horikoshi N, Osakabe A, Taguchi H, Tachiwana H, et al. Contribution of histone N-terminal tails to the structure and stability of nucleosomes. FEBS Open Bio. 2013;**3**(1):363-369

[5] Gillette TG, Hill JA. Readers, writers, and erasers: chromatin as the whiteboard of heart disease. Circulation Research. 2015;**116**(7):1245-1253

[6] Weber WW. Epigenetics. Comprehensive Medicinal Chemistry II. Vol. 1. Amsterdam, Netherlands: Elsevier; 2007. pp. 251-278

[7] Maunakea AK, Chepelev I, Cui K, Zhao K. Intragenic DNA methylation modulates alternative splicing by recruiting MeCP2 to promote exon recognition. Cell Research. 2013;**23**(11):1256-1269

[8] Carey N, Marques CJ, Reik W. DNA demethylases: a new epigenetic frontier in drug discovery. Drug Discovery Today. 2011;**16**(15-16):683-690

[9] Mahmood N, Rabbani SA. DNA methylation readers and cancer: Mechanistic and therapeutic applications. Frontiers in Oncology. 2019;**9**:489

[10] Blanco S, Frye M. Role of RNA methyltransferases in tissue renewal and pathology. Current Opinion in Cell Biology. 2014;**31**:1-7

[11] Yang Y, Hsu PJ, Chen YS, Yang YG. Dynamic transcriptomic m 6 A decoration: Writers, erasers, readers and functions in RNA metabolism. Cell Research. 2018;**28**(6):616-624

[12] Arango D, Sturgill D, Alhusaini N, Dillman AA, Sweet TJ, Hanson G, et al. Acetylation of cytidine in mRNA promotes translation efficiency. Cell. 2018;**175**(7):1872-1886

[13] Smith BC, Denu JM. Chemical mechanisms of histone lysine and arginine modifications. Biochim Biophy Acta (BBA)-Gene Regulatory Mechanisms. 2009;**1789**(1):45-57

[14] Tsukada YI, Fang J, Erdjument-Bromage H, Warren ME, Borchers CH, Tempst P, et al. Histone demethylation by a family of JmjC domain-containing proteins. Nature. 2006;**439**(7078):811-816

[15] Yun M, Wu J, Workman JL, Li B. Readers of histone modifications. Cell Research. 2011;**21**(4):564-578

[16] Portela A, Esteller M. Epigenetic modifications and human disease. Nature Biotechnology. 2010;**28**(10):1057

[17] Mulero-Navarro S, Esteller M. Chromatin remodeling factor CHD5 is silenced by promoter CpG island hypermethylation in human cancer. Epigenetics. 2008;**3**(4):210-215

[18] Ito Y, Koessler T, Ibrahim AE, Rai S, Vowler SL, Abu-Amero S, et al. Somatically acquired hypomethylation of IGF2 in breast and colorectal cancer. Human Molecular Genetics. 2008;**17**(17):2633-2643

[19] Sun XJ, Man N, Tan Y, Nimer SD, Wang L. The role of histone

acetyltransferases in normal and malignant hematopoiesis. Frontiers in Oncology. 2015;**5**:108

[20] Ropero S, Esteller M. The role of histone deacetylases (HDACs) in human cancer. Molecular Oncology. 2007;**1**(1):19-25

[21] National Cancer Institute. Types of Cancer Treatment. 2017. Available from: https://www.cancer.gov/about-cancer/treatment/types

[22] Ross JS, Schenkein DP, Pietrusko R, Rolfe M, Linette GP, Stec J, et al. Targeted therapies for cancer 2004. American Journal of Clinical Pathology. 2004;**122**(4):598-609

[23] Lee YT, Tan YJ, Oon CE. Molecular targeted therapy: Treating cancer with specificity. European Journal of Pharmacology. 2018;**834**:188-196

[24] Hanahan D, Weinberg RA. Hallmarks of cancer: the next generation. Cell. 2011;**144**(5):646-674

[25] Troiani T, Martinelli E, Capasso A, Morgillo F, Orditura M, De Vita F, et al. Targeting EGFR in pancreatic cancer treatment. Current Drug Targets. 2012;**13**(6):802-810

[26] Prabhu L, Wei H, Chen L, Demir Ö, Sandusky G, Sun E, et al. Adapting AlphaLISA high throughput screen to discover a novel small-molecule inhibitor targeting protein arginine methyltransferase 5 in pancreatic and colorectal cancers. Oncotarget. 2017;**8**(25):39963

[27] Suda K, Mitsudomi T. Successes and limitations of targeted cancer therapy in lung cancer. In: Successes and Limitations of Targeted Cancer Therapy. Vol. 41. Basel, Switzerland: Karger Publishers; 2014. pp. 62-77

[28] Nwibo DD, Levi CA, Nwibo MI. Small molecule drugs; down but not out: A future for medical research and therapeutics. IOSR Journal of Dental and Medical Sciences (IOSR-JDMS). 2015;**14**:70-77

[29] Lavanya V, Mohamed Adil AA, Ahmed N, Rishi AK, Jamal S. Small molecule inhibitors as emerging cancer therapeutics. Integrative Cancer Science and Therapeutics. 2014;**1**(3):39-46

[30] Capdeville R, Silberman S, Dimitrijevic S. Imatinib: The first 3 years. European Journal of Cancer. 2002;**38**:S77-S82

[31] Eckschlager T, Plch J, Stiborova M, Hrabeta J. Histone deacetylase inhibitors as anticancer drugs. International Journal of Molecular Sciences. 2017;**18**(7):1414

[32] Hauser AT, Robaa D, Jung M. Epigenetic small molecule modulators of histone and DNA methylation. Current Opinion in Chemical Biology. 2018;**45**:73-85

[33] Allfrey VG, Faulkner R, Mirsky AE. Acetylation and methylation of histones and their possible role in the regulation of RNA synthesis. Proceedings of the National Academy of Sciences. 1964;**51**(5):786-794

[34] Murray K. The occurrence of iε-N-methyl lysine in histones. The Biochemist. 1964;**3**(1):10-15

[35] Shi Y, Lan F, Matson C, Mulligan P, Whetstine JR, Cole PA, et al. Histone demethylation mediated by the nuclear amine oxidase homolog LSD1. Cell. 2004;**119**(7):941-953

[36] Dillon SC, Zhang X, Trievel RC, Cheng X. The SET-domain protein superfamily: Protein lysine methyltransferases. Genome Biology. 2005;**6**(8):227

[37] Feng Q, Wang H, Ng HH, Erdjument-Bromage H, Tempst P,

Struhl K, et al. Methylation of H3-lysine 79 is mediated by a new family of HMTases without a SET domain. Current Biology. 2002;**12**(12):1052-1058

[38] Ng HH, Feng Q, Wang H, Erdjument-Bromage H, Tempst P, Zhang Y, et al. Lysine methylation within the globular domain of histone H3 by Dot1 is important for telomeric silencing and Sir protein association. Genes & Development. 2002;**16**(12):1518-1527

[39] van Leeuwen F, Gafken PR, Gottschling DE. Dot1p modulates silencing in yeast by methylation of the nucleosome core. Cell. 2002;**109**(6):745-756

[40] Wood A, Shilatifard A. Posttranslational modifications of histones by methylation. In: Advances in protein chemistry. Vol. 67. Cambridge, Massachusetts: Academic Press; 2004. pp. 201-222

[41] Trievel RC, Beach BM, Dirk LM, Houtz RL, Hurley JH. Structure and catalytic mechanism of a SET domain protein methyltransferase. Cell. 2002;**111**(1):91-103

[42] Kouzarides T. Chromatin modifications and their function. Cell. 2007;**128**(4):693-705

[43] Rea S, Eisenhaber F, O'Carroll D, Strahl BD, Sun ZW, Schmid M, et al. Regulation of chromatin structure by site-specific histone H3 methyltransferases. Nature. 2000;**406**(6796):593-599

[44] Ng HH, Robert F, Young RA, Struhl K. Targeted recruitment of Set1 histone methylase by elongating Pol II provides a localized mark and memory of recent transcriptional activity. Molecular Cell. 2003;**11**(3):709-719

[45] Krogan NJ, Dover J, Wood A, Schneider J, Heidt J, Boateng MA, et al. The Paf1 complex is required for histone H3 methylation by COMPASS and Dot1p: Linking transcriptional elongation to histone methylation. Molecular Cell. 2003;**11**(3):721-729

[46] Rayasam GV, Wendling O, Angrand PO, Mark M, Niederreither K, Song L, et al. NSD1 is essential for early post-implantation development and has a catalytically active SET domain. The EMBO Journal. 2003;**22**(12):3153-3163

[47] Lu T, Jackson MW, Wang B, Yang M, Chance M, Miyagi M, et al. Regulation of NF-κB by NSD1/FBXL11-dependent reversible lysine methylation of p65. Proceedings of the National Academy of Sciences. 2010;**107**:46-51

[48] Lu T, Yang M, Huang D, Ghosh G, Stark GR. Role of lysine methylation of NF-κB in differential gene regulation. Proceedings of the National Academy of Sciences. 2013;**110**(33):13510-13515

[49] Lu T, Stark GR. NF-κB: Regulation by methylation. Cancer Research. 2015;**75**(18):3692-3695

[50] Stark GR, Wang Y, Lu T. Lysine methylation of promoter-bound transcription factors and relevance to cancer. Review. Cell Research. 2011;**21**:375-380

[51] Rodriguez-Paredes M, Martinez de Paz A, Simó-Riudalbas L, Sayols S, Moutinho C, Moran S, et al. Gene amplification of the histone methyltransferase SETDB1 contributes to human lung tumorigenesis. Oncogene. 2014;**33**(21):2807-2813

[52] Dodge JE, Kang YK, Beppu H, Lei H, Li E. Histone H3-K9 methyltransferase ESET is essential for early development. Molecular and Cellular Biology. 2004;**24**(6):2478-2486

[53] Xiao B, Jing C, Wilson JR, Walker PA, Vasisht N, Kelly G, et al. Structure and catalytic mechanism of

the human histone methyltransferase SET7/9. Nature. 2003;**421**(6923):652-656

[54] Kouskouti A, Scheer E, Staub A, Tora L, Talianidis I. Gene-specific modulation of TAF10 function by SET9-mediated methylation. Molecular Cell. 2004;**14**(2):175-182

[55] Chuikov S, Kurash JK, Wilson JR, Xiao B, Justin N, Ivanov GS, et al. Regulation of p53 activity through lysine methylation. Nature. 2004;**432**(7015):353-360

[56] Völkel P, Angrand PO. The control of histone lysine methylation in epigenetic regulation. Biochimie. 2007;**89**(1):1-20

[57] Li J, Zhu S, Ke XX, Cui H. Role of several histone lysine methyltransferases in tumor development. Biomed Report. 2016;**4**(3):293-299

[58] Ding J, Li T, Wang X, Zhao E, Choi JH, Yang L, et al. The histone H3 methyltransferase G9A epigenetically activates the serine-glycine synthesis pathway to sustain cancer cell survival and proliferation. Cell Metabolism. 2013;**18**(6):896-907

[59] Dong C, Wu Y, Yao J, Wang Y, Yu Y, Rychahou PG, et al. G9a interacts with Snail and is critical for Snail-mediated E-cadherin repression in human breast cancer. The Journal of Clinical Investigation. 2012;**122**(4):1469-1486

[60] Chen MW, Hua KT, Kao HJ, Chi CC, Wei LH, Johansson G, et al. H3K9 histone methyltransferase G9a promotes lung cancer invasion and metastasis by silencing the cell adhesion molecule Ep-CAM. Cancer Research. 2010;**70**(20):7830-7840

[61] Hua KT, Wang MY, Chen MW, Wei LH, Chen CK, Ko CH, et al. The H3K9 methyltransferase G9a is a marker of aggressive ovarian cancer that promotes peritoneal metastasis. Molecular Cancer. 2014;**13**(1):189

[62] Cho S, Park JS, Kang YK. Dual functions of histone-lysine N-methyltransferase Setdb1 protein at promyelocytic leukemia-nuclear body (PML-NB) maintaining PML-NB structure and regulating the expression of its associated genes. The Journal of Biological Chemistry. 2011;**286**(47):41115-41124

[63] Ceol CJ, Houvras Y, Jane-Valbuena J, Bilodeau S, Orlando DA, Battisti V, et al. The histone methyltransferase SETDB1 is recurrently amplified in melanoma and accelerates its onset. Nature. 2011;**471**(7339):513-517

[64] Lee JK, Kim KC. DZNep, inhibitor of S-adenosylhomocysteine hydrolase, down-regulates expression of SETDB1 H3K9me3 HMTase in human lung cancer cells. Biochemical and Biophysical Research Communications. 2013;**438**(4):647-652

[65] Spyropoulou A, Gargalionis A, Dalagiorgou G, Adamopoulos C, Papavassiliou KA, Lea RW, et al. Role of histone lysine methyltransferases SUV39H1 and SETDB1 in gliomagenesis: Modulation of cell proliferation, migration, and colony formation. NeuroMolecular Medicine. 2014;**16**(1):70-82

[66] Sun Y, Wei M, Ren SC, Chen R, Xu WD, Wang FB, et al. Histone methyltransferase SETDB1 is required for prostate cancer cell proliferation, migration and invasion. Asian Journal of Andrology. 2014;**16**(2):319

[67] Simon JA, Lange CA. Roles of the EZH2 histone methyltransferase in cancer epigenetics. Mutation Research, Fundamental and Molecular Mechanisms of Mutagenesis. 2008;**647**(1-2):21-29

[68] Holm K, Grabau D, Lövgren K, Aradottir S, Gruvberger-Saal S, Howlin J,

et al. Global H3K27 trimethylation and EZH2 abundance in breast tumor subtypes. Molecular Oncology. 2012;**6**(5):494-506

[69] Xu K, Wu ZJ, Groner AC, He HH, Cai C, Lis RT, et al. EZH2 oncogenic activity in castration-resistant prostate cancer cells is Polycomb-independent. Science. 2012;**338**(6113):1465-1469

[70] Xie L, Zhang Z, Tan Z, He R, Zeng X, Xie Y, et al. MicroRNA-124 inhibits proliferation and induces apoptosis by directly repressing EZH2 in gastric cancer. Molecular and Cellular Biochemistry. 2014;**392**(1-2):153-159

[71] Pekowska A, Benoukraf T, Zacarias-Cabeza J, Belhocine M, Koch F, Holota H, et al. H3K4 tri-methylation provides an epigenetic signature of active enhancers. The EMBO Journal. 2011;**30**(20):4198-4210

[72] Peserico A, Germani A, Sanese P, Barbosa AJ, Di Virgilio V, Fittipaldi R, et al. A SMYD3 small-molecule inhibitor impairing cancer cell growth. Journal of Cellular Physiology. 2015;**230**(10):2447-2460

[73] Hamamoto R, Silva FP, Tsuge M, Nishidate T, Katagiri T, Nakamura Y, et al. Enhanced SMYD3 expression is essential for the growth of breast cancer cells. Cancer Science. 2006;**97**(2):113-118

[74] Liu C, Wang C, Wang K, Liu L, Shen Q, Yan K, et al. SMYD3 as an oncogenic driver in prostate cancer by stimulation of androgen receptor transcription. Journal of the National Cancer Institute. 2013;**105**(22):1719-1728

[75] Chiam K, Ricciardelli C, Bianco-Miotto T. Epigenetic biomarkers in prostate cancer: Current and future uses. Cancer Letters. 2014;**342**(2):248-256

[76] Berdasco M, Ropero S, Setien F, Fraga MF, Lapunzina P, Losson R, et al. Epigenetic inactivation of the Sotos overgrowth syndrome gene histone methyltransferase NSD1 in human neuroblastoma and glioma. Proceedings of the National Academy of Sciences. 2009;**106**(51):21830-21835

[77] Yokoyama Y, Matsumoto A, Hieda M, Shinchi Y, Ogihara E, Hamada M, et al. Loss of histone H4K20 trimethylation predicts poor prognosis in breast cancer and is associated with invasive activity. Breast Cancer Research. 2014;**16**(3):R66

[78] Nguyen AT, Zhang Y. The diverse functions of Dot1 and H3K79 methylation. Genes & Development. 2011;**25**(13):1345-1358

[79] Okada Y, Feng Q, Lin Y, Jiang Q, Li Y, Coffield VM, et al. hDOT1L links histone methylation to leukemogenesis. Cell. 2005;**121**(2):167-178

[80] Kim W, Kim R, Park G, Park JW, Kim JE. Deficiency of H3K79 histone methyltransferase Dot1-like protein (DOT1L) inhibits cell proliferation. The Journal of Biological Chemistry. 2012;**287**(8):5588-5599

[81] Tewary SK, Zheng YG, Ho MC. Protein arginine methyltransferases: insights into the enzyme structure and mechanism at the atomic level. Cellular and Molecular Life Sciences. 2019;**76**(15):2917-2932

[82] Yang Y, Bedford MT. Protein arginine methyltransferases and cancer. Nature Reviews. Cancer. 2013;**13**(1):37-50

[83] Di Lorenzo A, Bedford MT. Histone arginine methylation. FEBS Letters. 2011;**585**(13):2024-2031

[84] Bedford MT, Clarke SG. Protein arginine methylation in mammals: who, what, and why. Molecular Cell. 2009;**33**(1):1-13

[85] Najbauer J, Johnson BA, Young AL, Aswad DW. Peptides with sequences similar to glycine, arginine-rich motifs in proteins interacting with RNA are efficiently recognized by methyltransferase(s) modifying arginine in numerous proteins. The Journal of Biological Chemistry. 1993;**268**(14):10501-10509

[86] Cheng D, Cote J, Shaaban S, Bedford MT. The arginine methyltransferase CARM1 regulates the coupling of transcription and mRNA processing. Molecular Cell. 2007;**25**(1):71-83

[87] Lee J, Bedford MT. PABP1 identified as an arginine methyltransferase substrate using high-density protein arrays. EMBO Reports. 2002;**3**(3):268-273

[88] Branscombe TL, Frankel A, Lee JH, Cook JR, Yang Z, Pestka S, et al. PRMT5 (Janus kinase-binding protein 1) catalyzes the formation of symmetric dimethylarginine residues in proteins. The Journal of Biological Chemistry. 2001;**276**(35):32971-32976

[89] Lin WJ, Gary JD, Yang MC, Clarke S, Herschman HR. The mammalian immediate-early TIS21 protein and the leukemia-associated BTG1 protein interact with a protein-arginine N-methyltransferase. The Journal of Biological Chemistry. 1996;**271**(25):15034-15044

[90] Tang J, Frankel A, Cook RJ, Kim S, Paik WK, Williams KR, et al. PRMT1 is the predominant type I protein arginine methyltransferase in mammalian cells. The Journal of Biological Chemistry. 2000;**275**(11):7723-7730

[91] Le Romancer M, Treilleux I, Leconte N, Robin-Lespinasse Y, Sentis S, Bouchekioua-Bouzaghou K, et al. Regulation of estrogen rapid signaling through arginine methylation by PRMT1. Molecular Cell. 2008;**31**(2):212-221

[92] Le Romancer M, Treilleux I, Bouchekioua-Bouzaghou K, Sentis S, Corbo L. Methylation, a key step for nongenomic estrogen signaling in breast tumors. Steroids. 2010;**75**(8-9):560-564

[93] Cha B, Kim W, Kim YK, Hwang BN, Park SY, Yoon JW, et al. Methylation by protein arginine methyltransferase 1 increases stability of Axin, a negative regulator of Wnt signaling. Oncogene. 2011;**30**(20):2379-2389

[94] Polakis P. Drugging Wnt signalling in cancer. The EMBO Journal. 2012;**31**(12):2737-2746

[95] Boisvert FM, Rhie A, Richard S, Doherty AJ. The GAR motif of 53BP1 is arginine methylated by PRMT1 and is necessary for 53BP1 DNA binding activity. Cell Cycle. 2005;**4**(12):1834-1841

[96] Yu Z, Vogel G, Coulombe Y, Dubeau D, Spehalski E, Hebert J, et al. The MRE11 GAR motif regulates DNA double-strand break processing and ATR activation. Cell Research. 2012;**22**(2):305-320

[97] Kuo LJ, Yang LX. Gamma-H2AX—A novel biomarker for DNA double-strand breaks. In Vivo. 2008;**22**(3):305-309

[98] Mitchell TR, Glenfield K, Jeyanthan K, Zhu XD. Arginine methylation regulates telomere length and stability. Molecular and Cellular Biology. 2009;**29**(18):4918-4934

[99] Frietze S, Lupien M, Silver PA, Brown M. CARM1 regulates estrogen-stimulated breast cancer growth through up-regulation of E2F1. Cancer Research. 2008;**68**(1):301-306

[100] Ou CY, LaBonte MJ, Manegold PC, So AY, Ianculescu I, Gerke DS, et al. A coactivator role of CARM1 in the dysregulation of beta-catenin activity in colorectal cancer cell growth and gene

expression. Molecular Cancer Research. 2011;**9**(5):660-670

[101] Fauquier L, Duboe C, Jore C, Trouche D, Vandel L. Dual role of the arginine methyltransferase CARM1 in the regulation of c-Fos target genes. The FASEB Journal. 2008;**22**(9):3337-3347

[102] Hou Z, Peng H, Ayyanathan K, Yan KP, Langer EM, Longmore GD, et al. The LIM protein AJUBA recruits protein arginine methyltransferase 5 to mediate SNAIL-dependent transcriptional repression. Molecular and Cellular Biology. 2008;**28**(10):3198-3207

[103] Jansson M, Durant ST, Cho EC, Sheahan S, Edelmann M, Kessler B, et al. Arginine methylation regulates the p53 response. Nature Cell Biology. 2008;**10**(12):1431-1439

[104] Scoumanne A, Zhang J, Chen X. PRMT5 is required for cell-cycle progression and p53 tumor suppressor function. Nucleic Acids Research. 2009;**37**(15):4965-4976

[105] Cho EC, Zheng S, Munro S, Liu G, Carr SM, Moehlenbrink J, et al. Arginine methylation controls growth regulation by E2F-1. The EMBO Journal. 2012;**31**(7):1785-1797

[106] Wei H, Wang B, Miyagi M, She Y, Gopalan B, Huang DB, et al. PRMT5 dimethylates R30 of the p65 subunit to activate NF-κB. Proceedings of the National Academy of Sciences. 2013;**110**(33):13516-13521

[107] Shailesh H, Zakaria ZZ, Baiocchi R, Sif S. Protein arginine methyltransferase 5 (PRMT5) dysregulation in cancer. Oncotarget. 2018;**9**(94):36705-36718

[108] Neault M, Mallette FA, Vogel G, Michaud-Levesque J, Richard S. Ablation of PRMT6 reveals a role as a negative transcriptional regulator of the p53 tumor suppressor. Nucleic Acids Research. 2012;**40**(19):9513-9521

[109] Hughes JP, Rees S, Kalindjian SB, Philpott KL. Principles of early drug discovery. British Journal of Pharmacology. 2011;**162**(6):1239-1249

[110] Yang Y, Adelstein SJ, Kassis AI. Target discovery from data mining approaches. Drug Discovery Today. 2012;**17**:S16-S23

[111] Janzen WP. Screening technologies for small molecule discovery: The state of the art. Chemistry & Biology. 2014;**21**(9):1162-1170

[112] Gul S. Epigenetic assays for chemical biology and drug discovery. Clinical Epigenetics. 2017;**9**(1):41

[113] Yasgar A, Jadhav A, Simeonov A, Coussens NP. AlphaScreen-based assays: Ultra-high-throughput screening for small-molecule inhibitors of challenging enzymes and protein-protein interactions. Methods in Molecular Biology. 2016;**1439**:77-98

[114] Prabhu L, Chen L, Wei H, Demir Ö, Safa A, Zeng L, et al. Development of an AlphaLISA high throughput technique to screen for small molecule inhibitors targeting protein arginine methyltransferases. Molecular BioSystems. 2017;**13**(12):2509-2520

[115] Beaudet L, Rodriguez-Suarez R, Venne MH, Caron M, Bédard J, Brechler V, et al. AlphaLISA immunoassays: The no-wash alternative to ELISAs for research and drug discovery. Nature Methods. 2008;**5**(12):A10

[116] Zhang JH, Chung TD, Oldenburg KR. A simple statistical parameter for use in evaluation and validation of high throughput screening assays. Journal of Biomolecular Screening. 1999;**4**(2):67-73

[117] Pappano WN, Guo J, He Y, Ferguson D, Jagadeeswaran S, Osterling DJ, et al. The histone

methyltransferase inhibitor A-366 uncovers a role for G9a/GLP in the epigenetics of leukemia. PLoS One. 2015;**10**(7):e0131716

[118] Verma SK, Knight SD. Recent progress in the discovery of small-molecule inhibitors of the HMT EZH2 for the treatment of cancer. Future Medicinal Chemistry. 2013;**5**(14):1661-1670

[119] Simard JR, Plant M, Emkey R, Yu V. Development and implementation of a high-throughput AlphaLISA assay for identifying inhibitors of EZH2 methyltransferase. Assay and Drug Development Technologies. 2013;**11**(3):152-162

[120] Song Y, Madahar V, Liao J. Development of FRET assay into quantitative and high-throughput screening technology platforms for protein–protein interactions. Annals of Biomedical Engineering. 2011;**39**(4):1224-1234

[121] Bajar BT, Wang ES, Zhang S, Lin MZ, Chu J. A guide to fluorescent protein FRET pairs. Sensors. 2016;**16**(9):1488

[122] Glickman JF, Wu X, Mercuri R, Illy C, Bowen BR, He Y, et al. A comparison of ALPHAScreen, TR-FRET, and TRF as assay methods for FXR nuclear receptors. Journal of Biomolecular Screening. 2002;**7**(1):3-10

[123] Liu W, Cui Y, Ren W, Irudayaraj J. Epigenetic biomarker screening by FLIM-FRET for combination therapy in ER+ breast cancer. Clinical Epigenetics. 2019;**11**(1):16

[124] Machleidt T, Robers MB, Hermanson SB, Dudek JM, Bi K. TR-FRET cellular assays for interrogating posttranslational modifications of histone H3. Journal of Biomolecular Screening. 2011;**16**(10):1236-1246

[125] Seifert MH, Wolf K, Vitt D. Virtual high-throughput in silico screening. Biosilico. 2003;**1**(4):143-149

[126] Heinke R, Carlino L, Kannan S, Jung M, Sippl W. Computer-and structure-based lead design for epigenetic targets. Bioorganic & Medicinal Chemistry. 2011;**19**(12):3605-3615

[127] Yang SY. Pharmacophore modeling and applications in drug discovery: Challenges and recent advances. Drug Discovery Today. 2010;**15**(11-12):444-450

[128] Lu W, Zhang R, Jiang H, Zhang H, Luo C. Computer-aided drug design in epigenetics. Frontiers in Chemistry. 2018;**6**:57

[129] Zhou R, Xie Y, Hu H, Hu G, Patel VS, Zhang J, et al. Molecular mechanism underlying PRMT1 dimerization for SAM binding and methylase activity. Journal of Chemical Information and Modeling. 2015;**55**(12):2623-2632

[130] Vaswani RG, Gehling VS, Dakin LA, Cook AS, Nasveschuk CG, Duplessis M, et al. Identification of (R)-N-((4-Methoxy-6-methyl-2-oxo-1, 2-dihydropyridin-3-yl) methyl)-2-methyl-1-(1-(1-(2, 2, 2-trifluoroethyl) piperidin-4-yl) ethyl)-1 H-indole-3-carboxamide (CPI-1205), a potent and selective inhibitor of histone methyltransferase EZH2, suitable for phase I clinical trials for B-Cell lymphomas. Journal of Medicinal Chemistry. 2016;**59**(21):9928-9941

[131] Taplin M, Hussain A, Shah S, Shore ND, Edenfield JW, Sartor OA, et al. Phase Ib results of ProSTAR: CPI-1205, EZH2 inhibitor, combined with enzalutamide (E) or abiraterone/prednisone (A/P) in patients with

metastatic castration-resistant prostate cancer (mCRPC). Cancer Research. 2019;**79**(13 Suppl):CT094

[132] Yap TA, Winter JN, Giulino-Roth L, Longley J, Lopez J, Michot JM, et al. Phase I study of the novel enhancer of zeste homolog 2 (EZH2) inhibitor GSK2816126 in patients with advanced hematologic and solid tumors. Clinical Cancer Research. 2019;**25**(24):7331-7339

[133] Gulati N, Béguelin W, Giulino-Roth L. Enhancer of zeste homolog 2 (EZH2) inhibitors. Leukemia & Lymphoma. London, UK. 2018;**59**(7):1574-1585

[134] Qi W, Chan H, Teng L, Li L, Chuai S, Zhang R, et al. Selective inhibition of Ezh2 by a small molecule inhibitor blocks tumor cells proliferation. Proceedings of the National Academy of Sciences. 2012;**109**(52):21360-21365

[135] Campbell JE, Kuntz KW, Knutson SK, Warholic NM, Keilhack H, Wigle TJ, et al. EPZ011989, a potent, orally-available EZH2 inhibitor with robust *in vivo* activity. ACS Medicinal Chemistry Letters. 2015;**6**(5):491-495

[136] Konze KD, Ma A, Li F, Barsyte-Lovejoy D, Parton T, MacNevin CJ, et al. An orally bioavailable chemical probe of the lysine methyltransferases EZH2 and EZH1. ACS Chemical Biology. 2013;**8**(6):1324-1334

[137] Xu B, On DM, Ma A, Parton T, Konze KD, Pattenden SG, et al. Selective inhibition of EZH2 and EZH1 enzymatic activity by a small molecule suppresses MLL-rearranged leukemia. Blood. 2015;**125**(2):346-357

[138] Daigle SR, Olhava EJ, Therkelsen CA, Basavapathruni A, Jin L, Boriack-Sjodin PA, et al. Potent inhibition of DOT1L as treatment of MLL-fusion leukemia. Blood. 2013;**122**(6):1017-1025

[139] Chen L, Deshpande AJ, Banka D, Bernt KM, Dias S, Buske C, et al. Abrogation of MLL–AF10 and CALM–AF10-mediated transformation through genetic inactivation or pharmacological inhibition of the H3K79 methyltransferase Dot1l. Leukemia. 2013;**27**(4):813-822

[140] Wong M, Polly P, Liu T. The histone methyltransferase DOT1L: Regulatory functions and a cancer therapy target. American Journal of Cancer Research. 2015;**5**(9):2823-2837

[141] Song Y, Wu F, Wu J. Targeting histone methylation for cancer therapy: Enzymes, inhibitors, biological activity and perspectives. Journal of Hematology & Oncology. 2016;**9**(1):49

[142] Bonday ZQ, Cortez GS, Grogan MJ, Antonysamy S, Weichert K, Bocchinfuso WP, et al. LLY-283, a potent and selective inhibitor of arginine methyltransferase 5, PRMT5, with antitumor activity. ACS Medicinal Chemistry Letters. 2018;**9**(7):612-617

[143] Li KK, Huang K, Kondengaden S, Wooten J, Reyhanfard H, Qing Z, et al. Histone methyltransferase inhibitors for cancer therapy. In: Epigenetic technological applications. Academic Press; 2015. pp. 363-395

[144] Zhou Z, Feng Z, Hu D, Yang P, Gur M, Bahar I, et al. A novel small-molecule antagonizes PRMT5-mediated KLF4 methylation for targeted therapy. eBioMedicine. 2019;**44**:98-111

[145] Chan-Penebre E, Kuplast KG, Majer CR, Boriack-Sjodin PA, Wigle TJ, Johnston LD, et al. A selective inhibitor of PRMT5 with in vivo and in vitro potency in MCL models. Nature Chemical Biology. 2015;**11**(6):432

Chapter 2

IL10 as Cancer Biomarker

Maria Teresa Gonzalez-Garza, Delia Elva Cruz-Vega and Carmen Maldonado-Bernal

Abstract

Chronic inflammation can trigger events that would induce the malignant transformation of cells and carcinogenesis. Cytokines play a crucial role and can control the development and multiplication of cancerous cells. However, clinical data present controversy about the participation of these proteins in the establishment and development of cancer. Interleukin 10 (IL-10), a potent anti-inflammatory cytokine, has been the subject of multiple studies. Several studies have reported that IL-10 has pro- and antitumor effects. Elevated levels of IL-10 are associated with increased tumor growth with poor prognosis and drug resistance. However, this cytokine has both tumor-promoting and tumor-inhibiting properties. *In vitro* and *in vivo* studies report mechanisms by which IL-10 expression downregulates class I, which results in the control of the metastatic disease. IL-10 also inhibits tumorigenesis via downregulation of other cytokines. The variation observed could be the result of concentration ranges of this protein, genetic polymorphism, or both. The value obtained may serve as a biomarker indicative of tumor development and its prognosis.

Keywords: interleukin 10, IL-10, IL10 polymorphism, cancer biomarker

1. Introduction

The immune system is responsible for monitoring and getting rid of molecules or cells outside the body that can be potentially malignant. This system is constituted by cells that can act by themselves or the synthesis of molecules capable of inducing the destruction of strange agents or invading cells. In addition, these cells synthesize proteins called cytokines, which are not only capable of destroying invading cells; they activate other cells of the same immune system, which makes the system efficient. In a coordinated way, the synthesis of anti-inflammatory cytokines begins that will stop the inflammatory process and prevent the damage from spreading in healthy tissue. In the case of cancer, the cells will have nonnormal characteristics due to the changes they undergo during their transformation. The immune system works to eliminate these cells; however, for reasons not well established yet, at some point, the immune system fails, and the malignant cells survive and establish [1]. Even when the production of anti-inflammatory cytokines is present, the levels of pro- and anti-inflammatory cytokines have an imbalance that prevents completing the final objective. An increase of anti-inflammatory cytokines, such as interleukin 10 (IL-10), has been associated with a poor prognosis and considered as a biomarker for cancer disease. This chapter presents evidence that shows alterations in the serum levels of IL-10 in cancer patients, the participation of the cancerous tumor in the synthesis of this cytokine, and its possible relationship with polymorphisms in the gene promoter, the gene of this protein.

2. Interleukin 10 (IL-10)

IL-10 is an important regulatory cytokine with a potent anti-inflammatory effect. In humans, it is encoded by the IL10 gene [2]. It presents polymorphisms (SNPs), most of them within the promoter regions, and has been proposed as responsible for the altered function, by dysregulating their expression. Several groups report associations between polymorphism and cancer risk [3–7]. It is a helical cytokine and exists in solution predominantly as a homodimer, composed of two polypeptide chains of 160 amino acids, each with a molecular weight of 20,6419 kD [8].

IL-10 was initially thought to be produced only by T helper (Th2) cells but is now known to be made by a variety of cell types [9]. It is primarily produced by monocytes upon PD-1 triggering in these cells and, to a lesser extent, lymphocytes type 2 T helper cells (TH2), mast cells, CD4+CD25+Foxp3+ regulatory T cells, and in a specific subset of activated T cells and B cells (**Figure 1**) [10]. IL-10 expression is minimal in unstimulated tissues and seems to require triggering [11].

Cytokine signals are generated through a receptor complex consisting of two IL-10 receptor-1 and two IL-10 receptor-2 proteins. After IL-10 binding, it induces STAT3 signaling via the phosphorylation of the cytoplasmic tails of IL-10 receptor 1 + IL-10 receptor 2 by JAK1 and Tyk2, respectively (**Figure 2**) [12, 13].

IL-10 expression is regulated at the transcriptional and posttranscriptional levels. Extensive IL-10 locus remodeling in monocytes upon the stimulation of Toll-like receptor (TLR) or Fc receptor pathways was described. Induction involves ERK1/2, p38, and NF-κB signaling and transcriptional activation via promoter binding of

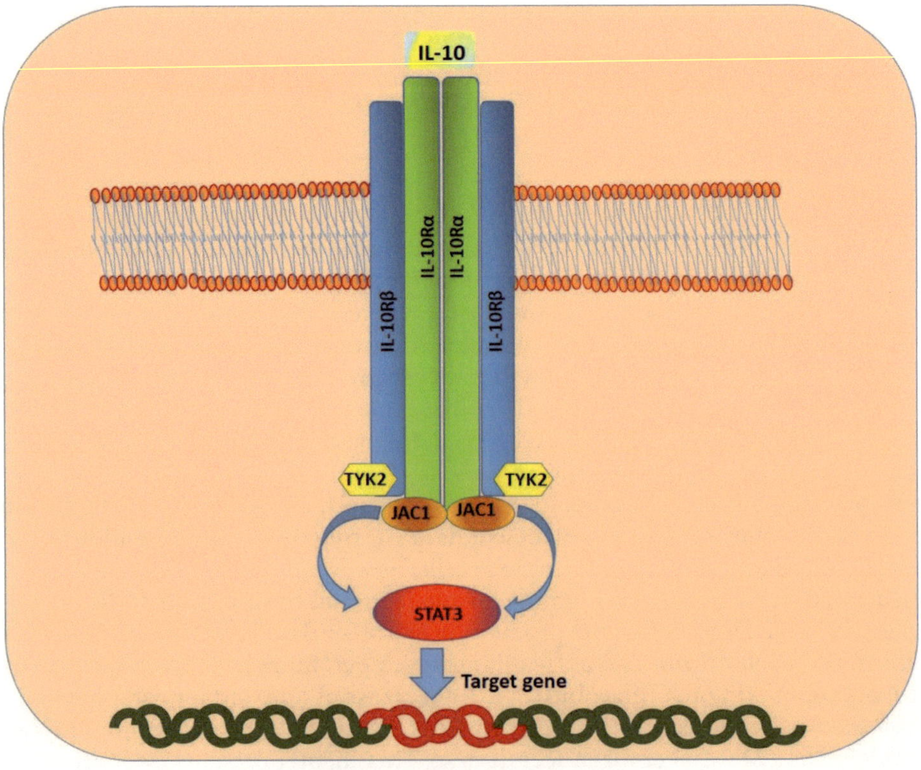

Figure 1.
IL-10R homodimers bind to form in a tetrameric heterodimer after IL-10 binds to its receptor α. It downstream signaling through STAT3 until target genes.

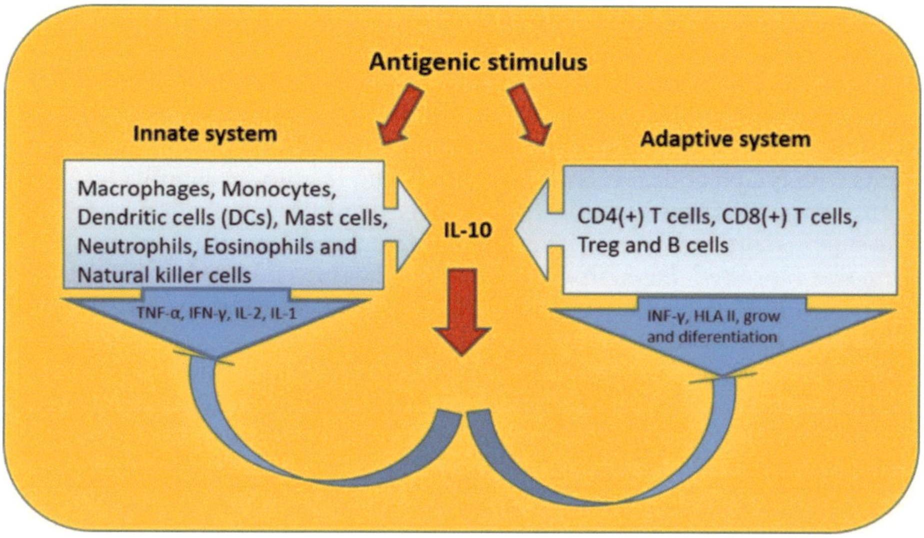

Figure 2.
After antigenic stimulus on cells from innate and adaptive system, the IL-10 is expressed from these cells. To avoid severe danger from pro-inflammatory cytokines and reactive radicals, IL-10 acts as anti-inflammatory cytokine by blocking its expression.

the transcription factors NF-κB and AP-1; other regulation as a complex of multiple transcriptional factors has been described, such as GATA-3, E4BP4, MAF, and Blimp [14, 15]. These reports are allowing the possibility that transcriptional regulatory machinery could be specific to certain cell types [16, 17]. In addition, the regulation of IL-10 production depending on the TLR2 or TLR4-stimulated in BM-derived macrophages presents different stability profiles for the IL10 mRNA [18].

It has the ability to inhibit activation and effector function of T cells, monocytes, and macrophages. It regulates the growth and differentiation of several cells such as B cells, NK cells, cytotoxic, and helper T cells, as well as mast cells, granulocytes, dendritic cells, keratinocytes, and endothelial cells (**Figure 1**).

Discovered in 1991, IL-10 was initially reported to suppress cytokine secretion, antigen presentation, and CD4+ T cell activation. IL-10 is crucial for controlling these T-cell responses, as IFNγ [19–22]. Further investigations have shown that IL-10 predominantly inhibits the synthesis of the pro-inflammatory cytokines IL-1, IL12, tumor necrosis factor (TNFα), and gamma Interferon (IFNγ) by stimulated monocytes/macrophages [23–25]. IL-10 is crucial for controlling these T-cell responses, as IFNγ-secreting and blocking proliferation [22, 26–28].

The pivotal role of autocrine IL-10 and the interaction with CD28 in the induction of T cell are to initiate peripheral tolerance as an immunoregulatory mechanism controlling antigen-specific T cell responses [21].

In addition, several effects have been reported: it downregulates the expression of Th1 cytokines, MHC class II antigens, dendritic cells, and co-stimulatory molecules on macrophages [29].

Biphasic effects have been reported on B cells. It prevents apoptosis in germinal B cells but induces apoptosis on B-chronic lymphocytic leukemia cells, enhances proliferation induced by CD40L, and promotes differentiation of B cells to become plasma cells secreting IgM, IgG, and IgA immunoglobulins [30–34].

IL-10 appears to have considerable importance in the development of human cancer and its immune escape. These have suggested that it could serve as a biomarker for prognostic diseases or as a target for treatment. Two factors should be considered: high levels of this cytokine in the system, and genetic polymorphisms.

3. IL-10 serum levels on cancer patients

Considering their possible role in the development and establishment of malignant cells, the first studies conducted to detect serum IL-10 levels in cancer patients, reported a higher concentration than in healthy subjects. In melanoma patients with lymph node metastases, stages III and IV showed significantly high concentration with respect to a healthy subject. *In vitro* determination performed on the supernatant of primary malignant melanoma cultures, IL-I0 mRNA, and protein was expressed. Later, in a meta-analysis that included melanoma patients, high expression of serous IL-10 leads to an adverse survival and correlated with worse outcomes in cancer patients [35–39].

On serum samples of 90 patients with gastric cancer, high IL-10 levels were associated with a worse prognosis independent of the gastric-stage patients and pancreatic cancer [40]. Similar observations were reported on another group of patients with a pancreatic and gastric cancer stage (IV). In the same study, patients with colon and renal carcinoma IL-10 levels did not significantly differ from controls [41]. *In vitro* study, supernatants of pancreatic tumors primary cultures, high concentration of IL-10 was detected [42].

Similar clinical findings on sera and tissues samples from lung cancer patients were report; samples with high levels were found on patients in stages III and IV, and less in stages II and I. The increased IL-10 levels correlate with a poor prognosis. On lung tumor tissues samples from those patients, IL10 concentration showed than the higher expression, presented lower survival rates [43].

Samples from breast cancer from patients, who underwent surgery as well as peritumoral normal breast tissue, were analyzed. Correlation between the IL-10 expressions of breast cancer tissue showed poor prognosis. No IL-10 was detected on normal tissue samples [44]. Determination of IL-10 on patients with breast cancer and early breast cancer showed that it could be usefully associated with other cytokines as biomarkers to discriminating advanced cancer, reported that IL-10 is significantly upregulated. These data could be used discerning between the two stages. [45].

Hodgkin's disease presented sera elevated IL-10 levels on range 4.5–225.6 pg/ml, suggesting that IL-10 could be an independent prognostic factor and correlates to poor survival [46]. Lymph nodes from pediatric patients with Hodgkin's disease express high levels of IL-10 mRNA where there were associated with an unfavorable prognosis [47, 48]. For the study of sera levels in 153 patients with Non-Hodgkin's disease, IL-10 was detectable with a similar frequency in all subtypes and all clinical stages. Nevertheless, high levels correlate with poor prognosis. Patients with stage IV disease and detectable serum IL-10 had a particularly poor prognosis [49, 50]. Additional information on sera levels of IL-10 is shown in **Table 1**.

IL-10 protein or mRNA appears to be an important component of the tumor micro-environment in a range of human cancer types, as renal cell carcinoma [68]. The role of macrophages in the regulation of tumor cell proliferation, invasion, angiogenesis, or immune control does not always have a positive effect; in fact, it has shown a negative effect. The secretion of IL-10 inhibits the inflammatory response [69–72] and also has been suggested that the detection of IL-10 into and surrounding the tumor may be derived directly from the tumor cells; *in vitro* studies reveal that melanoma cells themselves are the primary origin of IL-10 in tumor specimens *in vivo* [35]. Nevertheless, Mocellin *et al*. report evidence about immunostimulating anticancer properties, suggesting IL-10 over-expression within the tumor micro-environment and it may catalyze cancer immune rejection [73].

IL-10 and IL10R were quantified in sera and surgical specimens, although no significant serum IL-10 elevation was found. On surgical lung tumor cells, IL-10

Disease	Patients IL-10 levels	Healthy donor	References
Melanoma	15–480 pg/ml	<3.0 pg/ml	[35]
	8.75 pg/ml	<3.0 pg/ml	[39]
	24.3 ng/ml	3.4 ng/ml	[41]
Gastric cancer	6.3 ng/ml	3.4 ng/ml	[41]
	12.5 pg/ml	4.0 pg/ml	[40]
	27.52 pg/ml	<12 np/ml	[51]
	19.6 pg/ml	9.2 pg/ml	[52]
	>21.0 pg/ml	<3.0 pg/ml	[53]
Pancreatic cancer	6.8 ng/ml	3.4 ng/ml	[41]
	>10.0 pg/ml	ND	[54]
	>9.8 pg/ml	3.0 pg/ml	[55]
Colorectal cancer	97.36 ng/l	24.53 ng/l	[56]
	16.09 pg/ml	5.1 pg/ml	[57]
Hepatic cancer	12 pg/ml	6.3 pg/ml	[58]
Hodgkin lymphoma	61.5 pg/ml	No detectable	[46]
	>10 pg/ml	7.1 pg/ml	[59]
	>10 pg/ml	ND	[60]
	>10 pg/ml	ND	[61]
	26.79 pg/ml	ND	[62]
Non-Hodgkin lymphoma	>7.98 pg/ml	<5.0 pg/ml	[50]
Lung cancer	>38.16 pg/ml	32.55 pg/ml	[43]
	21.4 pg/ml	9.2 pg/ml	[63]
Multiple myeloma	201.96 pg/ml	ND	[64]
	2.39 ± 0.82 ng/ml	(0.34 ± 0.15 ng/ml)	[65]
B-cell lymphoma	26.0 pg/ml	18.0 pg/ml	[66]
Chronic lymphocytic leukemia	74 pg/ml	<13.68 pg/ml	[67]

Table 1.
Determination of IL-10 levels in serum from cancer patients.

expression was considered as a prognostic factor on nonsmall-cell lung cancer surgical specimens. In addition to an immunohistochemistry study on human lung surgery, a positive correlation between IL-10 and IL-10 receptor expressions was related to the lung tumor diameter. Interestingly, IL-10R was mainly expressed on the surface of Foxp-3þ T-regulatory lymphocytes infiltrating the tumor [74, 75].

4. IL10 polymorphims related to the development and prognosis of cancer

Single nucleotide polymorphisms (SNPs) has been described on IL10 promoter, where adenine was substituted by guanine at −1082 bp (rs1800896). Thymine was replaced by cytosine at −819 bp (rs1800871) and adenine by cytosine at −592 bp (rs1800872). All of those contribute to the variation in protein expression [76]. The IL10 production have a hereditary component estimated in 75%, suggesting that clinical outcome imparted by IL10 genetic variants may be mediated by effects on the tumor micro-environment composition or modulation [47]. The possibility that SNPs participate in the development, establishment, and the prognosis of cancer has been investigated by numerous research groups and includes several group malignances.

Eastern European patients with breast cancer, IL10 −1082A > G, −819 T > C, −592A > C polymorphisms, and phased haplotypes have not revealed a prognostic value [77]. Nevertheless, another study report 592C > A polymorphisms could modify disease-free and overall survival in women with lymph node-positive breast cancer [78]. In a Chinese Han population study, the −1082AA genotype was associated with a significantly increase risk of lymph node involvement and larger tumor size at the time of diagnosis [79]. After meta-analysis, it showed that IL10 rs1800896 and rs1800871 polymorphisms had no association with breast cancer risk, while rs1800872 polymorphism had a decreased risk of breast cancer in Caucasians [3]. However, another meta-analysis suggests that IL10 rs1800871 and rs1800872 polymorphisms might contribute to breast cancer susceptibility in the overall population, but not by ethnicity [6].

Chinese men, diagnostic with prostate cancer, do not show significant differences in (−1082A/G, −819 T/C, and −592A/C) SNPs between patients and control subjects [80]. Meta-analysis performed with a Caucasian and Asiatic population suggests that there is no association between IL10 gene rs1800896, rs1800871, and rs1800872 polymorphisms and prostate cancer [81]. A study looking for the participation of variant alleles at both −819 and −592 polymorphisms was modestly associated with the advanced stages of prostate cancer [82, 83]. Other meta-analysis reports that rs1800896 polymorphism is associated with a decreased risk of prostate cancer [84].

In a meta-analysis including 26 studies designed to search the risk of skin cancer and IL10 polymorphism, the results show that there is not a significant association of −1082G > A or −592C > A and risk to skin cancer. Nevertheless, it suggested a potential association between −819C > T polymorphism and decreased risk of skin cancer [38]. A meta-analysis carried out for possible association between polymorphism and melanoma did not find an association between skin cancer risk and the −592A/C or IL-10-1082G/A. However, there was a correlation between IL10 −819T/C polymorphisms and skin cancer [85].

Association between IL10 −1082A/G, −592C/A, and −819T/C gene polymorphisms and risk of lung cancer was also investigated by meta-analysis, but until now, there are inconsistent results: on Asian populations, IL10 −1082A/G and −819T/C polymorphisms might have a significant association with the risk of lung cancer [86]. Another meta-analysis suggests that the polymorphism associated with a risk factor for lung cancer was IL10 −592A > C polymorphism, especially among Asians and Caucasians. In contrast, the IL10 −819 T > C and −1082A > G polymorphisms are not significantly associated with an increased risk of lung cancer [87].

Cervical cancer associated with a polymorphism at this time is not conclusive: −1082 polymorphism was suggested as a marker of genetic susceptibility to cervical cancer among Japanese women but was not significantly increased in Zimbabwean women or Korean women [88]. In a meta-analysis, including 17 publications of Asian, African, and Caucasian populations, it did not find a significant association between the polymorphism and cervical cancer risk [89]. Other meta-analysis looking for association between −1082 G/A polymorphism and cervical cancer risk, including the same population, report as well that there is no association [90].

Association between rs1800896 polymorphism and head and neck cancer risk and its clinical stages in Caucasian and Asiatic evaluated by meta-analysis gave a significant association with head and neck cancer risk but not with the clinical

Disease	Population	Polymorphism	Association	Reference
Breast cancer	Eastern European	IL10 −1082A/G, IL10 −592A, IL10 −819C	No prognostic value	[77]
	Eastern European	IL10 −592C > A	Associated with survival	[78]
	Chinese Han	IL10 −1082AA	Associated with cancer risk	[79]
	Chinese Han	rs1800896, rs1800871	No associated with cancer risk	[3]
	Caucasian	rs1800872	Associated with cancer risk	[3]
Prostate	Chinese men study	IL10 −1082A/G, IL10 −592A/C, IL10 −819 T/C	No associated with cancer risk	[80]
	Caucasian, African-Americans, and Asiatic	rs1800896	Associated with reduced cancer risk	[84]
	Caucasian and Asiatic	rs1800896, rs1800871, rs1800872	No association with risk cancer	[81]
	Caucasian, African-Americans, and Asiatic	IL10-1082 A4G, IL10-819 C4, IL10-592 C4A	No association with cancer risk	[82]
	Caucasian and Asiatic	IL10--592A > C	No association with cancer risk	[83]
Skin cancer	Caucasian, African-Americans, and Asiatic	IL10 −1082A/G, IL10-592A, IL10-819C	No associated with cancer skin risk	[82]
	Caucasian, African-Americans, and Asiatic	IL10 −592A/C, IL10 −1082G/A	No associated with cancer risk	[85]
Lung cancer	Asiatic	IL10 −1082A/G, IL10-592A, IL10-819C	Associated with cancer risk	[86]
	Caucasian	IL10 −1082A/G, IL10-592A, IL10-819C	No association with cancer risk	[86]
	Caucasian	IL10 −592A > C	Associated with cancer risk	[87]
	Caucasian and Asiatic	IL10 −819 T > C, IL10 −1082A > G	No associated with cancer risk	[87]
Cervix cancer	Japanese women	IL10 −1081	Associated with cancer risk	[88]
	Zimbabwean women and Korean women	IL10 −1082	No associated with risk	[88]
	Caucasian, African-Americans, and Asiatic	IL10 −1082A > G	No associated with risk	[89]
	Caucasian, African-Americans, and Asiatic	IL10 −1082 G/A	No associated with cancer risk	[90]
Head and neck cancer	Caucasian and Asiatic	rs1800896	Associated with cancer risk	[91]
	Caucasian, and Asiatic	IL10 −1082A > G, IL10 −819 T > C	Associated with cancer risk	[92]

Disease	Population	Polymorphism	Association	Reference
Gastric cancer	Mexican population	IL10 −819	Associated with risk	[93]
	Mexican population	IL10 −592C/A, IL10 −1082A/G	No associated with risk	[93]
Oral mucosa cancer	Indian population	IL10-592 A/C	Associated with cancer risk	[94]
Colorectal cancer	Caucasian and Asiatic	IL10819T > C	Associated with cancer risk	[95]
	Caucasian and Asiatic	rs1800871 rs1800872	No associated with cancer risk	[95]
	Caucasian and Asiatic	IL10 −1082A > G, IL10 −592C > A	No associated with cancer risk	[95]
Pediatric Hodgkin's disease	Caucasian	IL10-592AA	Pronostic marker	[96]
	Brazilian	IL10 −1082GG	Unfavorable prognosis	[47]
Acute myeloid leukemia	Egyptian	IL10-819	Associated with risk	[97]
	Chinese Han	IL-10-819, −592	Associated with risk	[98]
	Sudanese	IL10 −1082G/A	Associated with risk	[7]

Table 2.
Relationship of IL10 polymorphism and cancer risk.

stages [91]. Other analysis reports significant associations between the IL10 −1082A > G and IL10 −819 T > C polymorphism and increased risks of head and neck cancer similar population [92].

Other studies on the relation between risk or prognosis polymorphisms in cancer have been performed. In there, a possible association with gastric cancer showed a significant association with IL10-819 on the Mexican population. Nevertheless, no significant association was found for IL10 −592C/A (rs1800872) and IL10 −1082A/G (rs1800896) [93]. Looking for a possible predispose to oral squamous cell carcinoma (−592), A/C polymorphism was significantly associated with reduced risk [94]. In colorectal cancer IL10 −819 T > C, polymorphism was associated with significantly increased risk [95].

In a clinical study with child Hokdkin disease, −1082GG genotype was associated with lower IL10 mRNA expression. Nevertheless, genotypes of the −592 SNP showed no association with IL10 mRNA expression. However, −1082AACAG genotypes, ATA haplotype, and the presence of the −592AA genotype were associated with unfavorable prognosis [47, 96].

Genotypic variants of IL10 (−1082G/A) polymorphism in adult Sudanese patients with acute myeloid leukemia were investigated as a possible risk factor. In there, no association between IL10 (−1082G/A) and acute myeloid leukemia was detected [7]. Nevertheless, in the Egyptian population, −819 polymorphism was associated with enhanced risk [97]. In the Chinese population, the −819A allele frequencies in the AML group were higher than in the controls [98]. In pediatric patients, Classical Hodgkin lymphoma −1082AA/AG, −592CC genotypes, and ATA haplotype were associated with unfavorable prognosis; interestingly, −1082 was associated with low IL10 mRNA expression [46].

Unfortunately, to date, the results are controversial; the relationship of polymorphism with the presence of cancer and/or the possible risk of developing cancer is shown in **Table 2**.

5. Conclusions

High concentrations of IL-10 in the serum of cancer patients seem to correspond not only to the expression of this protein by immune cells. The evidence shows that the cancer cell is capable of synthesizing it, which would cause an imbalance in the homeostasis of the immune system.

Besides, the presence of polymorphisms suggested the possibility that some of them could be involved in the regulation of the activity of IL10; this gave rise to numerous studies seeking opportunities to explore for cancer risks or implications in the development, establishment, and survival of the cancer cell. The relationship between polymorphisms and the risk and prevalence of different types of cancer had evaluated by meta-analysis. Unfortunately, until now, the results are not conclusive.

Nevertheless, the fact is that IL-10 can exert the antitumor effect by mechanisms such as the activation of natural killer cells (NK), lymphocytes T, macrophages, and nitric oxide; its high concentration shows the deregulation of the immune system, where a high level of IL10 allows the tumor to escape. Nevertheless, the fact that IL-10 can exert the antitumor effect by mechanisms such as the activation of natural killer cells, lymphocytes T, macrophages, and nitric oxide results controversial. Its high concentration induces the deregulation of the immune system, where a high level of IL-10 allows the tumor escape. In some cases, it could be propose as a biomarker for patient lifespan or chemotherapy respond.

Because of this, it is essential to study not only the mechanisms that allow this high expression of interleukin IL-10, but its effect on tumor cells and also. It is important to consider its relationship with other cytokines.

Conflict of interest

The authors declare that they have no competing interests.

Author details

Maria Teresa Gonzalez-Garza*, Delia Elva Cruz-Vega and Carmen Maldonado-Bernal
Laboratorio de Investigación en Inmunología y Proteómica, Hospital Infantil de México Federico Gómez, Mexico City, Mexico

*Address all correspondence to: mtgonzalezgarza@itesm.mx

References

[1] de Visser KE, Eichten A, Coussens LM. Paradoxical roles of the immune system during cancer development. Nature Reviews Cancer. 2006;**6**:24-37. DOI: 10.1038/nrc1782

[2] Jordan WJ, Eskdale J, Boniotto M, Lennon GP, Peat J, Campbell JD, et al. Human IL-19 regulates immunity through auto-induction of IL-19 and production of IL-10. European Journal of Immunology. 2005;**35**:1576-1582. DOI: 10.1002/eji.200425317

[3] Dai ZJ, Wang XJ, Zhao Y, Ma XB, Kang HF, Min WL, et al. Effects of interleukin-10 polymorphisms (rs1800896, rs1800871, and rs1800872) on breast cancer risk: Evidence from an updated meta-analysis. Genetic Testing and Molecular Biomarkers. 2014;**18**: 439-445. DOI: 10.1089/gtmb.2014.0012

[4] Fei C, Yao XM, Sun Y, Gu XZ, Yu LQ, Lai X. Interleukin-10 polymorphisms associated with susceptibility to acute myeloid leukemia. Genetics and Molecular Research. 2015;**14**:925-930. DOI: 10.4238/2015

[5] Yang Y, Fa X. Role of IL-10 gene polymorphisms on the susceptibility for esophageal cancer and its association with environmental factors. International Journal of Clinical and Experimental Pathology. 2015;**8**:9580-9585

[6] Moghimi M, Ahrar H, Karimi-Zarchi M, Aghili K, Salari M, Zare-Shehneh M, et al. Association of IL-10 rs1800871 and rs1800872 polymorphisms with breast cancer risk: A systematic review and meta-analysis. Asian Pacific Journal of Cancer Prevention. 2018;**19**:3353-3359. DOI: 10.31557/APJCP.2018.19.12.3353

[7] Sharif OM, Hassan R, Mohammed Basbaeen AA, Mohmed AH, Ibrahim IK. Interleukin-10 (1082G/A) polymorphism is associated with susceptibility of acute myeloid leukemia patients in Sudanese population. Asian Pacific Journal of Cancer Prevention. 2019;**20**:1939-1943. DOI: 10.31557/APJCP.2019.20.7.1939

[8] Vieira P, de Waal-Malefyt R, Dang MN, Johnson KE, Kastelein R, Fiorentino DF, et al. Isolation and expression of human cytokine synthesis inhibitory factor cDNA clones: Homology to Epstein-Barr virus open reading frame BCRFI. Proceedings of the National Academy of Sciences of the United States of America. 1991;**88**:1172-1176. DOI: 10.1073/pnas.88.4.1172

[9] Trinchieri G. Interleukin-10 production by effector T cells: Th1 cells show self control. The Journal of Experimental Medicine. 2007;**204**: 239-243. DOI: 10.1084/jem.20070104

[10] Said EA, Dupuy FP, Trautmann L, Zhang Y, Shi Y, El-Far M, et al. Programmed death-1-induced interleukin-10 production by monocytes impairs CD4+ T cell activation during HIV infection. Nature Medicine. 2010;**16**:452-459. DOI: 10.1038/nm.2106

[11] Li X, Mai J, Virtue A, Yin Y, Gong R, Sha X, et al. IL-35 is a novel responsive anti-inflammatory cytokine--a new system of categorizing anti-inflammatory cytokines. PLoS One. 2012;**7**(3):e33628. DOI: 10.1371/journal.pone.0033628

[12] Donnelly RP, Dickensheets H, Finbloom DS. The interleukin-10 signal transduction pathway and regulation of gene expression in mononuclear phagocytes. Journal of Interferon & Cytokine Research. 1999;**19**:563-573. DOI: 10.1089/107999099313695

[13] Josephson K, Logsdon NJ, Walter MR. Crystal structure of the IL-10/IL-10R1 complex reveals a shared

receptor binding site. Immunity. 2001;**15**:35-46. DOI: 10.1016/s1074-7613(01)00169-8

[14] Saraiva M, O'Garra A. The regulation of IL-10 production by immune cells. Nature Reviews Immunology. 2010;**10**:170-181. DOI: 10.1038/nri2711

[15] Gabryšová L, Howes A, Saraiva M, O'Garra A. The regulation of IL-10 expression. Current Topics in Microbiology and Immunology. 2014;**380**:157-190. DOI: 10.1007/978-3-662-43492-5_8

[16] Kubo M, Motomura Y. Transcriptional regulation of the anti-inflammatory cytokine IL-10 in acquired immune cells. Frontiers in Immunology. 2012;**3**:275. DOI: 10.3389/fimmu.2012.00275

[17] MacKenzie KF, Pattison MJ, Arthur JS. Transcriptional regulation of IL-10 and its cell-specific role in vivo. Critical Reviews in Immunology. 2014;**34**:315-345. DOI: 10.1615/critrevimmunol.2014010694

[18] Teixeira-Coelho M, Guedes J, Ferreirinha P, Howes A, Pedrosa J, Rodrigues F, et al. Differential post-transcriptional regulation of IL-10 by TLR2 and TLR4-activated macrophages. European Journal of Immunology. 2014;**44**:856-866. DOI: 10.1002/eji.201343734

[19] Moore KW, Rousset F, Banchereau J. Evolving principles in immunopathology: Interleukin 10 and its relationship to Epstein-Barr virus protein BCRF1. Seminars in Immunopathology. 1991;**13**:157-166. DOI: 10.1007/bf00201466

[20] de Waal Malefyt R, Abrams J, Bennett B, Figdor CG, de Vries JE. Interleukin 10(IL-10) inhibits cytokine synthesis by human monocytes: An autoregulatory role of IL-10 produced by monocytes. The Journal of Experimental Medicine. 1991;**174**: 1209-1220. DOI: 10.1084/jem.174.5.1209

[21] Akdis CA, Joss A, Akdis M, Blaser K. Mechanism of IL-10-induced T cell inactivation in allergic inflammation and normal response to allergens. International Archives of Allergy and Immunology. 2001;**124**:180-182. DOI: 10.1159/000053704

[22] Joss A, Akdis M, Faith A, Blaser K, Akdis CA. IL-10 directly acts on T cells by specifically altering the CD28 co-stimulation pathway. European Journal of Immunology. 2000;**30**: 1683-1690. DOI: 10.1002/1521-4141(200006)30:6<1683:AID-IMMU1683>3.0.CO;2-A

[23] Opp MR, Smith EM, Hughes TK Jr. Interleukin-10 (cytokine synthesis inhibitory factor) acts in the central nervous system of rats to reduce sleep. Journal of Neuroimmunology. 1995;**60**:165-168. DOI: 10.1016/0165-5728(95)00066-b

[24] Aste-Amezaga M, Ma X, Sartori A, Trinchieri G. Molecular mechanisms of the induction of IL-12 and its inhibition by IL-10. Journal of Immunology. 1998;**160**:5936-5944

[25] Varma TK, Toliver-Kinsky TE, Lin CY, Koutrouvelis AP, Nichols JE, Sherwood ER. Cellular mechanisms that cause suppressed gamma interferon secretion in endotoxin-tolerant mice. Infection and Immunity. 2001;**69**:5249-5263. DOI: 10.1128/iai.69.9.5249-5263.2001

[26] Maynard CL, Weaver CT. Diversity in the contribution of interleukin-10 to T-cell-mediated immune regulation. Immunological Reviews. 2008;**226**:219-233. DOI: 10.1111/j.1600-065X.2008.00711.x

[27] Veenbergen S, Li P, Raatgeep HC, Lindenbergh-Kortleve DJ,

Simons-Oosterhuis Y, Farrel A, et al. IL-10 signaling in dendritic cells controls IL-1β-mediated IFNγ secretion by human CD4(+) T cells: Relevance to inflammatory bowel disease. Mucosal Immunology. 2019;**12**:1201-1211. DOI: 10.1038/s41385-019-0194-9

[28] Verma R, Balakrishnan L, Sharma K, Khan AA, Advani J, Gowda H, et al. A network map of interleukin-10 signaling pathway. Journal of Cell Communication and Signaling. 2016;**10**:61-67. DOI: 10.1007/s12079-015-0302-x

[29] McCarter MD, Baumgartner J, Escobar GA, Richter D, Lewis K, Robinson W, et al. Immunosuppressive dendritic and regulatory T cells are upregulated in melanoma patients. Annals of Surgical Oncology. 2007;**14**:2854-2860. DOI: 10.1245/s10434-007-9488-3

[30] Rousset F, Garcia E, Defrance T, Péronne C, Vezzio N, Hsu DH, et al. Interleukin 10 is a potent growth and differentiation factor for activated human B lymphocytes. Proceedings of the National Academy of Sciences of the United States of America. 1992;**89**:1890-1893. DOI: 10.1073/pnas.89.5.1890

[31] Armitage RJ, Macduff BM, Spriggs MK, Fanslow WC. Human B cell proliferation and Ig secretion induced by recombinant CD40 ligand are modulated by soluble cytokines. Journal of Immunology. 1993;**150**:3671-3680

[32] Briere F, Servet-Delprat C, Bridon JM, Saint-Remy JM, Banchereau J. Human interleukin 10 induces naive surface immunoglobulin D+ (sIgD+) B cells to secrete IgG1 and IgG3. The Journal of Experimental Medicine. 1994;**179**: 757-762. DOI: 10.1084/jem.179.2.757

[33] Itoh K, Hirohata S. The role of IL-10 in human B cell activation, proliferation, and differentiation. Journal of Immunology. 1995;**154**:4341-4350

[34] Moens L, Tangye SG. Cytokine-mediated regulation of plasma cell generation: IL-21 takes center stage. Frontiers in Immunology. 2014;**5**:65. DOI: 10.1007/s13277-014-2589-2

[35] Dummer W, Becker JC, Schwaaf A, Leverkus M, Moll T, Bröcker EB. Elevated serum levels of interleukin-10 in patients with metastatic malignant melanoma. Melanoma Research. 1995;**5**:67-68. DOI: 10.1097/00008390-199502000-00008

[36] Dummer W, Bastian BC, Ernst N, Schänzle C, Schwaaf A, Bröcker EB. Interleukin-10 production in malignant melanoma: Preferential detection of IL-10-secreting tumor cells in metastatic lesions. International Journal of Cancer. 1996;**66**:607-610. DOI: 10.1002/(SICI)1097-0215(19960529)66:5<607::AID-IJC4>3.0.CO;2-X

[37] Zhao H, Yang J, Yu Z, Shen H, Huang X, Zhang M, et al. Synthetic analysis of associations between IL-10 polymorphisms and skin cancer risk. Oncotarget. 2017;**9**:6728-6736. DOI: 10.18632/oncotarget.23385

[38] Zhao S, Wu D, Wu P, Wang Z, Huang J. Serum IL-10 predicts worse outcome in cancer patients: A meta-analysis. PLoS One. 2015;**10**:e0139598. DOI: 10.1371/journal.pone.0139598

[39] Nemunaitis J, Fong T, Shabe P, Martineau D, Ando D. Comparison of serum interleukin-10 (IL-10) levels between normal volunteers and patients with advanced melanoma. Cancer Investigation. 2001;**19**:239-247. DOI: 10.1081/cnv-100102550

[40] Ikeguchi M, Hatada T, Yamamoto M, Miyake T, Matsunaga T, Fukumoto Y, et al. Serum interleukin-6 and -10 levels in patients with gastric cancer. Gastric Cancer. 2009;**12**:95-100. DOI: 10.1007/s10120-009-0509-8

[41] Fortis C, Foppoli M, Gianotti L, Galli L, Citterio G, Consogno G, et al. Increased interleukin-10 serum levels in patients with solid tumours. Cancer Letters. 1996;**104**:1-5. DOI: 10.1016/0304-3835(96)04213-9

[42] Danilova AB, Danilov AO, Fakhrutdinova OL, Baldueva IA, Moiseenko VM. Laboratory evaluation of TGFbeta1, IL-10, VEGF levels in vivo and in vitro in patients with solid tumors. Voprosy Onkologii. 2011;**57**:759-766

[43] Hsu TI, Wang YC, Hung CY, Yu CH, Su WC, Chang WC, et al. Positive feedback regulation between IL10 and EGFR promotes lung cancer formation. Oncotarget. 2016;7:20840-20854. DOI: 10.18632/oncotarget.7894. 8-870915

[44] Bhattacharjee HK, Bansal VK, Nepal B, Srivastava S, Dinda AK, Misra MC. Is interleukin 10 (IL10) expression in breast cancer a marker of poor prognosis? Indian Journal of Surgical Oncology. 2016;7:320-325. DOI: 10.1007/s13193-016-0512-6

[45] Liu C, Sun B, Xu B, Meng X, Li L, Cong Y, et al. A panel containing PD-1, IL-2Rα, IL-10, and CA15-3 as a biomarker to discriminatebreast cancer from benign breast disease. Cancer Management and Research. 2018;**10**:1749-1761. DOI: 10.2147/CMAR.S160452

[46] Bohlen H, Kessler M, Sextro M, Diehl V, Tesch H. Poor clinical outcome of patients with Hodgkin's disease and elevated interleukin-10 serum levels. Clinical significance of interleukin-10 serum levels for Hodgkin's disease. Annals of Hematology. 2000;**79**:110-113. DOI: 10.1007/s002770050564

[47] Vera-Lozada G, Minnicelli C, Segges P, Stefanoff G, Kristcevic F, Ezpeleta J, et al. Interleukin 10 (IL10) proximal promoter polymorphisms beyond clinical response in classical Hodgkin lymphoma: Exploring the basis for the genetic control of the tumor microenvironment. Oncoimmunology. 2018;7:e1389821. DOI: 10.1080/2162402X.2017.1389821

[48] Hsi ED, Li H, Nixon AB, Schöder H, Bartlett NL, LeBlanc M, et al. Serum levels of TARC, MDC, IL-10, and soluble CD163 in Hodgkin lymphoma: A SWOG S0816 correlative study. Blood. 2019;**133**:1762-1765. DOI: 10.1182/blood-2018-0

[49] Blay JY, Burdin N, Rousset F, Lenoir G, Biron P, Philip T, et al. Serum interleukin-10 in non-Hodgkin's lymphoma: A prognostic factor. Blood. 1993;**82**:2169-2174

[50] Cortes J, Kurzrock R. Interleukin -10 in non-Hodgkin's lymphoma. Leukemia & Lymphoma. 1997;**26**:251-259. DOI: 10.3109/10428199709051774

[51] Shokrzadeh M, Mohammadpour A, Hoseini V, Abediankenari S, Ghassemi-Barghi N, Tabari YS. Serum cytokine of il-2, il-10 and il-12 levels in patients with stomach adenocarcinoma. Archives of Gastroenterology. 2018;**55**:385-389. DOI: 10.1590/S0004-2803.201800000-83

[52] De Vita F, Orditura M, Galizia G, Romano C, Infusino S, Auriemma A, et al. Serum interleukin-10 levels in patients with advanced gastrointestinal malignancies. Cancer. 1999;**86**:1936-1943

[53] Szaflarska A, Szczepanik A, Siedlar M, Czupryna A, Sierzega M, Popiela T, et al. Preoperative plasma level of IL-10 but not of proinflammatory cytokines is an independent prognostic factor in patients with gastric cancer. Anticancer Research. 2009;**29**:5005-5012

[54] Feng L, Qi Q, Wang P, Chen H, Chen Z, Meng Z, et al. Serum levels of IL-6, IL-8, and IL-10 are indicators

of prognosis in pancreatic cancer. The Journal of International Medical Research. 2018;**46**:5228-5236. DOI: 10.1177/0300060518800588

[55] Ebrahimi B, Tucker SL, Li D, Abbruzzese JL, Kurzrock R. Cytokines in pancreatic carcinoma: Correlation with phenotypic characteristics and prognosis. Cancer. 2004;**101**:2727-2736. DOI: 10.1002/cncr.20672

[56] Li B, Wang F, Ma C, Hao T, Geng L, Jiang H. Predictive value of IL-18 and IL-10 in the prognosis of patients with colorectal cancer. Oncology Letters. 2019;**18**:713-719. DOI: 10.3892/ol.2019.10338

[57] Stanilov N, Miteva L, Deliysky T, JovchevJ, StanilovaS. Advancedcolorectal cancer is associated with enhanced IL-23 and IL-10 serum levels. Labmedicine. 2010;**41**:159-163

[58] Chau GY, Wu CW, Lui WY, Chang TJ, Kao HL, Wu LH, et al. Serum interleukin-10 but not interleukin-6 is related to clinical outcome in patients with resectable hepatocellular carcinoma. Annals of Surgery. 2000;**231**:552-558

[59] Sarris AH, Kliche KO, Pethambaram P, Preti A, Tucker S, Jackow C, et al. Interleukin-10 levels are often elevated in serum of adults with Hodgkin's disease and are associated withinferior failure-free survival. Annals of Oncology. 1999;**10**:433-440. DOI: 10.1023/a:1008301602785

[60] Visco C, Vassilakopoulos TP, Kliche KO, Nadali G, Viviani S, Bonfante V, et al. Elevated serum levels of IL-10 are associated with inferior progression-free survival in patients with Hodgkin's disease treated with radiotherapy. Leukemia & Lymphoma. 2004;**45**:2085-2092. DOI: 10.1080/10428190410001712234

[61] Vassilakopoulos TP, Nadali G, Angelopoulou MK, Siakantaris MP, Dimopoulou MN, Kontopidou FN, et al. Serum interleukin-10 levels are an independent prognostic factor for patients with Hodgkin's lymphoma. Haematologica. 2001;**86**:274-281

[62] Viviani S, Notti P, Bonfante V, Verderio P, Valagussa P, Bonadonna G. Elevated pretreatment serum levels of Il-10 are associated with a poor prognosis in Hodgkin's disease, the Milan cancer institute experience. Medical Oncology. 2000;**17**:59-63. DOI: 10.1007/bf02826218

[63] De Vita F, Orditura M, Galizia G, Romano C, Roscigno A, Lieto E, et al. Serum interleukin-10 levels as a prognostic factor in advanced non-small cell lung cancer patients. Chest. 2000;**117**:365-373. DOI: 10.1378/chest.117.2.365

[64] Wang H, Wang L, Chi PD, Wang WD, Chen XQ, Geng QR, et al. High level of interleukin-10 in serum predicts poor prognosis in multiple myeloma. British Journal of Cancer. 2016;**114**:463-468. DOI: 10.1038/bjc.2016.11

[65] Shekarriz R, Janbabaei G, Abedian Kenari S. Prognostic value of IL-10 and its relationship with disease stage in Iranian patients with multiple myeloma. Asian Pacific Journal of Cancer Prevention. 2018;**19**:27-32. DOI: 10.22034/APJCP.2018.19.1.27

[66] Gupta M, Han JJ, Stenson M, Maurer M, Wellik L, Hu G, et al. Elevated serum IL-10 levels in diffuse large B-cell lymphoma: A mechanism of aberrant JAK2 activation. Blood. 2012;**119**:2844-2853. DOI: 10.1182/blood-2011-10-388538

[67] Fayad L, Keating MJ, Reuben JM, O'Brien S, Lee BN, Lerner S, et al. Interleukin-6 and interleukin-10 levels in chronic lymphocytic leukemia: Correlation with phenotypic characteristics and outcome. Blood.

2001;**97**:256-263. DOI: 10.1182/blood.v97.1.256

[68] Nakagomi H, Pisa P, Pisa EK, Yamamoto Y, Halapi E, Backlin K, et al. Lack of i international journal of cancer nterleukin-2 (IL-2) expression and selective expression of IL-10 mRNA in human renal cell carcinoma. International Journal of Cancer. 1995;**63**:366-371. DOI: 10.1002/ijc.2910630311

[69] Welsh TJ, Green RH, Richardson D, Waller DA, O'Byrne KJ, Bradding P. Macrophage and mast-cell invasion of tumor cell islets confers a marked survival advantage in non-small-cell lung cancer. Journal of Clinical Oncology. 2005;**23**:8959-8967. DOI: 10.1200/JCO.2005.01.4910

[70] Lewis CE, Pollard JW. Distinct role of macrophages in different tumor microenvironments. Cancer Research. 2006;**66**:605-612. DOI: 10.1158/0008-5472.CAN-05-4005

[71] Redente EF, Orlicky DJ, Bouchard RJ, Malkinson AM. Tumor signaling to the bone marrow changes the phenotype of monocytes and pulmonary macrophages during urethane-induced primary lung tumorigenesis in a/J mice. The American Journal of Pathology. 2007;**170**:693-708. DOI: 10.2353/ajpath.2007.060566

[72] Zeni E, Mazzetti L, Miotto D, Lo Cascio N, Maestrelli P, Querzoli P, et al. Macrophage expression of interleukin-10 is a prognostic factor in nonsmall cell lung cancer. The European Respiratory Journal. 2007;**30**:627-632. DOI: 10.1183/09031936.00129306

[73] Mocellin S, Marincola FM, Young HA. Interleukin-10 and the immune response against cancer: A counterpoint. Journal of Leukocyte Biology. 2005;**78**:1043-1051. DOI: 10.1189/jlb.0705358

[74] Hatanaka H, Abe Y, Kamiya T, Morino F, Nagata J, Tokunaga T, et al. Clinical implications of interleukin (IL)-10 induced by non-small-cell lung cancer. Annals of Oncology. 2000;**11**:815-819. DOI: 10.1023/a:1008375208574

[75] Vahl JM, Friedrich J, Mittler S, Trump S, Heim L, Kachler K, et al. Interleukin-10-regulated tumour tolerance in non-small cell lung cancer. British Journal of Cancer. 2017;**117**:1644-1655. DOI: 10.1038/bjc.2017.336

[76] Howell MW, Rose-zerilli MJ. Cytokine gene polymorphisms, cancer susceptibility and prognosis. Journal of Nutrition. 2007;**137**(Suppl 1):194-199

[77] Korobeinikova E, Myrzaliyeva D, Ugenskiene R, Raulinaityte D, Gedminaite J, Smigelskas K, et al. The prognostic value of IL10 and TNF alpha functional polymorphisms in premenopausal early-stage breast cancer patients. BMC Genetics. 2015;**16**:70. DOI: 10.1186/s12863-015-0234-8

[78] Knechtel G, Hofmann G, Gerger A, Renner W, Langsenlehner T, Szkandera J, et al. Analysis of common germline polymorphisms as prognostic factors in patients with lymph node-positive breast cancer. Journal of Cancer Research and Clinical Oncology. 2010;**136**:1813-1819. DOI: 10.1007/s00432-010-0839-2

[79] Kong F, Liu J, Liu Y, Song B, Wang H, Liu W. Association of interleukin-10 gene polymorphisms with breast cancer in a Chinese population. Journal of Experimental & Clinical Cancer Research. 2010;**29**:72. DOI: 10.1186/1756-9966-29-72

[80] Liu J, Song B, Bai X, Liu W, Li Z, Wang J, et al. Association of genetic polymorphisms in the interleukin-10 promoter with risk of prostate cancer

in Chinese. BMC Cancer. 2010;**10**:456. DOI: 10.1186/1471-2407-10-456

[81] Zou YF, Wang F, Feng XL, Tian YH, Tao JH, Pan FM, et al. Lack of association of IL-10 gene polymorphisms with prostate cancer: Evidence from 11,581 subjects. European Journal of Cancer. 2011;**47**:1072-1079. DOI: 10.1016/j.ejca.2010.11.034

[82] Shao N, Xu B, Mi YY, Hua LX. IL-10 polymorphisms and prostate cancer risk: A meta-analysis. Prostate Cancer and Prostatic Diseases. 2011;**14**:129-135. DOI: 10.1038/pcan.2011.6

[83] Men T, Yu C, Wang D, Liu F, Li J, Qi X, et al. The impact of interleukin-10 (IL-10) gene 4 polymorphisms on peripheral blood IL-10 variation and prostate cancer risk based on published studies. Oncotarget. 2017;**8**:45994-46005. DOI: 10.18632/oncotarget.17522

[84] Chen H, Tang J, Shen N, Ren K. Interleukin 10 gene rs1800896 polymorphism is associated with the risk of prostate cancer. Oncotarget. 2017;**8**:66204-66214. DOI: 10.18632/oncotarget.19857

[85] Wu N, Sun H, Sun Q, Cui M, Jiang R, Cong X. Associations between IL-10 polymorphisms and susceptibility to melanoma, basal cell carcinoma, and squamous cell carcinoma: A meta-analysis. Genetic Testing and Molecular Biomarkers. 2018;**22**:693-701. DOI: 10.1089/gtmb.2018.0172

[86] Liu L, Zheng F. IL-10 -1082A/G, -592C/a, and -819T/C polymorphisms in association with lung cancer susceptibility: A meta-analysis. Onco Targets Therapy. 2016;**9**:6083-6091. DOI: 10.2147/OTT.S118481

[87] Jafari-Nedooshan J, Moghimi M, Zare M, Heiranizadeh N, Morovati-Sharifabad M, Akbarian-Bafghi MJ, et al. Association of promoter region polymorphisms of IL-10 gene with susceptibility to lung cancer: Systematic review and meta-analysis. Asian Pacific Journal of Cancer Prevention. 2019;**20**:1951-1957. DOI: 10.31557/APJCP.2019.20.7.1951

[88] Wang Y, Liu XH, Li YH, Li O. The paradox of IL-10-mediated modulation in cervical cancer. Biomedical Reports. 2013;**1**:347-351. DOI: 10.3892/br.2013.69

[89] Guo C, Wen L, Song JK, Zeng WJ, Dan C, Niu YM, et al. Significant association between interleukin-10 gene polymorphisms and cervical cancer risk: A meta-analysis. Oncotarget. 2018;**9**:12365-12375. DOI: 10.18632/oncotarget.24193

[90] Zhang S, Kong YL, Li YL, Yin YW. Interleukin-10 gene −1082 G/a polymorphism in cervical cancer and cervical intraepithelial neoplasia: Meta-analysis. The Journal of International Medical Research. 2014;**42**:1193-1201. DOI: 10.1177/0300060514544388

[91] Huang W, Song J, Jia XW, Chen YX, Shi J, Jiang X. Interleukin-10 rs1800896 polymorphism is associated with increased head and neck cancer risk but not associated with its clinical stages. Oncotarget. 2017;**8**:37217-37224. DOI: 10.18632/oncotarget.16660

[92] Niu YM, Du XY, Cai HX, Zhang C, Yuan RX, Zeng XT, et al. Increased risks between Interleukin-10 gene polymorphisms and haplotype and head and neck cancer: A meta-analysis. Scientific Reports. 2015;**5**:17149. DOI: 10.1038/srep17149

[93] Martínez-Campos C, Torres-Poveda K, Camorlinga-Ponce M, Flores-Luna L, Maldonado-Bernal C, Madrid-Marina V, et al. Polymorphisms in IL-10 and TGF-β gene promoter are associated with lower risk to gastric cancer in a Mexican population. BMC Cancer. 2019;**19**:453. DOI: 10.1186/s12885-019-5627-z

[94] Singh PK, Ahmad MK, Kumar V, Gupta R, Kohli M, Jain A, et al. Genetic polymorphism of interleukin-10 (-A592C) among oral cancer with squamous cell carcinoma. Archives of Oral Biology. 2017;**77**:18-22. DOI: 10.1016/j.archoralbio.2016.12.011

[95] Mirjalili SA, Moghimi M, Aghili K, Jafari M, Abolbaghaei SM, Neamatzadeh H, et al. Association of promoter region polymorphisms of interleukin-10 gene with susceptibility to colorectal cancer: A systematic review and meta-analysis. Arquivos de Gastroenterologia. 2018;**55**:306-313. DOI: 10.1590/S0004-2803.201800000-66

[96] Hohaus S, Giachelia M, Di Febo A, Martini M, Massini G, Vannata B, et al. Polymorphism in cytokine genes as prognostic markers in Hodgkin's lymphoma. Annals of Oncology. 2007;**18**:1376-1381. DOI: 10.1093/annonc/mdm132

[97] Rashed R, Shafik RE, Shafik NF, Shafik HE. Associations of interleukin-10 gene polymorphisms with acute myeloid leukemia in human (Egypt). Journal of Cancer Research and Therapeutics. 2018;**14**:1083-1086. DOI: 10.4103/0973-1482.187367

[98] Yao CJ, Du W, Chen HB, Xiao S, Wang CH, Fan ZL. Associations of IL-10 gene polymorphisms with acute myeloid leukemia in Hunan, China. Asian Pacific Journal of Cancer Prevention. 2013;**14**:2439-2442. DOI: 10.7314/apjcp.2013.14.4.2439

Chapter 3

Ion Channels and Transporters as Cancer Biomarkers and Targets for Diagnostics with Antibodies

Jessica Iorio, Claudia Duranti and Elena Lastraioli

Abstract

Cancer is a highly heterogeneous disease in terms of both response to therapy and prognosis. The introduction of molecular tools and antibodies had a great impact on cancer management in recent years for both cancer diagnosis and therapy. Ion channels and transporters (ICT) are membrane proteins aberrantly expressed in several human cancers. ICT can now represent potential cancer biomarkers as well as targets for therapeutic and diagnostic purposes. In particular, we will discuss about the potential role of ICTs as biomarkers for solid cancers (evaluated either by immunohistochemistry or molecular biology techniques) and the potential use of antibodies for diagnosis.

Keywords: ion channels, antibodies, biomarkers, cancer, diagnosis

1. Introduction

Ion channels and transporters (ICTs) are emerging as potential cancer biomarkers. Indeed, ICTs are aberrantly expressed in several types of human cancers, and exert a relevant role in mediating interactions between tumor cells and tumor microenvironment. Such interactions drive different functions which in turn regulate neoplastic progression, such as cell proliferation and survival, cell invasiveness and pro-angiogenetic programs [1–3]. Moreover, due to their prevalent expression at the cell surface, ICTs represent good targets for antibodies, to be exploited for diagnostic purposes. Finally, being highly druggable molecules, ICTs may represent novel molecular targets for antineoplastic therapy [4, 5].

The expression and role of different ion channels in tumor cells and their different contribution to tumor progression has been thoroughly described elsewhere [6]. In this chapter, we will focus on the possibility of exploiting ICTs as cancer biomarkers, for diagnostic, prognostic or predictive purposes. Some examples, relative to either solid cancers or hematologic malignancies are provided. We will analyze the possibility of using ICT-targeting antibodies for either *in vitro* or *in vivo* cancer diagnosis.

2. Cancer diagnosis: a focus on antibody-based techniques

The technologies available to help physicians to detect and diagnose cancer has changed dramatically in recent years. In particular, the use of biomarkers has greatly improved diagnosis through their application for either *in vitro* diagnosis (on tumor specimens or in blood samples) or *in vivo* molecular imaging. According to the National Cancer Institute (NCI) definition (NCI Dictionary of Cancer Terms, http://www.cancer.gov/dictionary?cdrid=46636), a biomarker may be used either to help diagnosis, for example, to identify early stage cancers (Diagnostic) or to forecast how aggressive a condition is (Prognostic), or to predict how well a patient will respond to a define treatment (Predictive).

For the purposes of this chapter, we will briefly summarize the main techniques, either *in vitro* or *in vivo*, which take advantage of the use of biomarkers to obtain diagnostic, prognostic and predictive data on the cancer under study. Notably, most, although not all, of these techniques are based on the use of antibodies, targeting specific cancer-related biomarkers.

2.1 *In vitro* cancer diagnosis

2.1.1 Immunohistochemistry (IHC)

IHC represents an indispensable diagnostic tool to assess the presence or absence, as well as the amount, of a specific molecular tumor marker in a tissue. After appropriate assessment of categorical scoring system and proper validation of the immunohistochemical assay, a given marker can be proposed as a potential diagnostic or prognostic factor. Indeed, many of the cancer biomarkers routinely used in cancer diagnostics are based on this technique.

2.1.2 Flow cytometry (FC)

Using a multiparametric approach, FC immunophenotyping plays an indispensable role in the diagnosis and subclassification of leukemias, as well as for minimal residual disease detection. FC, in fact, provides a rapid and detailed determination of antigen expression profiles; these information along with morphologic assessment, allow to diagnose a particular type of leukemia and/or help in distinguishing from other subtypes. Also, the identification of specific antigens has prognostic and therapeutic relevance in acute leukemias. Moreover, FC immunophenotyping is useful to monitor response to therapy, recurrence and minimal residual disease.

While IHC and FC represent the standard of care in solid cancers and hematologic malignancies, respectively, some remarkable technological breakthroughs of the last 10 years have greatly contributed to improve cancer diagnostics through either the definition of "Omics profile" or the assessment of plasma-based cancer biomarkers:

2.1.3 Omics profiles

The study of tumor genomes using high throughput profiling strategies including (but not limited to) DNA copy number, DNA methylation, and transcriptome and whole-genome sequencing—technologies that may collectively be defined as "omics"—has led to identifying genes and pathways deregulated in cancer, hence revealing those that may be useful for the detection and management of disease. In the near future, such discoveries will lead to the discovery of novel diagnostic, prognostic and predictive markers that will ultimately improve patient outcomes.

2.2 *In vivo* cancer diagnosis: molecular imaging

Besides *ex vivo* procedures (either on surgical/bioptic samples or blood), cancer *diagnosis* is mainly based on imaging procedures, such as *computed tomography,* magnetic resonance imaging and positron emission tomography. The advent of molecular imaging techniques has progressively allowed more accurate *in vivo* visualization of cancer, based on specific biological and pathological processes. Antibody-based imaging is of great utility since the combination of tumor specificity and different imaging methodologies might improve cancer diagnosis, monitoring and follow up [7–11]. The diagnostic imaging approaches currently used in cancer has been improved by the application of antibodies, thanks to the accuracy that allows antibodies to precisely identifying their targets. Some practical examples of mAbs recognizing cancer-specific biomarkers that are approved by the FDA and/or EMA and are currently used in the clinical setting have been described elsewhere [12]. Monoclonal antibodies (mAbs) have several features (big size, slow pharmacokinetics and blood clearance, not complete penetration and accumulation in tumor tissue) that can delay the time point for imaging. A different class of antibodies (single chain Fragment variable, scFv) might be useful to overcome such limitations and due to the possibility of conjugating the recombinant proteins with fluorescent dyes, scFv antibodies have been proposed for use in imaging applications, especially for cancer diagnostics [8, 11, 13].

3. Ion channels and transporters with clinical relevance in solid cancer

An overview of the main ion channels and transporters expressed in different solid tumors is reported in **Figure 1**.

3.1 Potassium channels

K^+ channels are the class of ion channels mostly de-regulated in cancers. Among them, ***KCa 1.1*** channels (also known as BK channels, encoded by the *KCNMA1* gene) have shown a clinical relevance in breast (BC) and prostate cancer (PCa). In both tumor types, BK overexpression can be traced back to the amplification of the *KCNMA1* gene located in 10q22: in BC, the amplification is restricted to invasive ductal tumors, and is associated with high stage, high grade and unfavorable prognosis [14]. In BC, KCa 1.1 positively correlates with the expression of estrogen

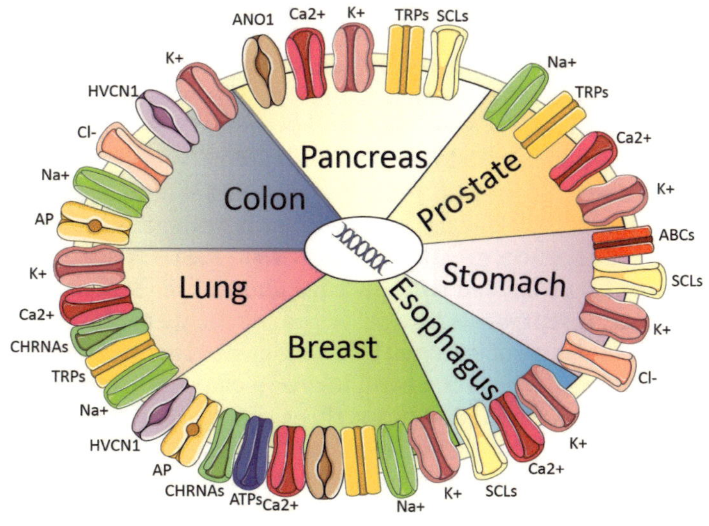

Figure 1.
Schematic representation of the main ICTs expressed in solid tumors.

receptors [15] and their levels are higher in BC metastatizing to brain [16]. In PCa, the *KCNMA1* gene is frequently amplified in late-stage tumors [17] and can be considered a potential biomarker [18]. Another Ca^{2+}-dependent K^+ channel often overexpressed in human cancers is ***KCa3.1*** (encoded by the *KCNN4* gene). $K_{Ca}3.1$ channels are upregulated in BC, especially in high grade tumors [19], in pancreatic cancer (pancreatic ductal adenocarcinoma, PDAC) [20], in colorectal cancer (CRC) [21] as well as in small cell lung cancer (SCLC) [22]. While the clinical relevance of $K_{Ca}3.1$ was hypothesized in CRC [23], although not validated [24], *KCNN4* hypomethylation turned out to be a negative prognostic factor in SCLC [22]. Kv channels are voltage-dependent K+ channels whose expression is often increased in cancer tissues [25]. For example, the expression of **Kv 1.3** (*KCNA3*), markedly increased in PCa in samples with Gleason score of 5–6 (GS5–6), but significantly decreased in the GS8–9 group. This malignancy grade-dependent K^+-channel expression pattern may provide a convenient marker to understand PCa progression level [26]. In PCa, Kv1.3 is mainly expressed in early stages of progression and down-regulated in high grade cancers [27]. Kv1.3 expression is lower in cancer compared with healthy pancreas. Kv1.3 downregulation could be traced back to promoter's methylation and was associated with the presence of metastases [28]. ***K2P9.1*** (KCNK9) belongs to the K2P family and genomic amplification of the gene was shown in a small fraction of BC [29]. **K2P5.1** (KCNK5) is a member of the same family and it was shown to be induced by estrogens in ER-positive BC cells; for this reason, it might represent a therapeutic target for ER-positive BCs [30]. The amplification of the *KCNK9* gene at the 8q23.4 locus justifies the over expression of $K_{2P}9.1$ channels in BC. The overexpression of another K2p channel ***K2p 2.1*** has been demonstrated in PCa and it was shown that it regulates cell proliferation [31]. The expression of inward rectifiers K^+ channels, in particular **Kir3.1** (KCNJ3) channels positively correlated with lymph node metastases in BC [32]. The voltage-gated K^+ channels (VGKC) appear to exert a pleiotropic role in colorectal cancer. In primary human samples, the transcripts of *KCNA3*, *KCNA5*, *KCNC1*, *KCNH1* [33–35], *KCNH2* [36] and *KCNK9* [37] have been detected. A relevant family of VGKC, whose most important members are Kv 10.1 and Kv 11.1 was shown to be highly represented in human cancers. **Kv10.1** (KCNH1) was expressed in esophageal squamous cell carcinoma (ESCC) compared with the corresponding normal tissue, it was associated with depth of invasion and represented an independent negative prognostic factor [38].

Kv11.1 (KCNH2) channels are expressed in gastric cancer (GC) cell lines and primary GCs. In GC cell lines, they regulate tumor proliferation [39]. Consistently, treatment with $K_v11.1$ blockers, like cisapride, and siRNA impairs tumor growth [40, 41]. It was also shown that the mean survival time was shorter in $K_v11.1$ positive patients thus $K_v11.1$ expression was proposed as an independent prognostic factor. We also showed that $K_v11.1$ regulates VEGF-A secretion, with a pathway similar to the one described in CRC [42]. *In vivo* analyses of xenografts obtained with GC cells demonstrated that the treatment with Bevacizumab and $K_v11.1$ blockers dramatically reduces greatly tumor growth. $K_v11.1$ is highly expressed in primary CRC and is associated with invasive phenotype [36]; moreover, along with Glut-1 absence, it represents a negative prognostic factor in TNM I and II CRC [43]. $K_v11.1$ expression is associated with chemosensitivity for several anti-tumor agents (such as vincristine, paclitaxel and hydroxy-camptothecin, doxorubicin). Such chemosensitivity is modulated by erythromycin that is also capable which, to inhibit $K_v11.1$ current [44]. $K_v11.1$ also regulates lung cancer (LC) cell proliferation [45]. $K_v11.1$ is expressed in precancerous and neoplastic lesions of the esophagus and it is associated with malignant progression [46]. $K_v11.1$ channel expression represents a negative prognostic factor in terms of ESCC patients' survival [47].

K_v11.1 are also expressed in PDAC cell lines and primary samples and it negatively affects patients' prognosis [48].

3.2 Sodium channels

Voltage-gated sodium channels (VGSC) were among the first channels to be demonstrated mis-expressed in BC and PCa. In particular, the predominant VGSC in BC is the "neonatal" splice variant of *SCN5A* (**nNaV1.5**), whose activity promotes metastatization [49–51]; consistently, the nNAv1.5 was up-regulated in metastatic BC samples [49, 50, 52]. On the whole, VGSC and in particular nNav1.5 could represent a good specific target for BC treatment. In CRC [53–55], the clinical relevance of Na_v 1.5 expression was established by IHC in CRC samples with respect to healthy colon. VGSC regulates invasiveness and it was shown that *SCNA5* gene modulates genes mediating, among others, cell migration and cell cycle control. Both nNa_v 1.5 and its "adult" counterpart are expressed in CRC and the local anesthetic Ropivacaine, blocks Na_v 1.5 variants [56]. PCa show an aberrant expression of **Nav1.7** (SCN9A), associated with a strong metastatic potential and its activity potentiates cell migration, crucial for the metastatic cascade [57]. Hence, Nav1.7 could represent a useful diagnostic marker [58]. A recent paper [59] showed that EGFR and Nav1.7 are expressed in NSCLC cells and that EGFR-mediated upregulation of *SCN9A* is necessary for the invasiveness of such cells. Nav1.7 has clinical relevance and might represent a novel target for therapy and/or a prognostic biomarker in NSCLC [59]. A recent multicenter study identified two single nucleotide polymorphisms of VGSC genes (*SCN4A*-rs2302237 and *SCN10A*-rs12632942) that were associated with oxaliplatin-induced peripheral neuropathy development [60].

3.3 Calcium channels

Calcium signal remodeling is one of the common features of proliferating cells, including cancer. Indeed many functional studies have provided different calcium signaling that can modulate cell proliferation and resistance to apoptosis [61–63]. Voltage-gated calcium channels (VGCC) that are involved in the regulation of BC cell proliferation. ***CACNA2D3*** gene (encoding the α2δ3 subunit of the voltage gated Ca^{2+} channel) is frequently up-regulated in BC, but in some metastatic cases, its expression is reduced [64]. The mechanisms of *CACNA2D3* contribution to the metastatic process has not being clarified yet. One possible mechanism for the overexpression of some calcium permeable ion channels is through the involvement of hormone receptors, such as ERα. Examples are **ORAI3** [65]. *CACNA2D3*, is frequently downregulated in primary BCs, as a result of methylation in CpG islands [64]. The influence of calcium channels in PCa has been known for over 30 years. Later research identified additional classes of channel proteins having an important regulatory role and affecting malignant transformation (reviewed in [66]). The expression of VGCC (mainly L-type) has been detected in the androgen-responsive LNCaP cells. In these cells Ca^{2+} currents are activated by androgens and mediate the androgen-induced effects [67]. Part of the Ca^{2+} effects depend on K^+ channels stimulation, for example, KCa3.1 blocking inhibits the proliferation of PCa cells [67]. An aberrant methylation of *CACNA2D1/3* gene (encoding the voltage-dependent calcium channel 2 subunit) was demonstrated in GC samples. *CACNA2D3* methylation is associated with diffuse type GC and shorter survival [68]. **ORAI1** and **STIM1**, belonging to the store operated calcium channels (SOC) family, are up-regulated in BC of the basal-like molecular subtype [69]. Moreover, another member of the same family, **STIM2**, is expressed at low levels in BC. Patients with high STIM1 and low STIM2 have unfavorable prognosis, suggesting that the SOC family has a role in aggressiveness and in the metastatic process [69]. **ORAI3** has recently been associated with ER-positive BC [65] and could represent a novel target for ER-positive BCs [70].

3.4 Transient receptor potential (TRP) channels

TRP channels are non-selective cation channels that can be activated by different stimuli such as pH variations, temperature and pressure among others [71, 72]. Since TRP channels are involved in migration and invasiveness, they contribute to the metastatic process in different tumors [73]. Ca^{2+} influx through TRPCs also occurs and promotes either cell proliferation or apoptosis, depending on TRPC subtype. **TRPC1** whose levels are high in BCs with low proliferation capacity, may not be the optimal target for therapies against aggressive BCs [74]. Significantly elevated (up to 200-fold) mRNA levels of ***TRPC6*** were shown in BC samples compared with paired control samples [74, 75], but no correlations with clinico-pathological features emerged [74]. A similar behavior characterizes TRPC1, whose expression levels decrease during the progression of PCa from androgen-dependent to androgen-independent phase [75]. TRPC6 is overexpressed in ESCC with respect to normal esophageal tissue at both protein and mRNA levels [76]. A recent report evidenced correlations of TRPC6 with T and staging and an association between *TRPC6* mRNA and poor prognosis [77]. **TRPV6** is up-regulated in PgR and ER-negative BCs [78]. Basal-like BCs with high TRPV6 mRNA levels are associated with poor survival [79]. *In vitro* data suggest that TRPV6 may be a potential therapeutic target [79]. TRPV6 is highly expressed in PCa and are associated with the Gleason score and metastatisation [80]. The expression of **TRPV4** is decreased by progesterone [81]. **TRPM7** is highly expressed in BC, and such over expression is associated with poor prognosis in terms of distant metastasis- and recurrence-free survival [82]. In accordance with these observation, *TRPM7* mRNA levels are higher in BC metastases with respect to primary tumors. Also, TRPM7 are overexpressed in pancreatic ductal adenocarcinomas and are associated with lymph node metastases [83]. TRPM7 mRNA and protein are also overexpressed in bladder cancer with respect to normal tissue and are associated with poor prognosis [84]. **TRPA1** is overexpressed also in SCLC patients compared with NSCLC and since it is associated with SCLC patients' survival representing a potential therapeutic target [85].

3.5 Chloride channels

Anoctamin 1 (**ANO1**), the calcium-activated chloride channel, is highly expressed in BC cell lines and primary BCs [86] and the 11q13 region is frequently amplified in BC and it is associated with grading and unfavorable outcome [86].

ANO1 was also shown to play an important role in controlling PDAC cell proliferation [87]. It has been shown that chloride channel accessory 1 and 2 genes (***CLCA1*** and ***CLCA2***) transcripts show widespread downregulation in CRC patients [88]. Therefore CLCA proteins could be tumor suppressors in CRC in analogy with what occurs in BC. **CLC1** is expressed in GC cells where it impairs cell proliferation and stimulates apoptosis, invasion and migration *in vitro* [89]. CLC1 overexpression in primary GC correlates with clinico-pathological parameters (lymph node involvement, stage, lymphatic and perineural invasion) as well as with poor prognosis [90]. **CLIC3** is not expressed in healthy pancreas while it is expressed in PanIN lesions [91] and in PDAC where it has a negative impact on patient survival.

3.6 Ligand-gated channels

The ligand-gated nicotinic acethylcholine receptors (**nAChRs**) are the channel type mostly studied in LC [92]. NSCLC shows altered expression of nicotinic subunits (mainly α1, α5 αvδ α7) compared with normal tissue. Moreover in NSCLC cells, nicotine has mitogenic effects of nicotine, mediated by α7-containing nAChRs [93]. Multiple genome-wide association studies (GWAS) have implicated the 15q25 nAChR gene cluster *CHRNA5-A3-B4* in nicotine dependence and LC [94]. The expression of the ***CHRNA5*** gene which encodes the α5-nAchR was increased in LC tissue and that the p.Asp398Asn polymorphism in the *CHRNA5* gene is associated with LC risk [92] and altered receptor function [95]. Additionally, the p.Asp398Asn polymorphism may influence α5 (CHRNA5) expression as well [92]. A α5-nAChR/HIF-1α/VEGF axis exists in LC and is involved in nicotine-induced tumor cell proliferation. This fact suggests that α5-nAChR may serve as a potential anticancer target in nicotine-associated LC [96].

3.7 Aquaporins (AQP)

AQP1 is expressed in BC and positively correlates with grading, histology, CK14 expression, smooth muscle actin expression, basal-like group and poor outcome, whereas it has significant negative correlation with ER status [97]. AQP1, **AQP3** and **AQP5** are expressed in CRC cell lines. AQP1 and AQP5 are expressed the early steps of CRC progression but also in liver metastases [98]. Moreover, AQP5 expression is associated with grading, nodal involvement and TNM stage [99]. AQP5 is expressed at significant levels in Lauren's intestinal type-GC, where it shows an apical localization [100], whereas AQP3 and **AQP4** are not overexpressed in GC. Shen et al. [101] showed that both AQP3 and AQP5 were overexpressed in GC and were associated with lymph node involvement. Moreover, AQP3 expression was higher in well differentiated tumors. AQP3 is also over-expressed in primary CRC with respect to healthy tissue, and its expression is positively regulated by EGF and is associated with lymph node involvement, metastasis and differentiation [102]. AQP3 and AQP5 are expressed in ESCC, while absent in healthy esophagus [103, 104]: the presence of the two aquaporins is associated with clinico-pathological features and their co-expression represents an independent negative prognostic factor. A recent microarray-based study demonstrated that reduced ***AQP9*** gene expression is related to absence of adjuvant chemotherapy response in CRC patients [38].

3.8 Transporters

The monocarboxylate transporter **SLC16A1** (encoded by the *SLC16A1* gene) is associated to basal-like BC, high histological grade, CK5, CK14, vimentin and Ki67. AQP1 along with SLC16A1 were shown to be associated with tumor aggressiveness of BC [105]. The voltage-gated proton channel Hv1 (**HVCN1**) overexpression in metastatic BC is associated with progression and unfavorable outcome [106]. The same occurs in CRC in which it is associated also with tumor size, lymph node involvement and stage [107]. In stage CRC, a low expression of **SLC7A1** (cationic amino-acid transporters-1, encoded by *SLC7A1* gene) is associated with shorter metastases-free survival [108].

The sodium proton exchanger 1 (**NHE1**, SLC9A1) interacts with EGFR and is involved in PDAC cell invasiveness [109]. It was shown that the Glucose Transporter 1 (**SLC2A1**, GLUT1) is expressed in BE-derived tumors in the late events of tumor progression [110]. SLC2A1 expression described also occurs in ESCC, where it represents a marker of poor prognosis [111]. Moreover, SLC2A1 expression increased after radiotherapy in ESCC patients [112]. The apical sodium-dependent bile acid transporters (**SLC10A2**), which mediate bile acid transport [113], are not expressed in the normal squamous epithelium of the esophagus [114], whereas their expression increases in Barrett's Esophagus, to decline in EA [115]. Divalent metal transporter1 (DMT1, **SLC11A2**) overexpression was associated with metastatization in EC [116]. One of the main causes of chemotherapy failure is drug efflux mediated by ATP-binding cassette transporters (ABC) [117]. It was recently shown that **ABCG2** together with V-ATPase are overexpressed in ESCC and are associated with grading, TNM stage and metastatization. **ABCB1** and ABCG2 are expressed in primary GC and GC cell lines [118] in which their expression is associated with tumor differentiation. ABCB1 expression is higher in diffuse type GC [119]. ABCG2 represents a target for a several chemotherapy drugs [120]: for example, cisplatin increases *ABCG2* mRNA *in vitro* and this is associated with patients' outcome [121]. In PDAC, **ABCB4, ABCB11, ABCC1, ABCC3, ABCC5, ABCC10** and ABCG2 are up-regulated, while **ABCA3, ABCC6**, CFTR (**ABCC7**) and **ABCC8** are down-regulated: such deregulation contributes to PDAC poor response to therapy [122]. The Solute Carrier transporters (SLC) is a family of transporters frequently deregulated in PDAC. **SLC7A5** (the L-type aminoacid transporter 1) are overexpressed in PDAC and are associated with molecular and clinico-pathological features (such as Ki-67, p53, CD34, CD98, VEGF size, stage) and prognosis [122]. **SLC22A3** and **SLC22A18** are up-regulated in PDAC with respect to healthy pancreas while **SLC22A1, SLC22A2, SLC22A11, SLC28A1, SLC28A3** and **SLC29A1** are down-regulated [122]. In particular, SLC28A1 overexpression was associated with poor overall survival whereas SLC22A3 and SLC29A3 overexpression was observed in patients treated with Gemcitabine with longer overall survival. PC patients with low expression of SMCT1 (**SLC5A8**) have poorer survival with respect to patients with high SLC5A8 levels [123]. The human equilibrative nucleoside transporter 1 (**SLC29A1**) is associated to longer time to progression and it was shown that it could predict gemcitabine effects in non-resectable PDAC patients, if evaluated in samples obtained by fine-needle aspiration [124]. Different conclusions were drawn when analyzing SLC29A1 expression in patients treated with chemo-radiotherapy [125]. In GC, **SLC7A5** overexpression was detected and it was found to be associated with clinico-pathological features such as size, lymph node involvement, TNM stage and local invasion [126]. **SLC16A1** was found to be expressed both in healthy stomach and GC, and it could be hypothesized a role in gastric physiology for this transporter [119]. In metastatic GC, **SLC16A3** is down-regulated [119] and is associated with intestinal type. 4F2hc (**SLC3A2**) was found to be over-expressed in GC cell lines and in primary GC, with no significant correlation with clinico-pathological features. Since the study was conducted on a small number of samples, it could not allow definitive conclusions [127].

4. Ion channels and transporters with clinical relevance in hematologic malignancies

As reported for solid tumors, a schematic overview of ion channels and transporters expressed in hematologic tumors is reported in **Figure 2**. Early evidence for the implication of K^+ channels in leukemia cell proliferation was obtained in the myeloblastic leukemia cell line ML-1 [128]. In leukemias, it was shown that **KCa3.1** might represent a useful target since its blockade impairs leukemic cells proliferation [129] while *KCNN4* overexpression was detected in follicular lymphomas [130]. A significant **Kv10.1** expression was detected in myelodysplastic syndromes, CML and almost half of a cohort of AML samples and blocking the channel results in the inhibition of both cell proliferation and migration. Smith

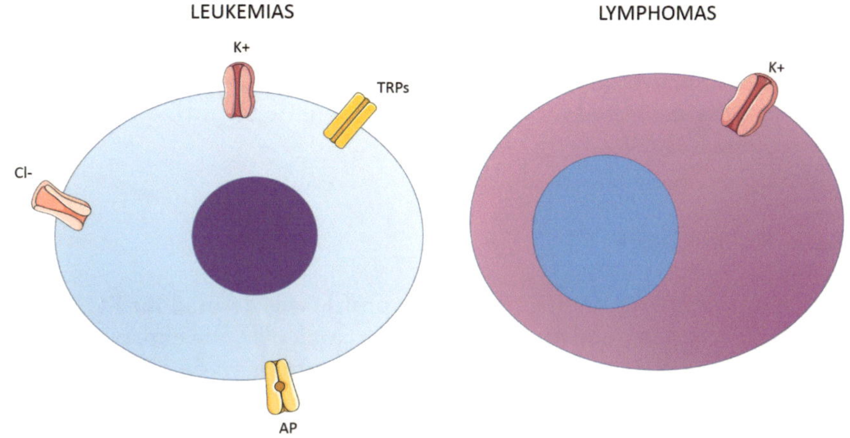

Figure 2.
Cartoon showing the main ICTs expressed in leukemias and lymphomas.

and colleagues [131] carried out an extensive study of the K+ channel transcripts in primary lymphocytes, leukemias (B-cell CLL) and several leukemic cell lines and they found only ***Kv11.1*** was significantly up-regulated. In AML cell lines (FLG 29.1, HL-60 and K562), it was shown that specific block of IKv11.1 led to G1 arrest and impaired their migration on fibronectin-containing ECM [132]. Kv11.1 was also overexpressed in circulating blasts from human AML, in which the block of the channel significantly decreased cell growth [132]. The *hsloBK* splice variant of ***gBK*** has been detected in gliomas [133] and the *herg1b* alternative transcript of *Kv11.1* is overexpressed in human leukemias and neuroblastomas [134, 135]. TWIK-related spinal cord K+ (**TRESK**) channels, members of the double-pore domain K+ channel family, are expressed in Jurkat cells [136] that also express TRPV5 and TRPV6, which were also detected in K562 cells. TRP channels control Ca^{2+} homeostasis in the context of malignant transformation [137] and it was shown that of TRPV5/TRPV6-like channels' activation mediate Ca^{2+} entry and the activation of Ca^{2+}/Calmodulin-dependent kinase II in irradiated K562 cells [138].

During the oxidative burst following activation of K562 cells non-selective cation channel TRPM2 are activated, thus activating **SK4** KCa channels. In parallel, the voltage-gated Cl-channel **ClC-3** is also activated. The overall effect is cell shrinkage because of the osmotic water loss determined KCl outflow [139, 140]. A similar volume-dependent regulation of leukemia cell apoptosis can be operated by volume-regulated chloride currents (**VRCC**). The volume-dependent regulatory mechanisms are accompanied by control of water levels suggesting it could represent an additional modulatory mechanism in the apoptotic cascade [141]. AQPs control osmotic fluxes in a variety of physiological conditions. For instance, AQP5 is overexpressed in CML cells, where it promotes cell proliferation and inhibits apoptosis, perhaps through an effect on cell volume control [142]. Expression of AQP5 increases in parallel with the development of resistance to imatinib mesylate [142].

5. Targeting ion channels and transporters for cancer diagnosis with antibodies

Recently, an antibody directed to a cancer-related ion channel (the purinergic receptor P2X7) was introduced into the clinical settings: it is a polyclonal antibody targeting a conformational epitope of the non-functional channel and it is likely to be approved as a first-generation therapy. Antibodies targeting ORAI1 were obtained using U2OS cells overexpressing human ORAI1 as immunogens. One of such antibodies impaired cell proliferation of T lymphocytes in peripheral blood [143, 144]. In 2014, a method for the isolation of functional antibodies against Nav1.7 was published [145].

6. Future perspectives

In a recent paper [146], an ICT molecular profile was defined for BC thus opening interesting perspectives in this field. In particular, the expression of 30 ion channel genes was shown to be associated with tumor grade. The authors were able of identifying a "IC30 gene signature" composed of 30 ion channel genes and demonstrated that IC30 might represent a prognostic biomarker predicting clinical outcome in BC, independently from clinical and pathological prognostic factors. The same approach was applied to LC and 37 ion channels genes were identified as differentially expressed in LC in comparison to healthy lung [147]. Moreover, 31 ion channel genes were identified as differentially expressed between lung adenocarcinoma and squamous-cell carcinoma samples, therefore the expression of such genes could be used for NSCLC molecular classification [147]. In NSCLC, it was shown that VDAC1 is an independent prognostic factor and it is associated with shorter overall survival [147]. VDAC1 was also found to be up-regulated in different types of carcinomas [148]. More recently, a paper describing gene expression profile in lymphomas demonstrated that *KCNN4* and *SLC2A1* genes are overexpressed in follicular lymphomas (FL) [130]. In particular, ***SLC2A1*** was proposed to be the hub of a functional network, connecting channels and transporters in FL. Moreover, relapsed FL had 38 differentially expressed ICT genes, among which **ATP9A**, **SLC2A1** and **KCNN4** were under-expressed. In the same paper, it was shown that diffuse large B Cell lymphoma (DLBCL) have a completely different pattern of K^+ channel encoding genes expression along with the overexpression of the fatty acid transporter-encoding gene **SLC27A1**.

Conflict of interest

The authors declare no conflict of interest.

Author details

Jessica Iorio, Claudia Duranti and Elena Lastraioli*
Department of Experimental and Clinical Medicine, Florence, Italy

*Address all correspondence to: elena.lastraioli@unifi.it

References

[1] Arcangeli A, Crociani O, Bencini L. Interaction of tumour cells with their microenvironment: Ion channels and cell adhesion molecules. A focus on pancreatic cancer. Philosophical Transactions of the Royal Society of London. Series B, Biological Sciences. 2014;**369**(1638):20130101. DOI: 10.1098/rstb.2013.0101

[2] Lastraioli E, Iorio J, Arcangeli A. Ion channel expression as promising cancer biomarker. Biochimica et Biophysica Acta. 2015;**1848**(10 Pt B):2685-2702. DOI: 10.1016/j.bbamem.2014.12.016

[3] Pedersen SF, Novak I, Alves F. Alternating pH landscapes shape epithelial cancer initiation and progression: Focus on pancreatic cancer. BioEssays. 2017;**39**(6):1-10. DOI: 10.1002/bies.201600253

[4] Arcangeli A, Crociani O, Lastraioli E. Targeting ion channels in cancer: A novel frontier in antineoplastic therapy. Current Medicinal Chemistry. 2009;**16**(1):66-93. DOI: 10.2174/092986709787002835

[5] Wulff H, Castle NA, Pardo LA. Voltage-gated potassium channels as therapeutic targets. Nature Reviews. Drug Discovery. 2009;**8**(12):982-1001. DOI: 10.1038/nrd2983

[6] Prevarskaya N, Skryma R, Shuba Y. Ion channels in cancer: Are cancer hallmarks oncochannelopathies? Physiological Reviews. 2018;**98**(2):559-621. DOI: 10.1152/physrev.00044.2016

[7] Kaur S, Venktaraman G, Jain M. Recent trends in antibody-based oncologic imaging. Cancer Letters. 2012;**315**:97-111. DOI: 10.1016/j.canlet.2011.10.017

[8] Xu W, Liu L, Brown NJ. Quantum dot-conjugated anti-GRP78 scFv inhibits cancer growth in mice. Molecules. 2012;**17**:796-808. DOI: 10.3390/molecules17010796

[9] Sharma SK, Wuest M, Way JD. Synthesis and pre-clinical evaluation of an (18)F-labeled single-chain antibody fragment for PET imaging of epithelial ovarian cancer. American Journal of Nuclear Medicine and Molecular Imaging. 2016;**6**:185-198

[10] Han D, Wu J, Han Y. A novel anti-PSMA human scFv has the potential to be used as a diagnostic tool in prostate cancer. Oncotarget. 2016;**7**:59471-59481. DOI: 10.18632/oncotarget.10697

[11] Mazzocco C, Fracasso G, Germain-Genevois C. In vivo imaging of prostate cancer using an anti-PSMA scFv fragment as a probe. Scientific Reports. 2016;**6**:23314. DOI: 10.1038/srep23314

[12] Duranti C, Arcangeli A. Ion channel targeting with antibodies and antibody fragments for cancer diagnosis. Antibodies. 2019;**8**(2):33. DOI: 10.3390/antib8020033

[13] Holliger P, Hudson PJ. Engineered antibody fragments and the rise of single domains. Nature Biotechnology. 2005;**23**:1126-1136. DOI: 10.1038/nbt1142

[14] Oeggerli M, Tian Y, Ruiz C. Role of KCNMA1 in breast cancer. PLoS One. 2012;**7**(8):e41664. DOI: 10.1371/journal.pone.0041664

[15] Brevet M, Ahidouch A, Sevestre H. Expression of K+ channels in normal and cancerous human breast. Histology and Histopathology. 2008;**23**(8):965-972. DOI: 10.14670/HH-23.965.

[16] Khaitan D, Sankpal UT, Weksler B. Role of KCNMA1 gene in breast cancer invasion and metastasis

to brain. BMC Cancer. 2009;**9**:258. DOI: 10.1186/1471-2407-9-258

[17] Bloch M, Ousingsawat J, Simon R. KCNMA1 gene amplification promotes tumor cell proliferation in human prostate cancer. Oncogene. 2007;**26**(17):2525-2534. DOI: 10.1038/sj.onc.1210036

[18] Altintas DM, Allioli N, Decaussin M. Differentially expressed androgen-regulated genes in androgen-sensitive tissues reveal potential biomarkers of early prostate cancer. PLoS One. 2013;**8**(6):e66278. DOI: 10.1371/journal.pone.0066278

[19] Haren N, Khorsi H, Faouzi M. Intermediate conductance Ca^{2+} activated K^{+} channels are expressed and functional in breast adenocarcinomas: Correlation with tumour grade and metastasis status. Histology and Histopathology. 2010;**25**(10):1247-1255. DOI: 10.14670/HH-25.1247.

[20] Bonito B, Sauter DR, Schwab A. $K_{Ca}3.1$ (IK) modulates pancreatic cancer cell migration, invasion and proliferation: Anomalous effects on TRAM-34. Pflügers Archiv. 2016;**468**(11-12):1865-1875. DOI: 10.1007/s00424-016-1891-9

[21] Lai W, Liu L, Zeng Y. KCNN4 channels participate in the EMT induced by PRL-3 in colorectal cancer. Medical Oncology. 2013;**30**:566. DOI: 10.1007/s12032-013-0566-z

[22] Bulk E, Ay AS, Hammadi M. Epigenetic dysregulation of KCa 3.1 channels induces poor prognosis in lung cancer. International Journal of Cancer. 2015;**137**(6):1306-1317. DOI: 10.1002/ijc.29490

[23] Pillozzi S, D'Amico M, Bartoli G. The combined activation of $K_{Ca}3.1$ and inhibition of $K_v11.1$/hERG1 currents contribute to overcome Cisplatin resistance in colorectal cancer cells. British Journal of Cancer. 2018;**118**(2):200-212. DOI: 10.1038/bjc.2017.392

[24] Muratori L, Petroni G, Antonuzzo L. hERG1 positivity and Glut-1 negativity identifies high-risk TNM stage I and II colorectal cancer patients, regardless of adjuvant chemotherapy. OncoTargets and Therapy. 2016;**9**:6325-6332. DOI: 10.2147/OTT.S114090

[25] Bielanska J, Hernández-Losa J, Pérez-Verdaguer M. Voltage-dependent potassium channels Kv1.3 and Kv1.5 in human cancer. Current Cancer Drug Targets. 2009;**9**(8):904-914. DOI: 10.3389/fphys.2013.00283

[26] Ohya S, Kimura K, Niwa S. Malignancy grade-dependent expression of K^{+}-channel subtypes in human prostate cancer. Journal of Pharmacological Sciences. 2009;**109**(1):148-151. DOI: 10.254/jphs.08208S

[27] Abdul M, Hoosein N. Reduced Kv1.3 potassium channel expression in human prostate cancer. The Journal of Membrane Biology. 2006;**214**(2):99-102. DOI: 10.1007/s00232-006-0065-7

[28] Brevet M, Fucks D, Chatelain D. Deregulation of 2 potassium channels in pancreas adenocarcinomas: Implication of KV1.3 gene promoter methylation. Pancreas. 2009;**38**(6):649-654. DOI: 10.1097/MPA.0b013e3181a56ebf

[29] Mu D, Chen L, Zhang X. Genomic amplification and oncogenic properties of the KCNK9 potassium channel gene. Cancer Cell. 2003;**3**(3):297-302. DOI: 10.1016/S1535-6108(03)00054-0

[30] Alvarez-Baron CP, Jonsson P, Thomas C. The two-pore domain potassium channel KCNK5: Induction by estrogen receptor alpha and role in proliferation of breast cancer cells. Molecular Endocrinology.

2011;**25**(8):1326-1336. DOI: 10.1210/me.2011-0045

[31] Voloshyna I, Besana A, Castillo M. TREK-1 is a novel molecular target in prostate cancer. Cancer Research. 2008;**68**(4):1197-1203. DOI: 10.1158/0008-5472.CAN-07-5163

[32] Stringer BK, Cooper AG, Shepard SB. Overexpression of the G-protein inwardly rectifying potassium channel 1 (GIRK1) in primary breast carcinomas correlates with axillary lymph node metastasis. Cancer Research. 2001;**61**(2):582-588

[33] Hemmerlein B, Weseloh RM, Mello de Queiroz F. Overexpression of Eag1 potassium channels in clinical tumours. Molecular Cancer. 2006;5(41):1-13. DOI: 10.1186/1476-4598-5-41

[34] Abdul M, Hoosein N. Voltage-gated potassium ion channels in colon cancer. Oncology Reports. 2002;**9**(5):961-964. DOI: 10.3892/or.9.5.961

[35] Ousingsawat J, Spitzner M, Puntheeranurak S. Expression of voltage-gated potassium channels in human and mouse colonic carcinoma. Clinical Cancer Research. 2007;**13**(3):824-831. DOI: 10.1158/1078-0432.CCR-06-1940

[36] Lastraioli E, Guasti L, Crociani O. herg1 gene and HERG1 protein are overexpressed in colorectal cancers and regulate cell invasion of tumor cells. Cancer Research. 2004;**64**(2):606-611. DOI: 10.1158/0008-5472.CAN-03-2360

[37] Kim CJ, Cho YG, Jeong SW. Altered expression of KCNK9 in colorectal cancers. APMIS. 2004;**112**(9):588-594. DOI: 10.1111/j.1600-0463.2004.apm1120905.x

[38] Ding XW, Wang XG, Luo HS. Expression and prognostic roles of Eag1 in resected esophageal squamous cell carcinomas. Digestive Diseases and Sciences. 2008;**53**(8):2039-2044. DOI: 10.1007/s10620-007-0116-7

[39] Lastraioli E, Gasperi Campani F, Taddei A. hERG1 channels are overexpressed in human gastric cancer and their activity regulates cell proliferation: A novel prognostic and therapeutic target? In: Proceedings of 6th IGCC; Yokohama. 2005. pp. 151-154

[40] Shao XD, Wu KC, Hao ZM. The potent inhibitory effects of cisapride, a specific blocker for human ether-a-go-go-related gene (HERG) channel, on gastric cancer cells. Cancer Biology & Therapy. 2005;**4**(3):295-301. DOI: 10.4161/cbt.4.3.1500

[41] Shao XD, Wu KC, Guo XZ. Expression and significance of HERG protein in gastric cancer. Cancer Biology & Therapy. 2008;**7**(1):45-50. DOI: 10.4161/cbt.7.1.5126

[42] Crociani O, Zanieri F, Pillozzi S. hERG1 channels modulate integrin signaling to trigger angiogenesis and tumor progression in colorectal cancer. Scientific Reports. 2013;**3**:3308. DOI: 10.1038/srep03308

[43] Lastraioli E, Bencini L, Bianchini E. hERG1 channels and Glut-1 as independent prognostic indicators of worse outcome in stage I and II colorectal cancer: A pilot study. Translational Oncology. 2012;**5**(2):105-112. DOI: 10.1593/tlo.11250

[44] Chen SZ, Jiang M, Zhen YS. HERG K+ channel expression-related chemosensitivity in cancer cells and its modulation by erythromycin. Cancer Chemotherapy and Pharmacology. 2005;**56**(2):212-220. DOI: 10.1007/s00280-004-0960-5

[45] Glassmeier G, Hempel K, Wulfsen I. Inhibition of HERG1 K+ channel protein expression decreases cell proliferation of human small cell lung cancer cells. Pflügers Archiv.

2012;**463**(2):365-376. DOI: 10.1007/s00424-011-1045-z

[46] Lastraioli E, Taddei A, Messerini L. hERG1 channels in human esophagus: Evidence for their aberrant expression in the malignant progression of Barrett's esophagus. Journal of Cellular Physiology. 2006;**209**(2):398-404. DOI: 10.1002/jcp.20748

[47] Ding XW, Luo HS, Luo B. Overexpression of hERG1 in resected esophageal squamous cell carcinomas: A marker for poor prognosis. Journal of Surgical Oncology. 2008;**97**(1):57-62. DOI: 10.1002/jso.20891

[48] Lastraioli E, Perrone G, Sette A. hERG1 channels drive tumour malignancy and may serve as prognostic factor in pancreatic ductal adenocarcinoma. British Journal of Cancer. 2015;**112**(6):1076-1087. DOI: 10.1038/bjc.2015.28

[49] Fraser SP, Diss JK, Chioni AM. Voltage-gated sodium channel expression and potentiation of human breast cancer metastasis. Clinical Cancer Research. 2005;**11**(15):5381-5389. DOI: 10.1158/1078-0432.CCR-05-0327

[50] Brackenbury WJ, Chioni AM, Diss JK. The neonatal splice variant of Nav1.5 potentiates in vitro invasive behaviour of MDA-MB-231 human breast cancer cells. Breast Cancer Research and Treatment. 2007;**101**(2):149-160. DOI: 10.1007/s10549-006-9281-1

[51] Gillet L, Roger S, Besson P. Voltage-gated sodium channel activity promotes cysteine cathepsin-dependent invasiveness and colony growth of human cancer cells. The Journal of Biological Chemistry. 2009;**284**(13):8680-8691. DOI: 10.1074/jbc.M806891200

[52] Chioni AM, Fraser SP, Pani F. A novel polyclonal antibody specific for the Na(v)1.5 voltage-gated Na(+) channel 'neonatal' splice form. Journal of Neuroscience Methods. 2005;**147**(2):88-98. DOI: 10.1016/j.jneumeth.2005.03.010

[53] Guzel RM, Ogmen K, Ilieva KM. Colorectal cancer invasiveness in vitro: Predominant contribution of neonatal Nav1.5 under normoxia and hypoxia. Journal of Cellular Physiology. 2019;**234**(5):6582-6593. DOI: 10.1002/jcp.27399

[54] Fairhurst C, Martin F, Watt I. Sodium channel-inhibiting drugs and cancer survival: Protocol for a cohort study using the CPRD primary care database. BMJ Open. 2016;**6**(9):e011661. DOI: 10.1136/bmjopen-2016-011661

[55] Roger S, Gillet L, Le Guennec JY. Voltage-gated sodium channels and cancer: Is excitability their primary role? Frontiers in Pharmacology. 2015;**6**:152. DOI: 10.3389/fphar.2015.00152

[56] Baptista-Hon DT, Robertson FM, Robertson GB. Potent inhibition by ropivacaine of metastatic colon cancer SW620 cell invasion and NaV1.5 channel function. British Journal of Anaesthesia. 2014;**113**(Suppl. 1):i39-i48. DOI: 10.1093/bja/aeu104

[57] Diss JK, Fraser SP, Djamgoz MB. Voltage-gated Na+ channels: Multiplicity of expression, plasticity, functional implications and pathophysiological aspects. European Biophysics Journal. 2004;**33**(3):180-193. DOI: 10.1007/s00249-004-0389-0

[58] Diss JK, Stewart D, Pani F. A potential novel marker for human prostate cancer: Voltage-gated sodium channel expression in vivo. Prostate Cancer and Prostatic Diseases. 2005;**8**(3):266-273. DOI: 10.1038/sj.pcan.4500796

[59] Campbell TM, Main MJ, Fitzgerald EM. Functional expression of the voltage-gated Na^+-channel Nav1.7 is necessary for EGF-mediated invasion in human non-small cell lung cancer cells. Journal of Cell Science. 2013;**126**(Pt 21):4939-4949. DOI: 10.1242/jcs.130013

[60] Argyriou AA, Cavaletti G, Antonacopoulou A. Voltage-gated sodium channel polymorphisms play a pivotal role in the development of oxaliplatin-induced peripheral neurotoxicity: Results from a prospective multicenter study. Cancer. 2013;**119**(19):3570-3577. DOI: 10.1002/cncr.28234

[61] Haustrate A, Hantute-Ghesquier A, Prevarskaya N. TRPV6 calcium channel regulation, downstream pathways, and therapeutic targeting in cancer. Cell Calcium. 2019;**80**:117-124. DOI: 10.1016/j.ceca.2019.04.006

[62] Fliniaux I, Germain E, Farfariello V, Prevarskaya N. TRPs and Ca^{2+} in cell death and survival. Cell Calcium. 2018;**69**:4-18. DOI: 10.1016/j.ceca.2017.07.002

[63] Iamshanova O, Fiorio Pla A, Prevarskaya N. Molecular mechanisms of tumour invasion: Regulation by calcium signals. The Journal of Physiology. 2017;**595**(10):3063-3075. DOI: 10.1113/JP272844

[64] Palmieri C, Rudraraju B, Monteverde M. Methylation of the calcium channel regulatory subunit α2δ-3 (CACNA2D3) predicts site-specific relapse in oestrogen receptor-positive primary breast carcinomas. British Journal of Cancer. 2012;**107**(2):375-381. DOI: 10.1038/bjc.2012.231

[65] Motiani RK, Zhang X, Harmon KE. Orai3 is an estrogen receptor α-regulated Ca^{2+} channel that promotes tumorigenesis. The FASEB Journal. 2013;**27**(1):63-75. DOI: 10.1096/fj.12-213801

[66] Shapovalov G, Skryma R, Prevarskaya N. Calcium channels and prostate cancer. Recent Patents on Anti-Cancer Drug Discovery. 2013;**8**(1):18-26. DOI: 10.2174/15748928113080100018

[67] Vanden Abeele F, Zholos A, Bidaux G. Ca^{2+}-independent phospholipase A2-dependent gating of TRPM8 by lysophospholipids. The Journal of Biological Chemistry. 2006;**281**(52):40174-40182. DOI: 10.1074/jbc.M605779200

[68] Wanajo A, Sasaki A, Nagasaki H. Methylation of the calcium channel-related gene, CACNA2D3, is frequent and a poor prognostic factor in gastric cancer. Gastroenterology. 2008;**135**(2):580-590. DOI: 10.1053/j.gastro.2008.05.041

[69] McAndrew D, Grice DM, Peters AA. ORAI1-mediated calcium influx in lactation and in breast cancer. Molecular Cancer Therapeutics. 2011;**10**(3):448-460. DOI: 10.1158/1535-7163.MCT-10-0923

[70] Faouzi M, Hague F, Potier M. Down-regulation of Orai3 arrests cell-cycle progression and induces apoptosis in breast cancer cells but not in normal breast epithelial cells. Journal of Cellular Physiology. 2011;**226**(2):542-551. DOI: 10.1002/jcp.22363

[71] Clapham DE. TRP channels as cellular sensors. Nature. 2003;**426**(6966):517-524. DOI: 10.1038/nature02196

[72] Nilius B, Owsianik G. The transient receptor potential family of ion channels. Genome Biology. 2011;**12**(3):218. DOI: 10.1186/gb-2011-12-3-218

[73] Canales J, Morales D, Blanco C. TR(i)P to cell migration:

New roles of TRP channels in mechanotransduction and cancer. Frontiers in Physiology. 2019;**10**:757. DOI: 10.3389/fphys.2019.00757

[74] Dhennin-Duthille I, Gautier M, Faouzi M. High expression of transient receptor potential channels in human breast cancer epithelial cells and tissues: Correlation with pathological parameters. Cellular Physiology and Biochemistry. 2011;**28**(5):813-822. DOI: 10.1159/000335795

[75] Nilius B. Transient receptor potential (TRP) cation channels: Rewarding unique proteins. Bulletin et Mémoires de l'Académie Royale de Médecine de Belgique. 2007;**162**(3-4):244-253

[76] Shi Y, Ding X, He ZH. Critical role of TRPC6 channels in G2 phase transition and the development of human oesophageal cancer. Gut. 2009;**58**(11):1443-1450. DOI: 10.1136/gut.2009.181735

[77] Zhang SS, Wen J, Yang F. High expression of transient potential receptor C6 correlated with poor prognosis in patients withesophageal squamous cell carcinoma. Medical Oncology. 2013;**30**(3):607. DOI: 10.1007/s12032-013-0607-7

[78] Bolanz KA, Hediger MA, Landowski CP. The role of TRPV6 in breast carcinogenesis. Molecular Cancer Therapeutics. 2008;**7**(2):271-279. DOI: 10.1158/1535-7163.MCT-07-0478

[79] Peters AA, Simpson PT, Bassett JJ. Calcium channel TRPV6 as a potential therapeutic target in estrogen receptor-negative breast cancer. Molecular Cancer Therapeutics. 2012;**11**(10):2158-2168. DOI: 10.1158/1535-7163.MCT-11-0965

[80] Fixemer T, Wissenbach U, Flockerzi V. Expression of the Ca^{2+}-selective cation channel TRPV6 in human prostate cancer: A novel prognostic marker for tumor progression. Oncogene. 2003;**22**(49):7858-7861. DOI: 10.1038/sj.onc.1206895

[81] Li C, Wu Y, Zhu Q. TRPV4 is involved in levonorgestrel-induced reduction in oviduct ciliary beating. The Journal of Pathology. 2019;**248**(1):77-87. DOI: 10.1002/path.5233

[82] Middelbeek J, Arthur J, Kuipers AJ, Henneman L. TRPM7 is required for breast tumor cell metastasis. Cancer Research. 2012;**72**(16):1-12. DOI: 10.1158/0008-5472.CAN-11-3863

[83] Rybarczyk P, Vanlaeys A, Brassart B. The transient receptor potential melastatin 7 channel regulates pancreatic cancer cell invasion through the Hsp90α/uPA/MMP2 pathway. Neoplasia. 2017;**19**(4):288-300. DOI: 10.1016/j.neo.2017.01.004

[84] Gao SL, Kong CZ, Zhang Z. TRPM7 is overexpressed in bladder cancer and promotes proliferation, migration, invasion and tumor growth. Oncology Reports. 2017;**38**(4):1967-1976. DOI: 10.3892/or.2017.5883

[85] Schaefer EA, Stohr S, Meister M. Stimulation of the chemosensory TRPA1 cation channel by volatile toxic substances promotes cell survival of small cell lung cancer cells. Biochemical Pharmacology. 2013;**85**(3):426-438. DOI: 10.1016/j.bcp.2012.11.019

[86] Britschgi A, Bill A, Brinkhaus H, Choudhury M, Gosling L, Wang S, et al. Bentires-AljCalcium-activated chloride channel ANO1 promotes breast cancer progression by activating EGFR and CAMK signaling. Proceedings of the National Academy of Sciences of the United States of America. 2013;**110**(11):E1026-E1034. DOI: 10.1073/pnas.1217072110

[87] Mazzone A, Eisenman ST, Strege PR. Inhibition of cell proliferation by a selective inhibitor of the Ca(2+)-activated Cl(−) channel, Ano1. Biochemical and Biophysical Research Communications. 2012;**427**(2):248-253. DOI: 10.1016/j.bbrc.2012.09.022

[88] Yang B, Cao L, Liu B. The transition from proliferation to differentiation in colorectal cancer is regulated by the calcium activated chloride channel A1. PLoS One. 2013;**8**(4):e60861. DOI: 10.1371/journal.pone.0060861

[89] Ma PF, Chen JQ, Wang Z. Function of chloride intracellular channel 1 in gastric cancer cells. World Journal of Gastroenterology. 2012;**18**(24):3070-3080. DOI: 10.3748/wjg.v18.i24.3070

[90] Chen CD, Wang CS, Huang YH. Overexpression of CLIC1 in human gastric carcinoma and its clinicopathological significance. Proteomics. 2007;**7**(1):155-167. DOI: 10.1002/pmic.200600663

[91] Dozynkiewicz MA, Jamieson NB, Macpherson I. Rab25 and CLIC3 collaborate to promote integrin recycling from late endosomes/lysosomes and drive cancer progression. Developmental Cell. 2012;**22**(1):131-145. DOI: 10.1016/j.devcel.2011.11.008

[92] Falvella FS, Galvan A, Colombo F. Promoter polymorphisms and transcript levels of nicotinic receptor CHRNA5. Journal of the National Cancer Institute. 2010;**102**(17):1366-1370. DOI: 10.1093/jnci/djq264

[93] Egleton RD, Brown KC, Dasgupta P. Nicotinic acetylcholine receptors in cancer: Multiple roles in proliferation and inhibition of apoptosis. Trends in Pharmacological Sciences. 2008;**29**(3):151-158. DOI: 10.1016/j.tips.2007.12.006

[94] Amos CI, Wu X, Broderick P. Genome-wide association scan of tag SNPs identifies a susceptibility locus for lung cancer at 15q25.1. Nature Genetics. 2008;**40**(5):616-622. DOI: 10.1038/ng.109

[95] George AA, Lucero LM, Damaj MI. Function of human α3β4α5 nicotinic acetylcholine receptors is reduced by the α5(D398N) variant. The Journal of Biological Chemistry. 2012;**287**(30):25151-25162. DOI: 10.1074/jbc.M112.379339

[96] Ma X, Jia Y, Zu S. α5 nicotinic acetylcholine receptor mediates nicotine-induced HIF-1α and VEGF expression in non-small cell lung cancer. Toxicology and Applied Pharmacology. 2014;**278**(2):172-179. DOI: 10.1016/j.taap.2014.04.023

[97] Otterbach F, Callies R, Adamzik M. Aquaporin 1 (AQP1) expression is a novel characteristic feature of a particularly aggressive subgroup of basal-like breast carcinomas. Breast Cancer Research and Treatment. 2010;**120**(1):67-76. DOI: 10.1007/s10549-009-0370-9

[98] Moon C, Soria JC, Jang SJ. Involvement of aquaporins in colorectal carcinogenesis. Oncogene. 2003;**22**(43):6699-6703. DOI: 10.1038/sj.onc.1206762

[99] Wang P, Zhang C, Yu P. Regulation of colon cancer cell migration and invasion by CLIC1-mediated RVD. Molecular and Cellular Biochemistry. 2012;**365**(1-2):313-321. DOI: 10.1007/s11010-012-1271-5

[100] Watanabe T, Fujii T, Oya T. Involvement of aquaporin-5 in differentiation of human gastric cancer cells. The Journal of Physiological Sciences. 2009;**59**(2):113-122. DOI: 10.1007/s12576-008-0017-3

[101] Shen L, Zhu Z, Huang Y. Expression profile of multiple

aquaporins in human gastric carcinoma and its clinical significance. Biomedicine & Pharmacotherapy. 2010;**64**(5):313-318. DOI: 10.1016/j.biopha.2009.12.003

[102] Li A, Lu D, Zhang Y. Critical role of aquaporin-3 in epidermal growth factor-induced migration of colorectal carcinoma cells and its clinical significance. Oncology Reports. 2013;**29**(2):535-540. DOI: 10.3892/or.2012.2144

[103] Kusayama M, Wada K, Nagata M. Critical role of aquaporin 3 on growth of human esophageal and oral squamous cell carcinoma. Cancer Science. 2011;**102**(6):1128-1136. DOI: 10.1111/j.1349-7006.2011.01927.x

[104] Liu S, Zhang S, Jiang H. Co-expression of AQP3 and AQP5 in esophageal squamous cell carcinoma correlates with aggressive tumor progression and poor prognosis. Medical Oncology. 2013;**30**(3):636. DOI: 10.1007/s12032-013-0636-2

[105] Pinheiro C, Albergaria A, Paredes J. Monocarboxylate transporter 1 is up-regulated in basal-like breast carcinoma. Histopathology. 2010;**56**(7):860-867. DOI: 10.1111/j.1365-2559.2010.03560.x

[106] Wang Y, Li SJ, Wu X. Clinicopathological and biological significance of human voltage-gated proton channel Hv1 protein overexpression in breast cancer. The Journal of Biological Chemistry. 2012;**287**(17):13877-13888. DOI: 10.1074/jbc.M112.345280

[107] Wang Y, Wu X, Li Q. Human voltage-gated proton channel hv1: A new potential biomarker for diagnosis and prognosis of colorectal cancer. PLoS One. 2013;**8**(8):e70550. DOI: 10.1371/journal.pone.0070550

[108] Iino I, Kikuchi H, Miyazaki S. Effect of miR-122 and its target gene cationic amino acid transporter 1 on colorectal liver metastasis. Cancer Science. 2013;**104**(5):624-630. DOI: 10.1111/cas.12122

[109] Cardone RA, Greco MR, Zeeberg K. A novel NHE1-centered signaling cassette drives epidermal growth factor receptor-dependent pancreatic tumor metastasis and is a target for combination therapy. Neoplasia. 2015;**17**(2):155-166. DOI: 10.1016/j.neo.2014.12.003

[110] Younes M, Ertan A, Lechago LV. Human erythrocyte glucose transporter (Glut1) is immunohistochemically detected as a late event during malignant progression in Barrett's metaplasia. Cancer Epidemiology, Biomarkers & Prevention. 1997;**6**(5):303-305

[111] Tohma T, Okazumi S, Makino H. Overexpression of glucose transporter 1 in esophageal squamous cell carcinomas: A marker for poor prognosis. Diseases of the Esophagus. 2005;**18**(3):185-189. DOI: 10.1111/j.1442-2050.2005.00489.x

[112] Doki Y, Takachi K, Ishikawa O. Reduced tumor vessel density and high expression of glucose transporter 1 suggest tumor hypoxia of squamous cell carcinoma of the esophagus surviving after radiotherapy. Surgery. 2005;**137**(5):536-544. DOI: 10.1016/j.surg.2005.01.008

[113] Alrefai WA, Gill RK. Bile acid transporters: Structure, function, regulation and pathophysiological implications. Pharmaceutical Research. 2007;**24**(10):1803-1823. DOI: 10.1007/s11095-007-9289-1

[114] Trauner M, Boyer JL. Bile salt transporters: Molecular characterization, function and regulation. Physiological

Reviews. 2003;**83**(2):633-671. DOI: 10.1016/j.surg.2005.01.008

[115] Dvorak K, Watts GS, Ramsey L. Expression of bile acid transporting proteins in Barrett's esophagus and esophageal adenocarcinoma. The American Journal of Gastroenterology. 2009;**104**(2):302-309. DOI: 10.1038/ajg.2008.85

[116] Boult J, Roberts Brookes MJ. Overexpression of cellular iron import proteins is associated with malignant progression of esophageal adenocarcinoma. Clinical Cancer Research. 2008;**14**(2):379-387. DOI: 10.1158/1078-0432.CCR-07-1054

[117] Mohelnikova-Duchonova B, Brynychova V, Oliverius M. Differences in transcript levels of ABC transporters between pancreatic adenocarcinoma and nonneoplastic tissues. Pancreas. 2013;**42**(4):707-716. DOI: 10.1097/MPA.0b013e318279b861

[118] Jiang Y, He Y, Li H. Expressions of putative cancer stem cell markers ABCB1, ABCG2, and CD133 are correlated with the degree of differentiation of gastric cancer. Gastric Cancer. 2012;**15**(4):440-450. DOI: 10.1007/s10120-012-0140-y

[119] Pinheiro C, Longatto-Filho A, Simões K. The prognostic value of CD147/EMMPRIN is associated with monocarboxylate transporter 1 co-expression in gastric cancer. European Journal of Cancer. 2009;**45**(13):2418-2424. DOI: 10.1016/j.ejca.2009.06.018

[120] Schnepf R, Zolk O. Effect of the ATP-binding cassette transporter ABCG2 on pharmacokinetics: Experimental findings and clinical implications. Expert Opinion on Drug Metabolism & Toxicology. 2013;**9**(3):287-306. DOI: 10.1517/17425255.2013.742063

[121] Zhang Q, Li K, Xu JH. Role of ABCG2 expression driven by cisplatin in platinum-containing chemotherapy for gastric cancer. World Journal of Gastroenterology. 2013;**19**(39):6630-6636. DOI: 10.3748/wjg.v19.i39.6630

[122] Kaira K, Sunose Y, Arakawa K. Prognostic significance of L-type amino-acid transporter 1 expression in surgically resected pancreatic cancer. British Journal of Cancer. 2012;**107**(4):632-638. DOI: 10.1038/bjc.2012.310

[123] Helm J, Coppola D, Ganapathy V. SLC5A8 nuclear translocation and loss of expression are associated with poor outcome in pancreatic ductal adenocarcinoma. Pancreas. 2012;**41**(6):904-909. DOI: 10.1097/MPA.0b013e31823f429f

[124] Eto K, Kawakami H, Kuwatani M. Human equilibrative nucleoside transporter 1 and Notch3 can predict gemcitabine effects in patients with unresectable pancreatic cancer. British Journal of Cancer. 2013;**108**(7):1488-1494. DOI: 10.1038/bjc.2013.108

[125] Kawada N, Uehara H, Katayama K. Human equilibrative nucleoside transporter 1 level does not predict prognosis in pancreatic cancer patients treated with neoadjuvant chemoradiation including gemcitabine. Journal of Hepato-Biliary-Pancreatic Sciences. 2012;**19**(6):717-722. DOI: 10.1007/s00534-012-0514-x

[126] Wang J, Chen X, Su L. LAT-1 functions as a promotor in gastric cancer associated with clinicopathologic features. Biomedicine & Pharmacotherapy. 2013;**67**(8):693-699. DOI: 10.1016/j.biopha.2013.05.003

[127] Yang Y, Toy W, Choong LY. Discovery of SLC3A2 cell membrane protein as a potential gastric cancer

biomarker: Implications in molecular imaging. Journal of Proteome Research. 2012;**11**(12):5736-5747. DOI: 10.1021/pr300555y

[128] Lu L, Yang T, Markakis D. Alterations in a voltage-gated K+ current during the differentiation of ML-1 human myeloblastic leukemia cells. The Journal of Membrane Biology. 1993;**132**:267-274. DOI: 10.1007/bf00235743

[129] Grössinger EM, Weiss L, Zierler S. Targeting proliferation of chronic lymphocytic leukemia (CLL) cells through KCa3.1 blockade. Leukemia. 2014;**28**(4):954-958. DOI: 10.1038/leu.2014.37

[130] Magi A, Masselli M, Sala C. The ion channels and transporters gene expression profile indicates a shift in excitability and metabolisms during malignant progression of follicular lymphoma. Scientific Reports. 2019;**9**(1):8586. DOI: 10.1038/s41598-019-44661-x

[131] Smith GAM, Tsui HW, Newell EW. Functional up-regulation of HERG K^+ channels in neoplastic hematopoietic cells. The Journal of Biological Chemistry. 2002;**277**(18): 528-534. DOI: 10.1074/jbc.M200592200

[132] Pillozzi S, Brizzi MF, Balzi M. HERG potassium channels are constitutively expressed in primary human acute myeloid leukemias and regulate cell proliferation of normal and leukemic hemopoietic progenitors. Leukemia. 2002;**16**(9):1791-1798. DOI: 10.1038/sj.leu.2402572

[133] Olsen ML, Weaver AK, Ritch PS. Modulation of glioma BK channels via erbB2. Journal of Neuroscience Research. 2005;**81**:179-189. DOI: 10.1002/jnr.20543

[134] Pillozzi S, Brizzi MF, Bernabei PA. VEGFR-1 (FLT-1), beta1 integrin, and hERG K+ channel form a macromolecular signaling complex in acute myeloid leukemia: Role in cell migration and clinical outcome. Blood. 2007;**110**:1238-1250. DOI: 10.1182/blood-2006-02-003772

[135] Crociani O, Guasti L, Balzi MA. Cell cycle-dependent expression of HERG1 and HERG1B isoforms in tumor cells. The Journal of Biological Chemistry. 2003;**278**:2947-2955. DOI: 10.1074/jbc.M210789200

[136] Pottosin II, Bonales-Alatorre E, Valencia-Cruz G. TRESK-like potassium channels in leukemic T cells. Pflügers Archiv. 2008;**456**(6):1037-1048. DOI: 10.1007/s00424-008-0481-x

[137] Vasil'eva IO, Neguliaev IA, Marakhova II. TRPV5 and TRPV6 calcium channels in human T cells. Tsitologiia. 2008;**50**(11):953-957

[138] Heise N, Palme D, Misovic M. Non-selective cation channel-mediated Ca2+entry and activation of Ca2+/calmodulin-dependent kinase II contribute to G2/M cell cycle arrest and survival of irradiated leukemia cells. Cellular Physiology and Biochemistry. 2010;**26**(4-5):597-608. DOI: 10.1159/000322327

[139] Kasinathan RS, Föller M, Lang C. Oxidation induces ClC-3-dependent anion channels in human leukaemia cells. FEBS Letters. 2007;**581**(28):5407-5412. DOI: 10.1016/j.febslet.2007.10.042

[140] Jiang B, Hattori N, Liu B. Expression of swelling- and/or pH-regulated chloride channels (ClC-2, 3, 4 and 5) in human leukemic and normal immune cells. Life Sciences. 2002;**70**(12):1383-1394. DOI: 10.1016/s0024-3205(01)01517-x

[141] Renaudo A, Watry V, Chassot AA. Inhibition of tumor cell proliferation by sigma ligands is associated with K+ channel inhibition

and p27kip1 accumulation. The Journal of Pharmacology and Experimental Therapeutics. 2004;**311**(3):1105-1114. DOI: 10.1124/jpet.104.072413

[142] Chae YK, Kang SK, Kim MS. Human AQP5 plays a role in the progression of chronic myelogenous leukemia (CML). PLoS One. 2008;**3**(7):e2594. DOI: 10.1371/journal.pone.0002594

[143] Lin FF, Elliott R, Colombero A. Generation and characterization of fully human monoclonal antibodies against human Orai1 for autoimmune disease. The Journal of Pharmacology and Experimental Therapeutics. 2013;**345**:225-238. DOI: 10.1124/jpet.112.202788

[144] Cox JH, Hussell S, Søndergaard H. Antibody-mediated targeting of the Orai1 calcium channel inhibits T cell function. PLoS One. 2013;**8**:e82944. DOI: 10.1371/journal.pone.0082944

[145] Lee JH, Park CK, Chen G. A monoclonal antibody that targets a NaV1.7 channel voltage sensor for pain and itch relief. Cell. 2014;**157**:1393-1404. DOI: 10.1016/j.cell.2014.03.064

[146] Ko JH, Ko EA, Gu W. Expression profiling of ion channel genes predicts clinical outcome in breast cancer. Molecular Cancer. 2013;**12**(1):106. DOI: 10.1186/1476-4598-12-106

[147] Grills C, Jitesh PV, Blayney J. Gene expression meta-analysis identifies VDAC1 as a predictor of poor outcome in early stage non-small cell lung cancer. PLoS One. 2011;**6**:e14635. DOI: 10.1371/journal.pone.0014635

[148] Ko JH, Gu W, Lim I. Expression profiling of mitochondrial voltage-dependent anion channel-1 associated genes predicts recurrence-free survival in human carcinomas. PLoS One. 2014;**9**:e110094. DOI: 10.1371/journal.pone.0110094

Chapter 4

Translational Perspective in Hepatocellular Carcinoma

Sivapatham Sundaresan and Palanirasu Rajapriya

Abstract

The burden of liver cancer is higher in Hispanics, African Americans, and Asians. Viral hepatitis (Hepatitis B and Hepatitis C viruses), non-alcoholic steatohepatitis (NASH), and alcoholic liver disease (ALD) are the most common etiological/risk factors for liver cancer. Approximately 80–90% of hepatocellular carcinoma (HCC) occurs in patients with underlying liver cirrhosis. Individuals with advanced cirrhosis represent a high-risk group for liver cancer. To fill the increasing gap between basic science and clinical research, translational research has been developed as an emerging technology. Basic science attempts to unravel the mechanisms of disease using tools (e.g., culture systems and animal models) that allow for easy manipulation of biological processes. Further, culture systems and animal models are useful to derive causal associations, but they generally do not include an endpoint directly applicable to clinical practice. Hence, development of new tools for early detection, including the evaluation of liquid biopsy, identification of tissue biomarkers of treatment response, execution of precision and enhancement of patient stratification in patients at risk for HCC development to enable chemoprevention clinical trials becomes important. It was identified as translational research has begun as an effective approach to facilitate the development of novel molecular-based biomarkers and to accelerate the implementation of laboratory discoveries into clinically applicable tools. Despite great advancement in diagnosis and management of HCC, the exact biology of the tumor remains poorly understood generally limiting the clinical outcome. Comprehensive analysis and characterization of the molecular mechanisms and subsequently individual prediction of corresponding prognostic traits would transform both diagnosis and treatment of HCC and is the key goal of modern medicine. To overcome the challenge and to accelerate the progress, a collaborative effort from various clinical research groups and translational approach is needed.

Keywords: biomarkers, clinical research, cancer, hepatocellular carcinoma and translational research

1. Introduction

Hepatocellular carcinoma (HCC) is a common form of liver cancer associated with high mortality rate [1]. It is estimated that approximately 750,000 new cases of HCC diagnosed per year worldwide which makes HCC as the fifth common cause of cancers affecting human [2]. Mortality rate of approximately 700,000 has been estimated annually due to HCC and it has been considered as the third common cause of death [3].

World Health Organization (WHO) reported that about one million people annually was diagnosed with HCC [4]. The major risk factors for developing HCC are viral infections, alcoholic liver diseases and nonalcoholic steatohepatitis (NASH) [5]. In most of the cases, HCC was diagnosed after the disease progresses, when survival rates are low [6]. Development of HCC is asymptomatic at early stages of the disease when current curative therapies are available [7]. Diagnosis of HCC is based on the combination of radiological, serological and histopathological criteria [8]. Almost 90% of the cases are diagnosed without the help of liver biopsy, as many non-invasive techniques such as serological examination and imaging techniques are used as standard diagnostic test for HCC [9]. Ultrasonography is the most widely used imaging test for screening because of its diagnostic accuracy, non-invasiveness, good acceptance by patients and moderate cost [10].

Because of a large variability in etiological and genetic backgrounds and the long-time development of the disease, HCC lesions are known to exhibit substantial intra-tumor and inter-tumor heterogeneity [11]. For the treatment stratification in HCC, tumor heterogeneity poses a significant challenge [12]. Non-invasive assessment of several tumor characteristics, such as cellularity, perfusion and oxygenation, can be performed using quantitative functional multiparametric magnetic resonance imaging (mpMRI), which can be also used for tumor characterization and for assessing the treatment response [13]. Although pathological and genetic heterogeneity in HCC lesions have been defined, imaging reports on HCC heterogeneity are extremely inadequate, with only one study reporting visual assessment of HCC heterogeneity on contrast-enhanced MRI, with no such study describing quantitative imaging measurements of HCC heterogeneity [14].

Nowadays, magnetic resonance imaging (MRI) analysis has been used to study the characterization of HCC lesions in biopsied or resected samples, and also it provides further information on tumor properties [15]. Without histological confirmation, HCC can be detected using imaging alone in most of the patients, [16], but histopathologic assessment has its own advantage over imaging analysis. Results of the study by Hectors et al. indicated that HCC patients could ultimately benefit from knowledge of about the correlation of imaging parameters with histopathological and genomics properties of HCC lesions [17].

Based on tumor burden, hepatic function and performance status, patient prognosis and treatment decisions are made [18]. Surgical resection and liver transplantation are generally recommended for HCC, but is indicated specifically for patients with early stage and well-preserved liver function [19]. For patients not suitable for curative treatment, transarterial chemoembolization (TACE) and transarterial radioembolization (TARE) may provide better loco-regional tumor control and increase patient survival [20]. It is commonly acknowledged as a palliative treatment option and improves survival in unresectable HCC.

Primary liver cancer or HCC imposes significant challenges to healthcare with huge unmet clinical needs. In males, it is the second leading cause of cancer-related mortality worldwide and 80% of HCC cases are found in the Asia-Pacific regions [21]. Although treatments such as surgical resection, liver transplantation or radiofrequency ablation are potentially curable options for early-stage HCC, recurrences remain the most common issue and limit the overall survival [22]. Survival may be prolonged by loco-regional therapy in intermediate stage HCC and by systemic therapies in advanced HCC [23]. Overall, when compared to other common cancers, clinical outcomes in HCC remain poor due to the lack of effective therapies [24]. It's intrinsically quite challenging to understand the biology of HCC as it is the common end-point of a number of etiologies with different molecular pathways. In addition to increasing the complexity, significant heterogeneity is also existent within the same tumor [25].

Treatment outcomes for the majority of patients with HCC have remained poor through the years. The overall 5-year survival rate for all patients with HCC has remained steady at 3–5% [26]. This results from two facts. The first major reason is that for most patients, diagnosis is made only when the disease is in advanced stage and inoperable, and the second reason is when the disease has very poor prognosis. Furthermore, cirrhosis of the liver is a major risk factor for HCC development [27]. In most of the cases, the cause of cirrhosis is mainly due to chronic hepatitis B or C virus infection, or heavy alcohol usage [28]. Other known risk factors may include hereditary hemochromatosis, α-1 antitrypsin deficiency, primary biliary cirrhosis, autoimmune hepatitis, smoking and aflatoxin exposure [29]. Regardless of the cause, the accompanying cirrhosis can independently cause death as well as complicate other treatments [30].

Because of the challenges faced by current and future populations due to HCC, treatment has been an ever-rising area of interest for research. So far there was no such improved results from cytotoxic therapies have been reported. Researchers' recent efforts have been mainly focused on a variety of proven tactics and techniques [30]. Reducing morbidity and mortality are the major concerns in the modern surgical era, as various studies have recommended that precise evaluation of liver function reserve is indispensable for prognosticating the occurrence of morbidities and mortalities [31]. A number of confounding variables and background liver changes pose a major challenge in clinical proteomics studies that target liver diseases and biomarker discovery. Fat accumulation, inflammation, necrosis, apoptosis, proliferation, fibrosis and viral replication can all occur simultaneously in liver injury [32]. In general, insulin resistance is associated with the pathogenesis of nonalcoholic fatty liver disease (NAFLD). A role of hepatic steatosis in the pathogenesis of chronic hepatitis C has also been studied, implying hepatitis C as a metabolic disease. As a result, there is a need for novel strategies and careful experimental design [32].

To improve our better understanding of the liver biology, integrative studies such as proteomics and basic cellular biology or other developing fields such as imaging studies and mouse models will play the most prominent role. The translation of basic discoveries into daily clinical practice will accelerate the ability to understand the underlying molecular dysfunction in human disease (such as signaling pathways, protein–protein interaction networks) [32]. A study by Li et al. showed how mouse models of liver disease can be used to provide valuable functional information. Therefore, it helps to improve the current concepts for better screening and prevention [33]. Conde-Vandellis et al., described that biomarker discovery revealed a powerful new path to study proteomic analysis of extracellular, circulating or urinary vesicles [34].

2. Biomarkers in HCC

Various circulating markers and tissue markers have been identified. Because of their low predictive accuracy and/or high cost, few biomarkers are acceptable for clinical utility [35]. Alpha-fetoprotein (AFP) was the first serologic assay for the detection and clinical follow-up of patients with HCC, which has been the standard tumor biomarker for HCC for many years [36]. Analysis of recent studies has indicated that AFP testing lacks adequate sensitivity and specificity for effective surveillance [37]. AFP levels were reported to be normal in up to 40% of patients with HCC, particularly during the early stage of the disease [38]. The combinational use of different biomarkers may enhance the detection sensitivity for the early detection of HCC. The tumor markers are most useful if utilized not only as confirmatory tests, but also as a part of routine follow-up [39].

Instead of simply utilizing a tumor marker test during the initial cancer evaluation, following the tumor marker levels serially against the background of clinical and other diagnostic findings will enhance the value of the tumor marker in providing information that could be used in therapeutic decisions and evaluation [39]. In recent years, many promising candidate biomarkers for HCC have been identified, but most of them have not been applied in the clinical diagnosis due to their limited practicability and high cost.

Discovering novel biomarkers that provide sensitive and specific detection of early stage disease when it is highly treatable is crucial [40]. In blood, the presence of low abundance and low molecular weight proteins and metabolites provide a potential and beneficial information, which also have great promise as a source of new biomarkers [41]. Unfortunately, they comprise less than 1 percent of the blood molecules, and in many cases exist in at two molar concentrations. The remainder of the proteins and peptides comprising the complex circulatory proteome range from 10 to 12 mg/mL to 10–3 mg/mL, spanning ten orders of magnitude, with a few high molecular weight proteins such as albumin and immunoglobulins accounting for 90% of total protein content [42].

It is quite difficult to detect and quantify low abundance, low molecular weight proteins and metabolites using conventional protein detection methods such as two dimensional gel electrophoresis (2-DGE), as they do not have the sensitivity and high resolution [43]. As the input volume is only a few microliters, it's also quite challenging for the moderately high-detection and sensitive modern mass spectrometers (at to molar concentration). And the complexity of protein mixture will influence the sensitivity and resolution [43]. The usual sample preparation steps for mass spectrometry (MS) experiments have several steps. MS experiments start with the depletion of high abundant proteins using commercially available immunoaffinity depletion columns. After depletion process, using size exclusion chromatography, ion exchange chromatography and/or isoelectric focusing it has been fractionized. However, as it has been recently shown that the vast majority of low abundance biomarkers are non-covalently and endogenously associated with the carrier proteins that are being removed, removal of abundant native high molecular weight proteins can significantly reduce the yield of candidate biomarkers [44]. Methods, such as size exclusion ultrafiltration under denaturing conditions, continuous elution denaturing electrophoresis or fractionation of serum by means of nano-porous substrates, have been proposed to solve this problem, but these methods are very time consuming, [45]. In the past, there has been no routine method for purifying and enriching low molecular mass peptides and metabolites from complex protein mixtures and biologic fluids in solution [46].

3. Translational research

In hepatology, HCC is an area that could benefit from translational research. In advanced-stage HCC, until 2016, sorafenib was the only systemic agent that can increase survival in patients [47]. In the meantime, four drugs, which include lenvatinib, regorafenib, cabozantinib and ramucirumab, have shown clinical efficacy either in first- or second-line therapy after phase 3 clinical trials [48]. Response rate of 14% for nivolumab and 17% for pembrolizumab was observed and they also increased the duration of response more than 1 year in half of the responders prompted the US Food and Drug Administration (FDA) approval of these two drugs under the accelerated program after single-arm phase 1/2 trials [49].

There are no other biomarkers except AFP that can identify the best responders to any other therapies, while the patients receiving ramucirumab in second-line therapy [48]. To identify an immune subclass in HCC resection specimens, translational research efforts played a prominent role. Its ability to predict response to immune-based therapies is still under investigation [50]. This is quite different with other tumor types where comprehensive molecular profiling of large sets of samples enabled the identification of robust predictive biomarkers of treatment response (e.g., BRAF mutations and response to vemurafenib in melanoma, and ALK rearrangements and response to crizotinib in lung cancer) [51]. These translational research initiatives helped coin the concept of "oncogene addiction," a term that describes a selective dependence of cancer cell growth for a certain genetic alteration. Some of these biomarkers are included in clinical practice guide-lines and FDA label [52].

As translational research established itself as a bridge between basic research and clinical practice, its application spread beyond cancer to disease in general and then to non-biomedical fields such as engineering [52]. Genome-wide association studies have shown that only a small fraction of an individual's risk for cancer can be predicted by their genetic constitution and that hundreds of genetic variants conspire to determine that risk [53]. Often, disease-related genetic variants do not alter protein-coding regions of the genome, and evidence is emerging to show that they influence cell physiology by altering non-coding RNAs with gene regulatory roles [54]. Additional layers of complexity have emerged from the sequencing of cancer genomes. These efforts have revealed large intra-individual heterogeneity in neoplasms of the same organ and histotype, i.e., each tumor has its own mutational profile [54]. Additionally, they have uncovered substantial intra-tumoral heterogeneity that complicates treatment decisions and calls into question the strategy of genotyping tumoral DNA using a single biopsy [55]. Altogether, this new understanding of cancer complexity is the driving force in the development of diagnostic tests for the molecular profiling of tumors, which may guide the choice of suitable personalized therapies for each patient [52].

4. Emerging methods in HCC

The stability of potential biomarkers poses a major challenge is greater over the complications associated with the harvest and enrichment of candidate biomarkers from complex natural protein mixtures (such as blood) [46]. Immediately after blood collection (e.g., by venipuncture), proteins that present in the serum are at risk of degradation by endogenous proteases or exogenous environmental proteases, such as proteases associated with the blood clotting process, enzymes shed from blood cells or associated with bacterial contaminants [56].

During transportation and storage, there is an increasing chance for the degradation of candidate diagnostic biomarkers in the blood. When the serum and other body fluids that are collected from a multiple institutions and different locations as large repositories where samples may be shipped without freezing, the fidelity of biomarkers becomes an even more important issue [46].

The fundamental and serious physiologic barriers upsetting biomarker discovery and measurement is the extremely low abundance (concentration) of candidate markers in blood and urine. Low limits of the biomarkers are very difficult to detect by mass spectrometry and conventional immunoassays. And also in the early stage of disease, the tissue contains a small proportion of the patient's tissue volume, thus generating a low amount of biomarkers [46].

The resident proteins such as albumin and immunoglobulins are the next hindrances, which account for greater than 90% of circulating plasma proteins, as it confound and mask the isolation of rare biomarkers. When compared to the rare biomarker, the resident proteins such as albumin exist in billion fold excess. The major problem is that the majority of low abundance biomarkers are non-covalently and endogenously associated with that resident proteins [46].

After blood or urine collection, the low abundance biomarkers are rapidly degraded by endogenous and exogenous proteinases. And also during transportation and storage of blood, candidate biomarkers are degraded which lead to serious false-positive and false-negative results [57].

Affinity bait hydrogel nanoparticles have been recently proposed in order to address these fundamental roadblocks to biomarker purification and preservation [58]. The nanoparticles contain a bait that targets classes of analytes. The nanoparticles simultaneously conduct molecular sieve chromatography and affinity chromatography, in one step, when it combined with a body fluid such as blood or urine [57]. The nanoparticles sequester all target molecules away from albumin association and completely exclude albumin [58]. It is proposed that proteins sequestered by the nanoparticles are eluted in small volumes, thus increasing their concentration, allowing analysis by a variety of techniques, such as mass spectrometry, western blotting and immunoassays [57, 58].

Author details

Sivapatham Sundaresan* and Palanirasu Rajapriya
Department of Medical Research, SRM MCH RC, SRM IST,
Kattankulathur-603203, Chengalpattu DT, Tamilnadu, India

*Address all correspondence to: ssunsrm@gmail.com

References

[1] Acharya SK. Epidemiology of hepatocellular carcinoma in India. Journal of clinical and experimental hepatology. 2014; 4: S27-33.

[2] Ferlay J, Shin HR, Bray F, Forman D, Mathers C, Parkin DM. Estimates of worldwide burden of cancer in 2008: GLOBOCAN 2008. Int J Cancer. 2010;127: 2893-2917.

[3] EASL–EORTC Clinical Practice Guideline Management of hepatocellular carcinoma. J Hepatol. 2012; 56:908-943.

[4] Abou-Alfa GK. Hepatocellular carcinoma: molecular biology and therapy. Semin Oncol. 2006;33:S79–S83.

[5] Kumari R, Sahu MK, Tripathy A, Uthansingh K, Behera M. Hepatocellular carcinoma treatment: hurdles, advances and prospects. Hepatic Oncology. 2018; 5:HEP08.

[6] Gomaa AI, Khan SA, Leen EL, Waked I, Taylor-Robinson SD. Diagnosis of hepatocellular carcinoma. World Journal of Gastroenterology. 2009; 21;15:1301.

[7] Hennedige T, Venkatesh SK. Imaging of hepatocellular carcinoma: diagnosis, staging and treatment monitoring. Cancer Imaging. 2012;12(3):530.

[8] Gomaa AI, Khan SA, Leen EL, Waked I, Taylor-Robinson SD. Diagnosis of hepatocellular carcinoma. World Journal of Gastroenterology. 2009;15(11):1301.

[9] Crissien AM, Frenette C. Current management of hepatocellular carcinoma. Gastroenterology & hepatology. 2014;10(3):153.

[10] Singh D, Das CJ, Baruah MP. Imaging of nonalcoholic fatty liver disease: A road less travelled. Indian J Endocrinol Metab. 2013;17:990-995.

[11] Anfuso B, El-Khobar KE, Sukowati CH, Tiribelli C. The multiple origin of cancer stem cells in hepatocellular carcinoma. Clin. Res. Hepatol. Gastroenterol. 2015;39 (Suppl 1):S92-97.

[12] Friemel J, et al. Intratumor heterogeneity in hepatocellular carcinoma. Clin. Cancer Res. 2015;21:1951-1961.

[13] Abramson RG, et al. MR Imaging Biomarkers in Oncology Clinical Trials. Magn. Reson. Imaging Clin. N. Am. 2016;24:11-29.

[14] Fujita N, et al. Hepatocellular carcinoma: clinical significance of signal heterogeneity in the hepatobiliary phase of gadoxetic acid-enhanced MR imaging. Eur. Radiol. 2015;25:211-220.

[15] Gillies RJ, Kinahan PE, Hricak H. Radiomics: Images Are More than Pictures, They Are Data. Radiology. 2016;278:563-577.

[16] McEvoy SH, et al. Hepatocellular carcinoma: illustrated guide to systematic radiologic diagnosis and staging according to guidelines of the American Association for the Study of Liver Diseases. Radiographics. 2013;33:1653-1668.

[17] Hectors SJ, et al. Intravoxel incoherent motion diffusion-weighted imaging of hepatocellular carcinoma: Is there a correlation with flow and perfusion metrics obtained with dynamic contrast-enhanced MRI? J. Magn. Reson. Imaging. 2016;44:856-864.

[18] Llovet JM, Brú C, Bruix J. Prognosis of hepatocellular carcinoma: the BCLC staging classification. Semin Liver Dis. 1999;19:329-38.

[19] Kow AW. Transplantation versus liver resection in patients with

hepatocellular carcinoma. Translational gastroenterology and hepatology. 2019;4.

[20] Carr BI. Review of therapies for intermediate and advanced stage hepatocellular carcinoma, not suitable for curative therapies: a rapidly changing landscape. Hepatoma research. 2019;5.

[21] Yang JD, Hainaut P, Gores GJ, Amadou A, Plymoth A, Roberts LR. A global view of hepatocellular carcinoma: trends, risk, prevention and management. Nature reviews Gastroenterology & hepatology. 2019; 22:1-6.

[22] Forner A, Llovet JM, Bruix J. Hepatocellular carcinoma. Lancet 2012; 379:1245-1255.

[23] Ogasawara S, Ooka Y, Koroki K et al. Switching to systemic therapy after locoregional treatment failure: Definition and best timing. Clinical and Molecular Hepatology. 2020;26(2):155-162.

[24] Chow, P.K.H., Gandhi, M., Tan, S.B. Asia-Pacific Hepatocellular Carcinoma Trials. Sirvenib: Selective Internal Radiation Therapy Versus Sorafenib in Aisa-Pacific Patients with Hepatocellular Carcinoma. J Clin Oncol. 2018;36:1913-1921.

[25] Lim C.J., Chow, P.K.H., Albani, S., Chew, V., et al. Multidimensional Analyses Reveal Distinct Immune Microenvironment in Hepatitis B Virus-Related Hepatocellular Carcinoma. Gut. 2019;68(5):916-27.

[26] Parkin DM, Bray F, Ferlay J, et al. Global cancer statistics. Cancer J Clin. 2005;55:74-108.

[27] Hussain SA, Ferry, El-Gazzaz, et al. Hepatocellular Carcinoma. Ann Oncol. 2001;12:161-172.

[28] Bosch FX, Ribes J, Cleries R, et al. Epidemiology of hepatocellular carcinoma. Clin Liver Dis. 2005;9:191-211.

[29] Farazi PA, Depinho RA. Hepatocellular carcinoma pathogenesis: from genes to environment. Nature Reviews. 2006;6:675-687.

[30] Kidner T, Dai M, Adusumilli PS, Fong Y. Advances in experimental and translational research in the treatment of hepatocellular carcinoma. Surgical oncology clinics of North America. 2008;17(2):377-89.

[31] De Lope CR, Tremosini S, Forner A, Reig M, Bruix J. Management of HCC. J Hepatol. 2012;56:S75-87.

[32] Beretta L. Liver proteomics applied to translational research in liver disease and cancer. Proteomics. Clinical applications. 2010;4(4):359.

[33] Li, Y. , Tang, Z.Y. , Hou, J.X. , 2011. Hepatocellular carcinoma: insight from animal models. Nat. Rev. Gastroenterol. Hepatol. 9, 32-43.

[34] Javier Conde-Vancells, Eva Rodriguez-Suarez, Nieves Embade, David Gil, Rune Matthiesen, Mikel Valle, Felix Elortza, Shelly C Lu, Jose M Mato, Juan M Falcon-Perez. Characterization and comprehensive proteome profiling of exosomes secreted by hepatocytes. J Proteome Res. 2008 ;7(12):5157-66.

[35] Bai DS, Dai Z, Zhou J et al. Capn4 overexpression underlies tumor invasion and metastasis after liver transplantation for hepatocellular carcinoma. Hepatology. 2009;49:460-470.

[36] Chen DS, Sung JL, Shed JC et al. Serum α-fetoprotein in the early stage of human hepatocellular carcinoma. Gastroenterology. 1984;86(6):1404-9.

[37] Singal A, Volk ML, Waljee A et al. Meta-analysis: surveillance with ultrasound for early-stage hepatocellular carcinoma in patients with cirrhosis. Aliment Pharmacol Ther. 2009;30:37-47.

[38] Barletta E, Tinessa V, Daniele B. Screening of hepatocellular carcinoma: role of the alpha-fetoprotein (AFP) and ultrasonography. Recenti Prog Med. 2005;96:295-299.

[39] Virji MA, Mercer DW, Herberman RB. Tumor markers in cancer diagnosis and prognosis. CA: a cancer journal for clinicians. 1988;38(2):104-26.

[40] Aebersold R, Anderson L, Caprioli R, et al. Perspective: a program to improve protein biomarker discovery for cancer. Journal of proteome research. 2005 8;4(4):1104-9.

[41] Espina V, Mehta AI, Winters ME et al. Protein microarrays: molecular profiling technologies for clinical specimens. Proteomics. 2003 ;3(11):2091-100.

[42] Anderson NL, Anderson NG. The human plasma proteome: history, character, and diagnostic prospects. Molecular & cellular proteomics. 2002 1;1(11):845-67.

[43] Conrads TP, Hood BL, Veenstra TD. Sampling and analytical strategies for biomarker discovery using mass spectrometry: Mass Spectrometry For Proteomics Analysis. Biotechniques. 2006; 40(6):799-805.

[44] Lowenthal MS, Mehta AI, Frogale K et al. Analysis of albumin-associated peptides and proteins from ovarian cancer patients. Clinical chemistry. 2005 1;51(10):1933-45.

[45] Camerini S, Polci ML, Liotta LA et al. A method for the selective isolation and enrichment of carrier protein-bound low-molecular weight proteins and peptides in the blood. Proteomics–Clinical Applications. 2007;1(2):176-84.

[46] Luchini A, Fredolini C, Espina BH et al. Nanoparticle technology: addressing the fundamental roadblocks to protein biomarker discovery. Current molecular medicine. 2010;10(2):133-41.

[47] European Association for the Study of the Liver. EASL Clinical Practice Guidelines: management of hepatocellular carcinoma. J Hepatol. 2018;69:182-236.

[48] Marrero JA, Kulik LM, Sirlin CB, et al. Diagnosis, staging, and management of hepatocellular carcinoma: 2018 Practice Guidance by the American Association for the Study of Liver Diseases. Hepatology. 2018;68:723-750.

[49] US Food and Drug Administration. Approved drugs. FDA grants accelerated approval to nivolumab for HCC previously treated with sorafenib. Available at: https://www.fda.gov/drugs/informationondrugs/approveddrugs/ucm577166.htm. Updated September 25, 2017. Accessed October 1, 2018.

[50] Sia D, Jiao Y, Martinez-Quetglas I, et al. Identification of an immune-specific class of hepatocellular carcinoma, based on molecular features. Gastroenterology. 2017;153:812-826.

[51] Von Felden J, Craig AJ, Villanueva A. The impact of Translational research in Hepatology. Clinical Liver Disease. 2019;13(1):29.

[52] Dragani TA, Castells A, Kulasingam V et al. Major milestones in translational oncology. BMC medicine. 2016;14(1):1-3.

[53] Galvan A, Ioannidis JP, Dragani TA. Beyond genome-wide association

studies: genetic heterogeneity and individual predisposition to cancer. Trends Genet. 2010;26:132-41.

[54] St Laurent G, Vyatkin Y, Kapranov P. Dark matter RNA illuminates the puzzle of genome-wide association studies. BMC Med. 2014;12:97.

[55] Parker NR, Khong P, Parkinson JF et al. Molecular heterogeneity in glioblastoma: potential clinical implications. Front Oncol. 2015;5:55.

[56] Schrohl AS, Würtz S, Kohn E et al. Banking of biological fluids for studies of disease-associated protein biomarkers. Molecular & Cellular Proteomics. 2008;7(10):2061-6.

[57] Fredolini C, Meani F, Reeder KA et al. Concentration and preservation of very low abundance biomarkers in urine, such as human growth hormone (hGH), by Cibacron Blue F3G-A loaded hydrogel particles. Nano research. 2008;1(6):502-18.

[58] Luchini A, Geho DH, Bishop B et al. Smart hydrogel particles: biomarker harvesting: one-step affinity purification, size exclusion, and protection against degradation. Nano letters. 2008;8(1):350-61.

Chapter 5

Chalcones: Potential Anticancer Agents

Adam McCluskey and Cecilia Russell

Abstract

Chalcones in their various guises have been considered either valid and critically important lead compounds in the development of novel anticancer agents or as pan assay interference compounds, PAINS. Medicinal chemistry is replete with exemplars from both "camps" progressing to clinical utility. Chalcones offer a simple starting point for the development of specific compounds with high levels of activity toward key biological targets. Chalcones have been shown to display a wide array of anticancer compounds. This chapter seeks to offer an overview of key examples in an effort to encourage further reading and research in development in this intriguing space.

Keywords: chalcones, biologically active, cancer, structure activity relationship data

1. Introduction

Arguably, cancer represents one of the most serious threats to human health. Its incidence is on the rise, and while there have been an increasing number of new drugs and new targets over the past 50 or so years, it is still responsible for multiple deaths across the globe [1]. The advent of targeted therapies arguably commenced with the discovery and clinical use of the protein kinase inhibitor imatinib [2]. Since this first report, there have been multiple novel protein kinase inhibitor-based drugs entering clinical use [3]. More recently, there has been a significant shift in treatment paradigms to the use of mono-clonal antibodies, with this market predicted to be >$US300 billion by 2030 [4]. Despite this, the survival rates for metastatic breast cancer (Stage IV, 5-year survival is <25%), for pancreatic cancer this is a more dire 7% [5]. Treatment of glioblastoma and other neurological cancers has not advanced in the past 3–4 decades [6, 7].

2. Biological activity of chalcones

Chalcones or analogues or derivatives of (*E*)-1,3-diphenyl-2-propene-1-one represent a very diverse array of molecules. This family of molecules are known to possess a myriad of biological activities spanning (but not limited to) antidiabetic, antimicrobial, antioxidant, anti-inflammatory, anticancer and chemopreventative properties [8]. A number of chalcones are in current clinical use, exemplified by the selected analogues shown in **Figure 1** and in other figures throughout this chapter.

IntechOpen

Note that the breadth of the potential applications of chalcones in cancer is expansive and beyond the scope of this chapter, the intent here is to supply a snapshot of chalcones and their targets to encourage further exploration, by the reader, of this area [8–10].

Despite the numerous examples of clinically used chalcones, they are often overlooked for lead development as a function of PAINS filtering [11]. We note the key role here of the medicinal chemist in understanding both the limitations of the lead scaffold, potential promiscuity and the nature of the biological screening conducted. If the scaffold limitations are understood, there is limited rationale in excluding a whole compound class, especially given the current utility of these analogues. However, vigilance is required in SAR examinations. We recommend the removal of PAINS filters from preliminary screening cascades and the introduction of robust orthogonal assay procedures to enable rapid identification of true lead compounds [12, 13]. In so doing, we believe that this will increase the attractiveness of chalcones as leads; potentially matching their use will greatly increase the attractiveness of chalcones as potential starting points for drug discovery [9, 14].

Historically, chalcones, for example **1–5**, have been used in a therapeutic environment for millennia. Typically, through the ingestion of plants and herbs, chalcones have been used in the treatment of a myriad of conditions, spanning but not limited to inflammation, diabetes, and the topic of this chapter, cancer [8, 15–18]. Metochalcone (**1**) and sofalcone (**2**) have been used in the treatment of ulcers and as mucoprotective agents, respectively (**Figure 1**) [15, 16].

Being able to switch between two chalconoid structures (**6a** and **6b**; **Figure 2**) in principle establishes two Michael acceptor possibilities for this class of compounds. It is important to recognize at this point that key researchers view these and molecules such as these as PAINS [11]. As such, caution should be used in determining absolute effects and ascribing them to specific compounds' actions in a

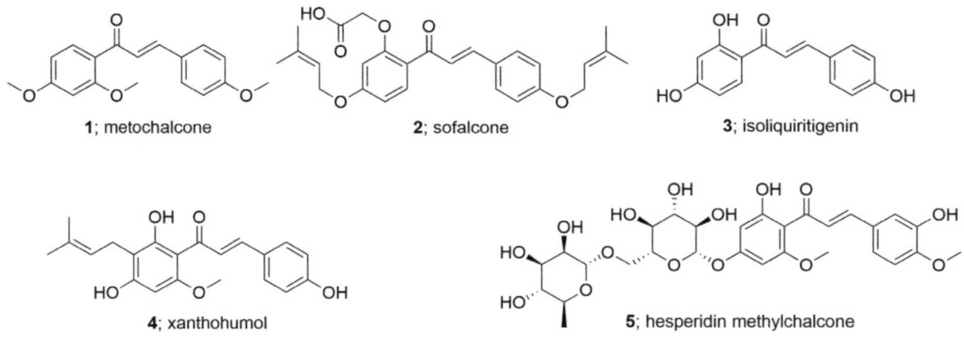

Figure 1.
Chemical structures of selected clinically used chalcones: metochalcone (1), sofalcone (2), isoliquiritigenin, xanthohumol (4) and hesperidin methylchalcone (5).

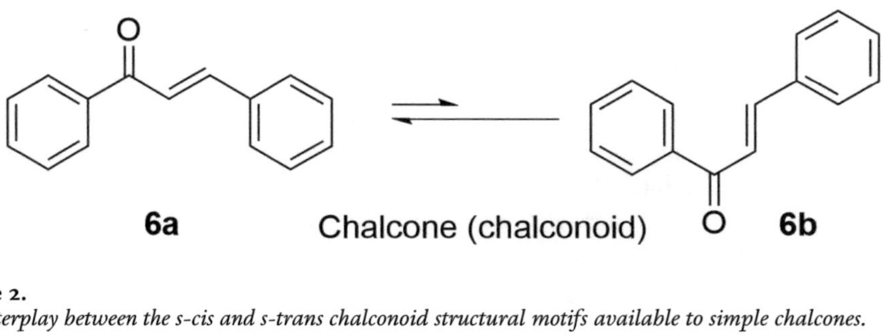

Figure 2.
The interplay between the s-cis and s-trans chalconoid structural motifs available to simple chalcones.

biological system. Clearly, Michael acceptors are generally biologically active. Michael acceptor-type compounds are known to be involved in cell signaling cascades and in many cases these compounds are capable of forming covalent attachments to the sulfhydryl of cysteine or other thiols to obtain the Michael adduct 7 (**Figure 3**), which may play an important role in their biological activities [19–23]. Interestingly, the past reservations about small molecules forming covalent linkages with proteins are subsiding with a wide variety of targeted drugs operating via a covalent interaction mode [24]. This may lead to a resurgence in the examination of chalcones as lead compounds.

Despite the PAINS expectation, there have been a large number of chalcones reported to elicit anticancer activity via specific cell signaling pathways. Of note are those analogues (**8–10**) that target the NF-kB pathway. It has been reported that the anticancer activity of 3-hydroxy-4,3′,4′,5′-tetramethoxychalcone (**9**) correlates with its NF-κB inhibitory activity. The reported mechanism of action requires interaction with the IKKb cysteines (46% inhibition; 10 μM) [23] proceeding via a JNK-mediated autophagy pathway triggering c-IAP (**Figure 4**) [25].

A key feature of chalcone **9** is its ability to synergize with existing clinical treatments. As a combination therapy, **9** and the TNF-related apoptosis-inducing ligand (TRAIL) or cisplatin significantly enhanced its cytotoxicity in lung cancer cells. This effect is mediated via the suppression of cellular FLICE (FADD-like IL-1b-converting enzyme)-inhibitory protein large (c-FLIPL) and cellular inhibitor of apoptosis proteins (c-IAPs), which in combination activate autophagy [26, 27].

Within the NF-κB activation pathway the Toll-like receptor 4 (TLR4) and myeloid differentiation 2 (MD2) regulate the downstream signal transduction, such as MAPK phosphorylation. In a LPS-acute lung injury model chalcone **10** inhibited the activity of MD2 reducing the inflammatory effects in this model [28].

The removal of purported PAINS is more frustrating with recent examples where promiscuous inhibitors were not removed or the filters demonstrated an

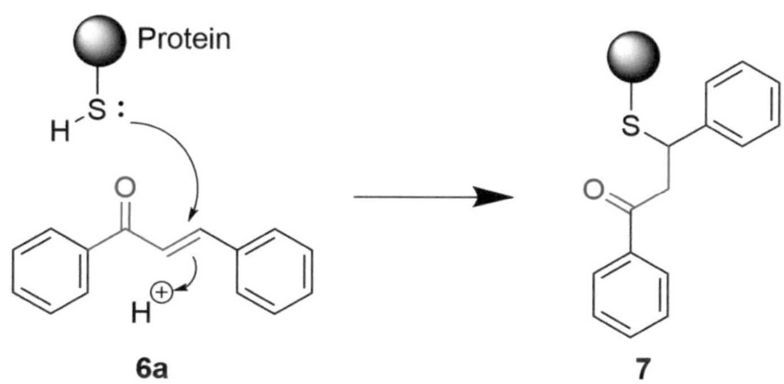

Figure 3.
*Michael addition of a chalcone (**6a**) with cysteine to form the Michael adduct 7.*

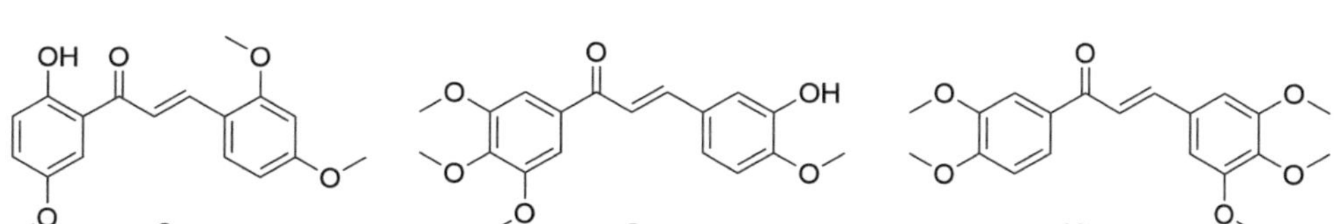

Figure 4.
Exemplar chalcones known to be NF-κB inhibitors [28].

oversensitivity toward key compound types. That is, these filters may reject non-promiscuous compounds [12, 29].

The use of bioisosteric replacements with chalcones has high prevalence. Commencing with 2,4,6-trimethoxychalcone (**11**) a simple H (**11**) to F (**12**) isosteric replacement effected a 2-fold potency increase against HeLa (cervical cancer), A498 (renal cancer), and HepG2 (hepatocellular carcinoma) cells, with retention of activity against the A549 (lung adenocarcinoma epithelial) and A375 (skin malignant melanoma) cell lines with IC_{50} values spanning 0.03–0.120 μM (**Table 1**) [30].

Isosteric replacements have not been limited to simple Grimm's isosteres, but they have been explored in nonclassical isostere space with the replacement of the central olefin with a small heterocyclic compound, such as the thiophene analogues shown in **Table 2**. These modified chalcones, for example, **14** developed from **13**, displayed good levels of cytotoxicity against a range of cancerous cell lines, with activities noted in the sub-μM to mid-nM range (0.160–0.510 μM) against HeLa,

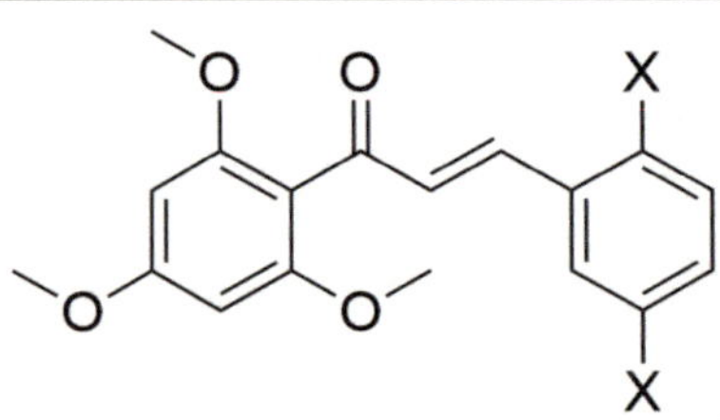

X	HeLa	A549	A498	A375	HepG2
11; H	0.134	0.134	0.067	0.067	0.134
12; F	0.060	0.120	0.030	0.060	0.060

Table 1.
*Effect of H to F bioisosteric modification on the cytotoxicity of a 2,4,6-trimethoxychalcone (**11**). IC_{50} values are expressed in μM.*

Compound	HeLa	Molt-4	CEM	L1210	FM3A
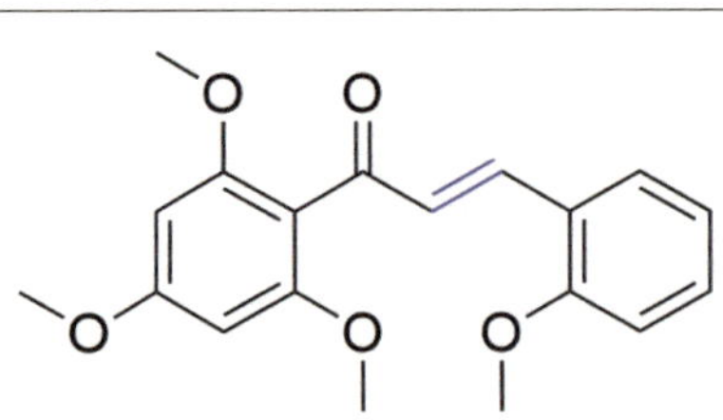	1.4	1.9	1.8	2.1	7.9
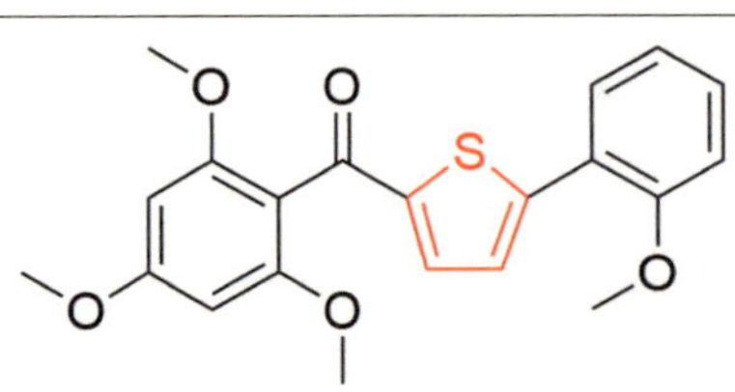	0.160	0.180	0.370	0.510	0.440

Table 2.
Bioisosterism represented by the replacing the double bond of the enone (blue) with a thiophene (red) [31]. IC_{50} values are expressed in μM.

Molt-4 (human T-lymphocyte), CEM (human T-lymphocyte), L1210 (murine leukemia), and FM3A cell lines (murine mammary carcinoma) (**Table 2**) [31].

2.1 Chalcone hybrids

The biological activity of chalcones, and study thereof is not limited to the parent structure, but has recently expanded to encapsulate hybrid (chimeric) molecules. These chimeras combine the cytotoxicity of the parent chalcone (**15**) and the biological activity of the second drug. Multiple chimeric partners have been reported including antibiotics (ciprofloxacin, **16**) linking through the N-aryl piperazine moiety. This allows access to the known inhibition of human DNA topoisomerase II, itself a known anticancer drug target (**Figure 5**) [32]. The chalcone-ciprofloxacin hybrid (**17**) inhibits human DNA topoisomerase II with potent in vitro anticancer activity against myriad of cancer cell lines [33–36].

Chalcones themselves are known to inhibit several anticancer targets, including thioredoxin reductase [21], and tubulin polymerization [37, 38]. Based on this there was an expectation (upheld) that chimeric molecules possessing a N-aryl piperazine and chalcone moieties would show higher potencies in the cell lines examined. Indeed, with these molecules considerable synergy arising from the combination of both partners was observed. Of the analogues reported, hybrid **17** displayed the highest activity against cervical cancer (Hela; IC_{50} = 190 nM) and gastric cancer (SGC7901; IC_{50} = 410 nM) cells (**Figure 5**). These data compare favorably with that reported for cisplatin in the same cell lines with IC_{50} values of 20 and 12 μM, respectively [32].

The introduction of an active warhead has been accomplished through the synthesis of a α-bromoacryloylamido chalcones (**Figure 6**). Analogues of this nature are expected to act as covalent modifiers of their target protein [39]. Intriguingly, this combines the once thought of anathema of a covalent inhibitor with a compound classified as a PAINS [11, 24]. Yet, compounds **18** and **19** exhibit the highest activity against tumor cell growth (IC_{50} < 1 μM) and 10- to 100-fold increases in potency relative to the corresponding amide derivatives. Preliminary mechanism of action studies support apoptosis induction via mitochondrial engagement and activation of caspase-3. The related amide-linked dithiocarbamate-chalcone (**20**) also exhibited excellent growth inhibition against SK-N-SH cells, with an IC_{50} value of 2.03 μM, with negligible toxicity toward the normal GES-1 cell line (IC_{50} > 50 mM). However, this effect is via G_0/G_1 arrest and progression through apoptosis. The nature of the linking and pendant moieties affects the compound mode of action [40].

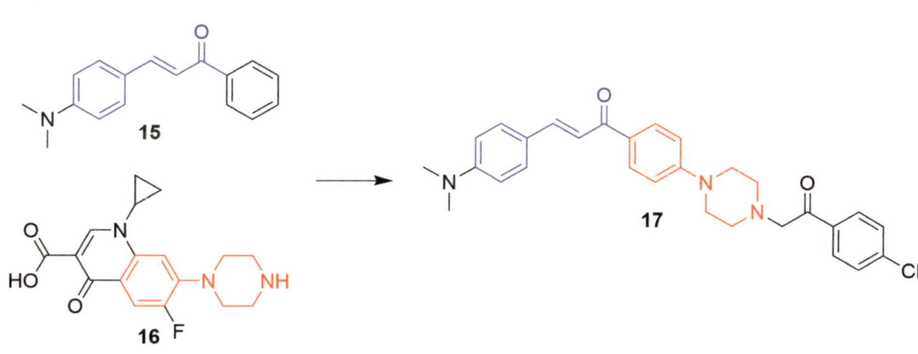

Figure 5.
Molecular hybrid obtained from the combination of chalcones (red) and N-aryl piperazine moiety (blue) [32].

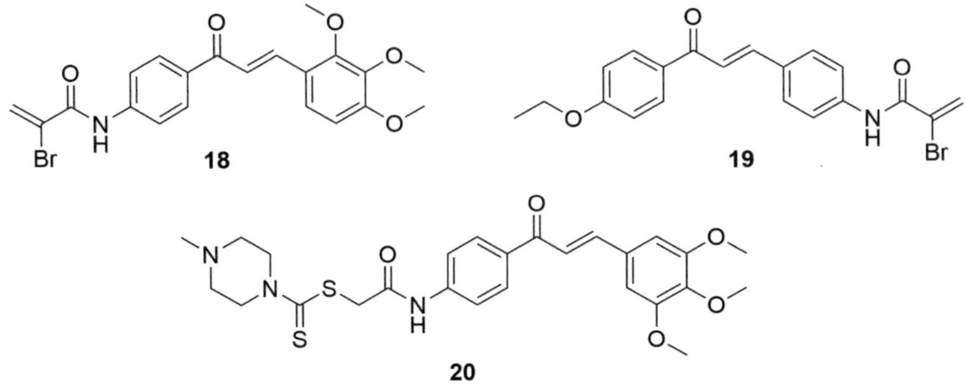

Figure 6.
Chemical structures of selected amide-linked chalcones bearing a covalently active warhead [40].

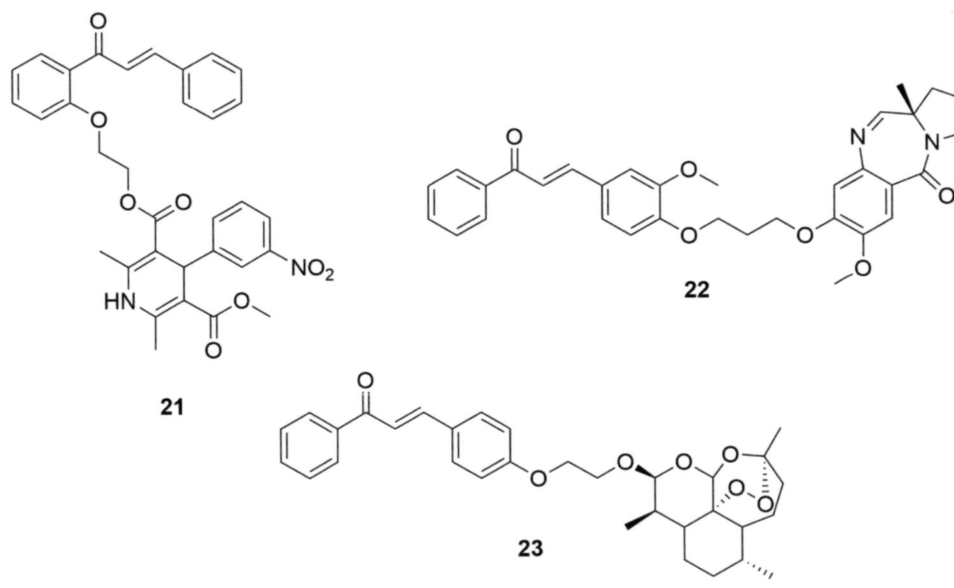

Figure 7.
Chemical structures of example chalcone hybrids linked though a diol linker [43].

Chalcones have been hybridized via an ethylene glycol (or related diol linker) linker (often used in medicinal chemistry to enhance solubility) (**Figure 7**) [41, 42]. Analogues such as the 1,4-dihydropyridyl-chalcones (**21–24**) show growth inhibition via an undetermined mechanism of action [43].

Access to chalcones can be via traditional solution phase synthesis approaches, but in some instances there are reports of the use of solid supports. With **22**, a supported intramolecular aza-Wittig reductive cyclization is utilized to afford a compound that showed high activity in the NCI-60 cell line panel. Acidity appears to be related to a high level of DNA binding as determined by thermal denaturing analysis [44, 45]. In keeping with the chimeric theme of this section, the inclusion of the dehydroartemisinin scaffold with and ethylene glycol spacer afforded **23,** which showed a 6-fold potency enhancement relative to the apparent dehydroartemisinin with an IC_{50} of 300 nM [46].

While amide linages have been reported in the development of chalcone hybridism, the use of an ester moiety has the added advantage of allowing a cellular esterase cleavage of the hybrid to afford the two parent drugs. In principle, this may allow the presentation of three different biologically active compounds simultaneously: the hybrid, the chalcone, and the co-drug. The ester approach to coupling compound pharmacophores has been elegantly demonstrated with chalcone hybrids leveraging the often-present hydroxyl moiety. This approach, obviously, can also afford the corresponding ether (versus ester) linked analogue, which is significantly more cleavage resistant. Within this coupled pharmacophore environment, chalcone-amidobenzothiazole chimeras **24** and **25** are 0.185–3.3 μM potent across a panel of cancer cell lines (**Figure 8**). These analogues induce cell cycle arrest at the G_2/M phase boundary [47]. Platinum incorporation into the amidobenzothiazole moiety with **26** also gave excellent anticancer activity across 21 cell lines, but no real potency boost relative to the parent chalcone, but the chimera did yield a different long-term treatment and mechanism of apoptosis induction pathway that may be beneficial, especially in the onset of resistance should this occur [48].

Like a significant number of other chimeric compounds, "click-approaches" have also been applied in the development of a series of chalcone-coumarin chimeras, for example, **27** and **28** (**Figure 9**). Gratifyingly, these chimeras displayed higher efficacy against HepG2 cells than etoposide combined with negligible toxicity toward normal cells. Molecular docking studies support, but do not confirm, that these hybrids may act through binding with both tubulin and falcipain [49].

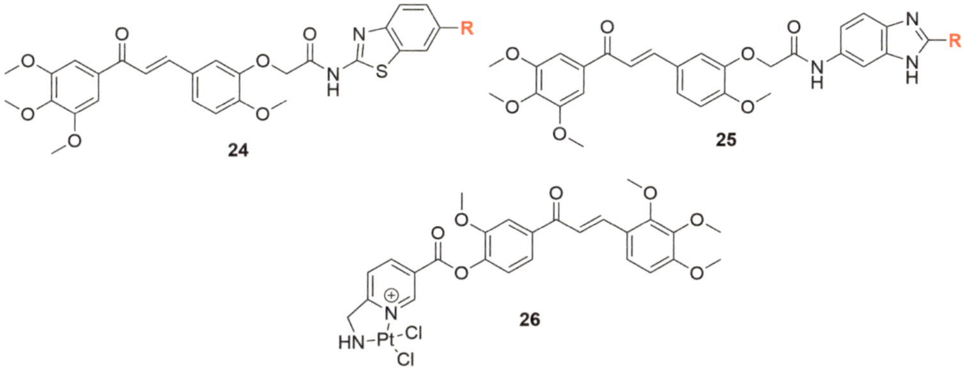

Figure 8.
Selected ester and ether-linked chalcones [47, 48].

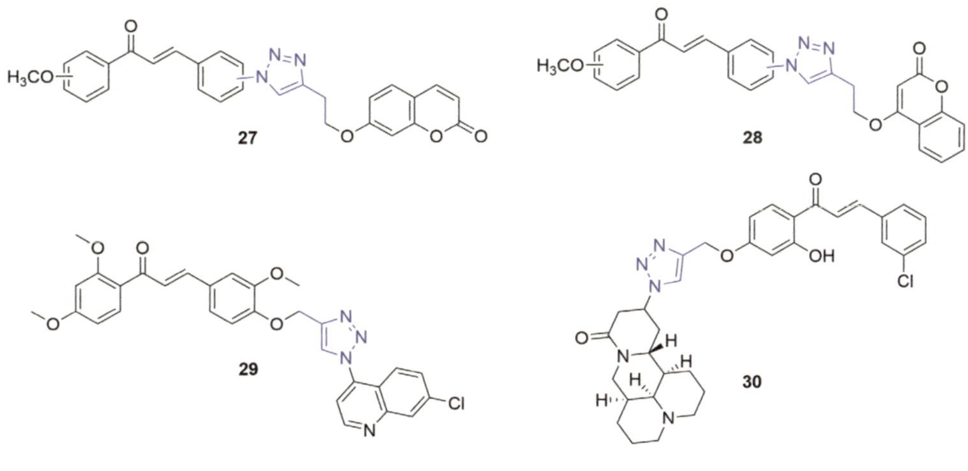

Figure 9.
Selected exemplars of Huisgen "click-linked" chalcone hybrid molecules [50].

Within this subset of click conjugates, **29** demonstrated higher efficacy than the archetypal cytotoxic agent 5-fluorouracil against four human cancer cell lines (A459 (lung), Bel-7402 (hepatocellular), HeLa (cervical), and MCF-7 (breast)) and low cytotoxicity to NIH3T3 normal cells. Chalcone **29** was synergistic with matrine against the A459 cell line demonstrating a favorable in vivo safety profile. Chalcone **29** has been reported as capable of effecting aa ca 90% tumor burden reduction in a A459 mouse xenograft model (10.0 mg/kg/day, 20 days, iv) without any apparent loss of body weight [50].

Continuation of the click-linked chalcone hybrids with β-lactams [51] revealed **30** as the most potent analogue within a discrete library. Of particular note was IC_{50} values < 1 μM against A549 and THP-1 (leukemia) cancer cells [52]. No other noteworthy analogue was reported.

Loch-Neckel et al. reported a further investigation of the mechanism of an analogue (**31**; **Figure 10**) [53]. In vitro and in vivo, it could inhibit glioma cell growth and induce mitochondrial apoptosis in U87-MG glioma cells via the inhibition of MDM2.

Several hybrids besides those discussed above have also been reported to exhibit potent anticancer activities (**Figure 11**). For example, β-carboline–chalcone (**32**) exhibits significant DNA binding interaction and DNA stabilization [54]. Imidazothiazole-chalcone (**33**) exhibits promising cytotoxicity with a microtubule destabilizing mechanism and could compete with colchicine [55, 56]. Anthraquinone-chalcone (**34**) shows high cytotoxicity in HeLa cells [57, 58]. The compound induces the activity of caspase-3 and caspase-8 in HeLa cells and has shown potent inhibition of MMP-2 secretion.

2.2 Inhibition of tubulin

Clinically, targeting microtubules—the multifunctional cytoskeletal proteins comprising α- and β-tubulin heterodimers—has provided considerable success in the treatment of multiple cancers. Archetypal microtubule-targeting compounds include the taxanes used in the treatment of metastatic pancreatic cancer [59], and vinca alkaloids in the treatment of hematological and lymphatic neoplasms [60].

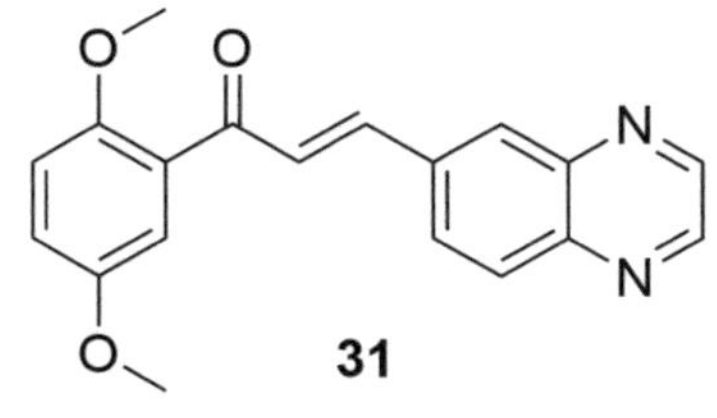

31

Figure 10.
Chemical structure of chalcone 31, (E)-1-(2,5-dimethoxyphenyl)-3-(quinoxalin-6-yl)prop-2-en-1-one [53].

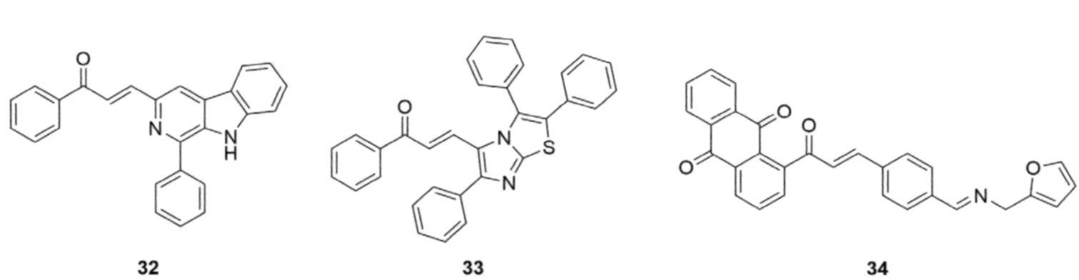

32 33 34

Figure 11.
Representatives of fused chalcone analogues [54].

However, the continued use of these agents, like a significant number of anticancer drugs, is limited by toxicity (here neurotoxicity) and drug resistance [61, 62]. In this target space, multiple natural and synthetic chalcones (**35-42**) have been reported with microtubule activity (**Figure 12**).

Given the current toxicity and resistance issues with the taxanes and vinca alkaloids, in combination with the decorated microtubule activity of chalcones, it is not surprising that the hybridization of these compound classes has been explored. Some groups have attempted to develop these combination drugs using rational drug design approaches. Niu approached this via molecular docking and high-correlation quantitative pharmacophore models (40 compounds with experimental data and 800 decoys to discriminate active versus inactive molecules) were generated using the SAR of known tubulin inhibitors [63]. Model validation followed by virtual screening identified ca. 1000 drug-like molecules that were pharmacophore matched. Ultimately, five differentially substituted (**43–47**) chalcones with diverse substituents and strong molecular interactions with the key amino acids in the tubulin-binding site were identified (**Figure 13**). Two compounds were of particular note, with **48** and **49** (**Figure 14**) demonstrating potent inhibitory activity against MCF-7 cells with IC_{50} values of 28 and 54 nM respectively [63].

Isolated from *Combretum caffrum*, Combretastatin A-4 is a microtubule-targeting natural product that has been further developed through imidazolone incorporation (**51**) (**Figure 15**) [64]. Evaluation in a broad-spectrum panel containing 53 human tumor cell lines spanning leukemia, non-small cell lung, colon,

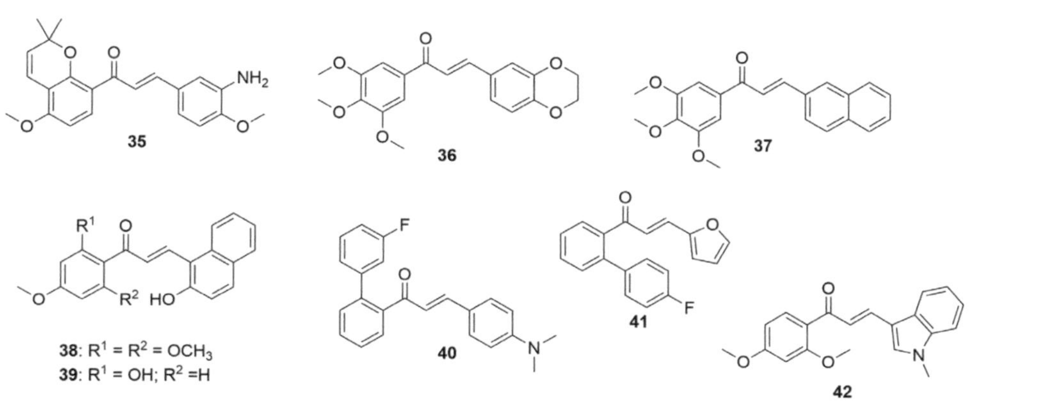

Figure 12.
Examples of natural and synthetic chalcones with reported biological activity against microtubules [60].

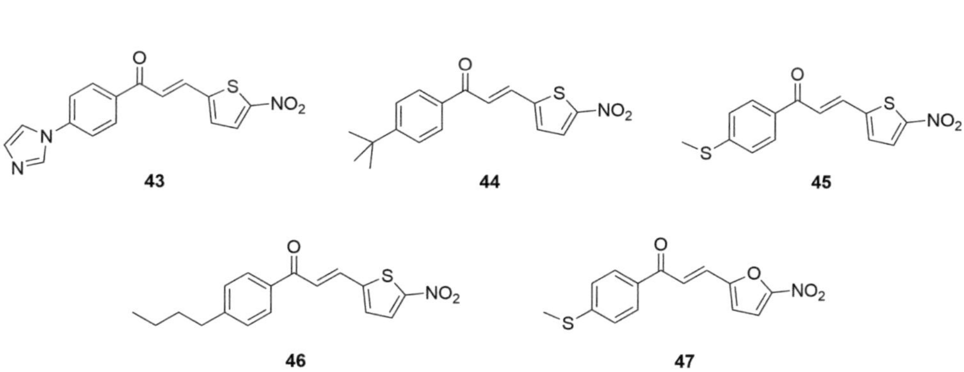

Figure 13.
Selected chalcones arising as hits from QSAR-based drug design strategy [63].

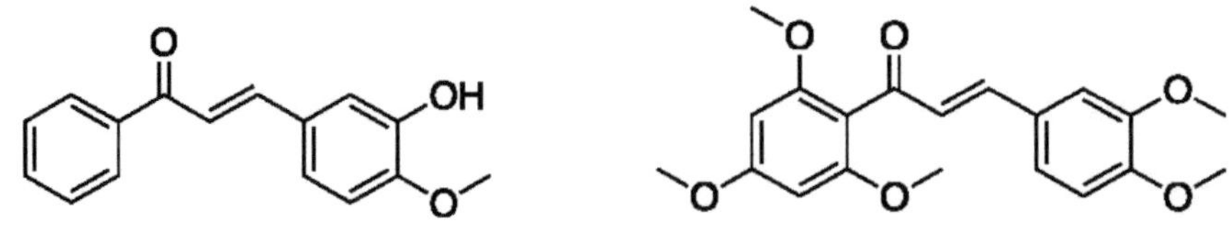

48 **49**

Figure 14.
*Chalcones with anticancer activity identified by integration of ligand-based pharmacophore screening and molecular docking studies [63]. Active against the breast cancer cell line, MCF-7 with IC_{50} = 28 and 54 nM, respectively (**48, 49**).*

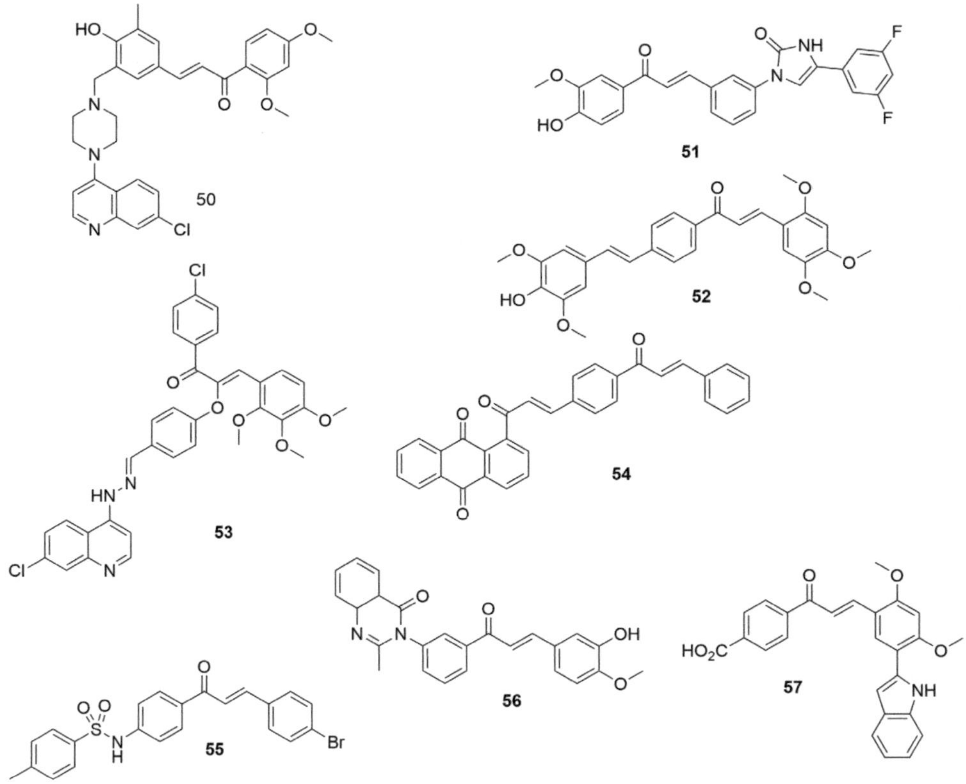

Figure 15.
Variety of linked chalcones including examples that induce apoptosis via the PI3K/Akt/mTOR pathway [64–67].

CNS, renal, prostate, ovarian, breast, and melanoma determined **51** showed good anticancer activity, with GI_{50} values ranging from 1.26 to 10.5 μM and arresting cells at G_2/M phase [65].

Other hybrids, for example, anthraquinone-chalcone (**54**), have high cytotoxicity toward HeLa cells but low toxicity to normal cells [66], as does the quinazolinone chalcone derivative (**56**), which induces mitochondria-dependent apoptosis and inhibits the PI3K/Akt/mTOR signaling pathway [67].

Chalcone modification afforded the amino-substituted **58** with subsequent examination of these analogues for their tubulin-binding, vascular-targeting, antitumor and antimetastatic activities revealing it to be the best compound in the series developed by Canela et al [68]. Chalcone **58** inhibited the proliferation of endothelial (HMEC-1, microvascular endothelial cell line-1; and BAEC, bovine aortic endothelial cells) and tumor (B16-F10.luc2, melanoma cells expressing firefly luciferase 2; Cem; and HeLa) cell lines with IC_{50} values of 1 and 4 nM [68]. The low solubility of **58** (0.016 mg/mL) was ameliorated through the incorporation of an amino acid-based pro-moiety with the L-Lysine-L-Proline derivative **59** approximately 2000x more soluble than **58** (**Figure 16**). Pro-drug **59** was effective in inhibiting tumor and endothelial cell proliferation, parent **58** was successfully released by the liver, and **59** demonstrated excellent in vivo anticancer activity in melanoma (10 mg/kg) and breast cancer models (15 mg/kg) by causing rapid intertumoral vascular shutdown and massive tumor necrosis [68].

Isolated from *Millettia pachycarpa*, millepachine (**60**) induces cell cycle arrest and apoptosis in human hepatocarcinoma cells in vitro and in vivo [69]. The development of amino-substituted-millepachines was explored in an effort to enhance the antiproliferative activity of the natural product lead (**Figure 17**). Millepachine derivative (**61**) exhibited excellent anticancer activity against a panel of drug-sensitive cancer cell lines and multidrug-resistant cancer cells. Studies support the inhibition of tubulin polymerization as the mechanism of action, by binding at the colchicine site [70–72]. More conformationally restrained analogues **62–65** and **68** in this amino-substituted series retained high levels of activity, again acting as anti-microtubule agents.

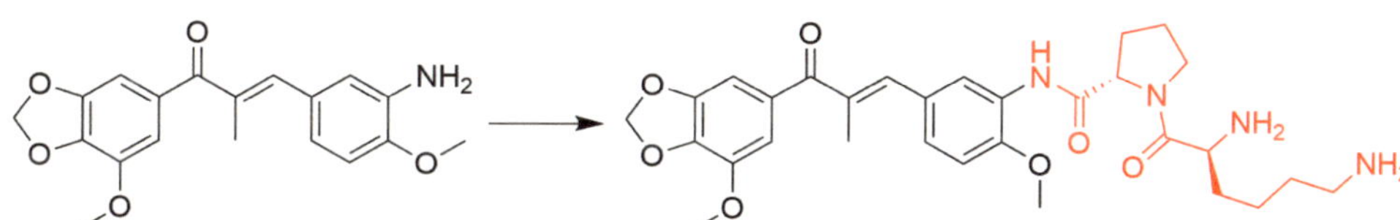

Figure 16.
Latentiation represented by the replacing the amine of 58 with an L-Lysine-L-Proline (red) [68].

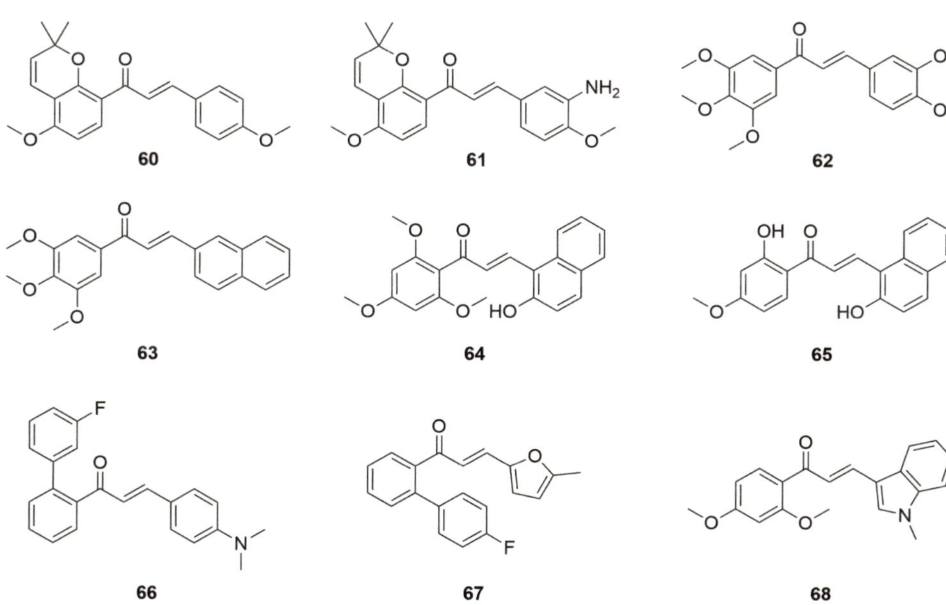

Figure 17.
Family of novel chalcones hypothesised to inhibit tubulin by binding at the colchicine site [70–72].

Novel o-aryl chalcone (**66**) showed potent cytotoxicity against several multidrug-resistant cancer cell lines (paclitaxel-resistant human ovarian carcinoma cells, vincristine-resistant human ileocecum carcinoma cells, and doxorubicin-resistant human breast carcinoma cells) in an extremely low nanomolar range. This has been shown to be G2/M phase cell cycle arrest effect, mediated by **66** binding to the colchicine site of tubulin as was observed with **62–65** and **68** [73], which is a key feature of anti-microtubule agents [74]. Acting via the colchicine-binding site [75], **67** was effective in mouse A549 xenograft models with no dose-limiting weight loss observed [37, 73]. An indole-chalcone (**68**), namely, IPP51, induced prometaphase arrest and the subsequent apoptosis of bladder cancer cells and showed a significant inhibition of tumor growth without a great loss in body weight [75].

Confirmation of the tubulin-binding target has been obtained with TUB091 (**58**), TUB092 (**69**), and TUB099 (**59**) series of compounds [68]. TUB092 (**70**) was soaked in the crystals of a protein complex comprising αβ-tubulin (T2) dimers, a stathmin-like protein RB3 (R), and tubulin tyrosine ligase (TTL) (**Figure 18**). The subsequent high-resolution cocrystal structure (2.4 Å) showed the chalcone bound with tubulin at the colchicine-binding site. The chalcone is organized such that the 1,3-benzodioxole ring of **69** is located in the β-tubulin residue-derived hydrophobic pocket, with a water-mediated hydrogen bond to the backbone carbonyl and amide of Gly237 and Cys241. The α,β-unsaturated ketone hydrogen bonds with Asp251 and two additional water-mediated hydrogen bonds are evident from the backbone carbonyls of Thr179 and Asn349 with the hydroxyl and methoxy groups. Optimization of lead solubility via L-Lys-L-Pro dipeptide incorporation yielded pro-drug **59** with a ca. 2000x solubility enhancement (31 mg/mL in PBS versus 0.016 mg/mL in PBS). **59** also inhibited primary tumor growth and spontaneous metastasis in mice (iv injection, 10 mg/kg, 5 days) with 90% or higher inhibition.

2.3 Miscellaneous chalcones

Chalcone-benzoxaborole (**70**), prepared from the intermediates 6-formylbenzoxaborole and the corresponding ketone, has recently been found to inhibit *Trypanosoma brucei* growth and possess antitrypanosomal activity (**Figure 19**) [76]. Boronic-chalcone (**71**) was described early in 2002 as a fluorescent probe for the detection of fluorides [77]. Boronic-chalcone hybrid (**71**) exhibits not only fluorescent properties but also other biological activity. Compound **71** has been reported as an antitumor agent targeting MDM2 oncoprotein [78]. Compound **72** can induce antitumor activity against malignant glioma cell lines both in vitro and in vivo [79]. Compound **73** exhibits potent anticancer activity (HCT116 cells, IC_{50} = 3.9 μM) together with proteasome inhibitory activity [80].

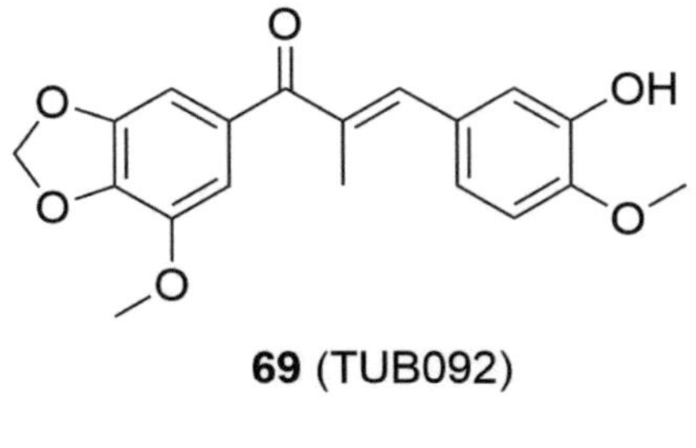

69 (TUB092)

Figure 18.
Chemical structure of TUB092 (69), which binds to tubulin at the colchicine site; this analogue is directly related to chalcones 58 and 59 (see **Figure 16***) [68].*

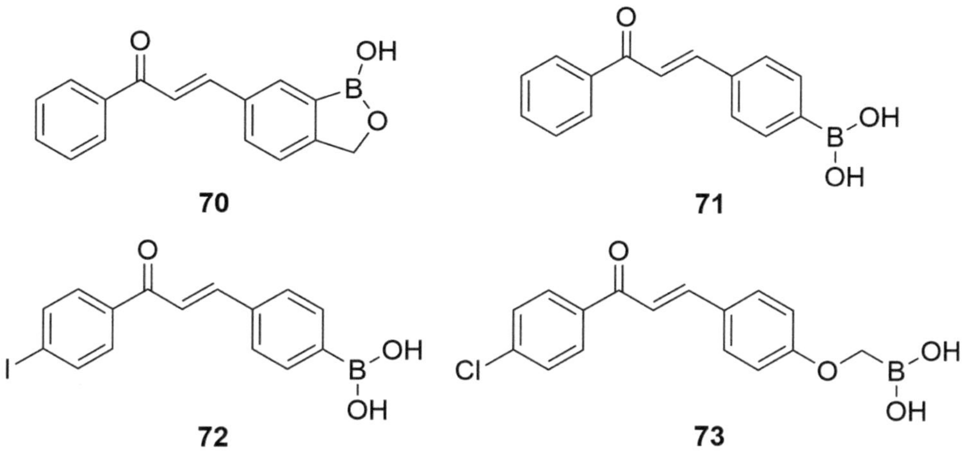

Figure 19.
Chemical structures of boron-containing chalcones [76–80].

2.4 Selected mechanism of action studies

Ducki et al. predicted tubulin to be the target of chalcone due to the similarity between chalcone and the β-tubulin inhibitor combretastatin A4 [81]. A 5D-QSAR model was used to conclude that the methyl group at the α-position made a sizable difference in the preferred conformation from s-cis (**74**) to s-trans (**75**) for tubulin binding. This theory explains the high potency of α-methyl chalcone (K562, IC_{50} = 0.21 nM; tubulin, IC_{50} = 0.46 μM) [81, 82]. In 1992, MDL-27048 (**76**) was the first chalcone found to have antimitotic activity [83]. This compound was bound to tubulin at the colchicine-binding site and inhibited tubulin polymerization. Based on a proposed binding model for MDL-27048 [83, 84], a virtual screening of 9720 natural compounds was carried out. Compound **77** has been found to show good inhibitory activity of tubulin polymerization [85]. Compounds **78**–**85** (**Figure 20**) have been designed and synthesized in later medicinal chemistry work. These compounds were originally predicted to bind to tubulin at the colchicine-binding site, which has been confirmed via in vitro competition binding assays [47, 75, 86–90]. Very recently, a series of novel indole-chalcone derivatives were synthesized and evaluated for their antiproliferative activity. Among these indole-chalcones, compound **81** has exhibited IC_{50} values of 3–9 nM against six cancer cell lines, with similar activities against resistant cancer cells, and low toxicity toward normal human cells. Molecular docking and mechanistic studies have demonstrated that this compound could bind to the colchicine-binding site, inhibit tubulin polymerization with an IC_{50} of 2.68 μM, arrest the cell cycle at the G2/M phase, induce apoptosis, and decrease the mitochondrial membrane potential (MMP). Moreover, this compound and its phosphate salt **82** with better water solubility have been shown to exhibit 66 and 70% in vivo antitumor inhibitory rates (ip, 30 mg/kg), respectively, without any apparent loss of body weight.

2.5 Targeting topoisomerase

Critically, the correct assembly of DNA is essential for cellular function. This assembly is in part governed by a series of topoisomerases (TOPOs), including TOPO-I and TOPO-II, which are responsible for the winding and unwinding of DNA. TOPO function is a critical process for DNA transcription and replication, and has been targeted as an anticancer strategy [91]. Several chalcones have shown

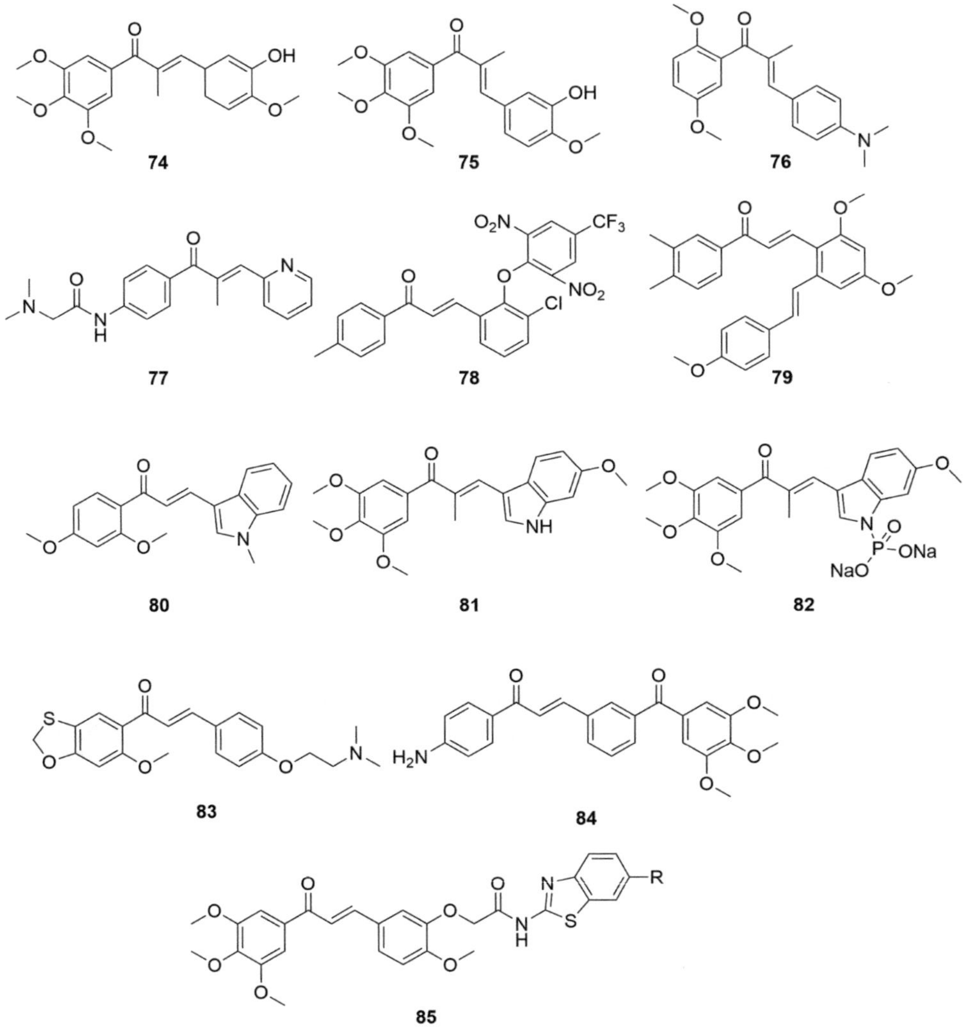

Figure 20.
Chalcones computationally predicted to target tubulin [81, 82].

TOPO inhibitory activity [92]. Chalcone **86** in addition to being a nonspecific inhibitor of TOPO-I/II also inhibits cathepsin. The observed cytotoxicity was comparable with camptothecin and etoposide. The correlations between TOPO inhibition and cytotoxicity was not reported [93]. Natural product-derived (isolated from *Angelica keiskei*) chalcone-based inhibitors of TOPO-II have also been reported by the Akihisa group with the most potent in the series, **87**, a more potent TOPO-II inhibitor than etoposide (a clinically used TOPO inhibitor) [93]. Other chalcone-based selective TOPO-II (versus TOPO-I) inhibitors such as **88** have been reported with high anticancer activity (**Figure 21**) [93, 94].

2.6 Estrogen receptor

In many cancers, the hormone receptor status is a governing factor in determining the treatment protocols. For example, in breast cancer key treatment drivers relate to the presence (or absence) of the estrogen, progesterone, and HER receptor subtypes. The first two receptors are sex-linked and act as transcription factors guiding the interplay between endogenous ligands such as 17β-estradiol. There are multiple clinical drugs that target aberrant ER activity to alleviate the symptoms of menopause, inflammation, and cancer [95].

Chalcone isoliquiritigen in (**89**) was isolated from liquorish root and displayed a concentration-dependent differential activity against ER-positive breast cancer cells (T-47D) (**Figure 22**). At low concentrations, **89** stimulates cell growth, at high dose it displays inhibitory activity; intriguingly, the activity at high concentration was noted as being ER concentration independent. In agreement with other studies, **89** was found to directly bind to the ER with low micromolar affinity. The related candidachalcone (**90**) is also an ER-responsive chalcone; and while not exact data were presented, it is suggested to be a mid-micromolar ER ligand [96, 97].

Gan et al. reported that chalcones **91** and **92** showed cellular TrxR inhibitory activity in a panel of Michael acceptor-type pharmacophores (**Figure 23**). MS analysis demonstrated that the most potent chalcone derivative (**92**) covalently modified TrxR at the selenocysteine residue U498 [21]. In 2015, Zhang et al. reported a series of chalcone analogues based on xanthohumol (**4**). Among them, compound **93** displayed good cytotoxicity against HeLa cells (IC_{50} = 1.4 μM),

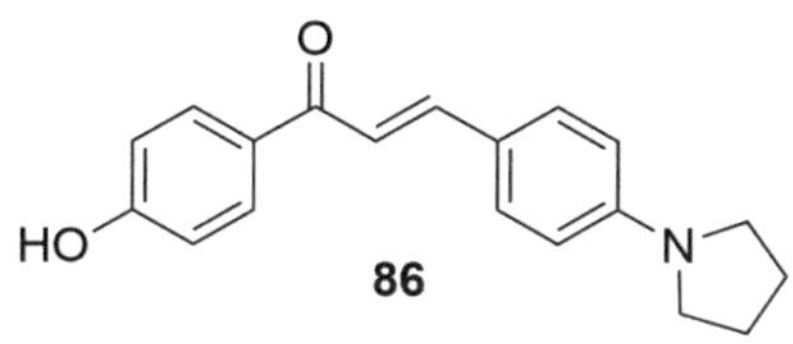

86

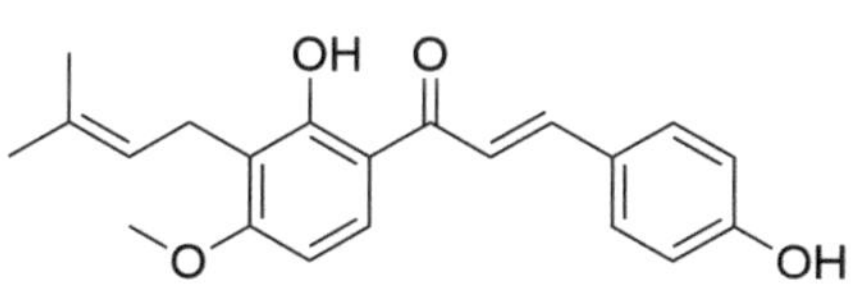

87

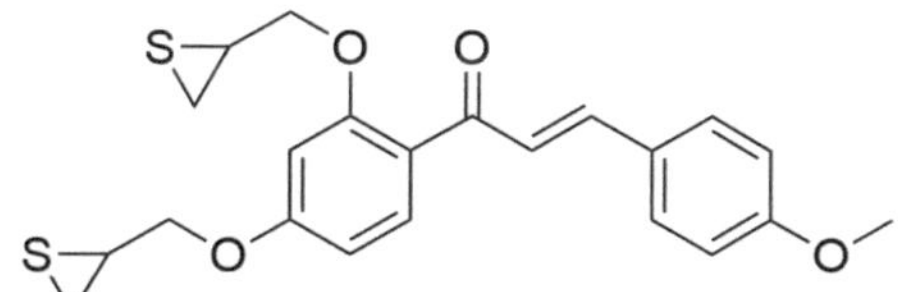

88

Figure 21.
Chemical structures of chalcones known to inhibit topoisomerases (TOPO) [93, 94].

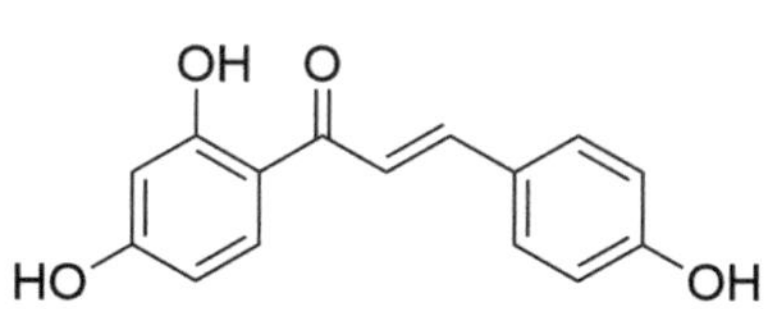

89; isoliquiritigenin

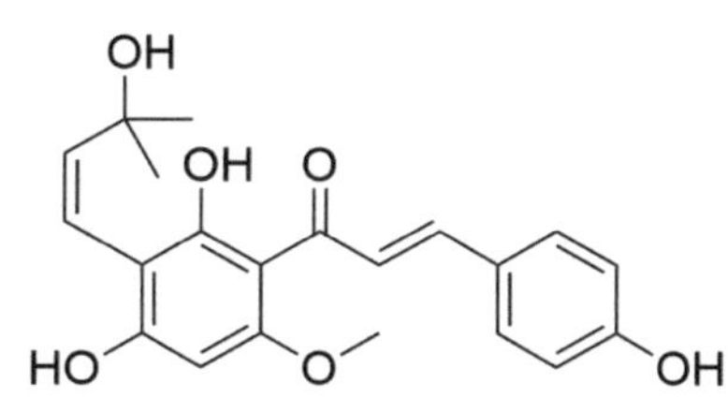

90

Figure 22.
Chalcone isokiquiriten (89) and an analogue (90) with activity against the ER-positive breast cancer cell line (T-47D) [96, 97].

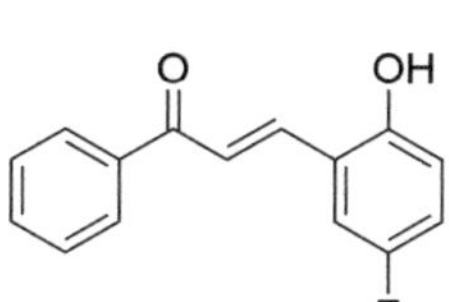

91

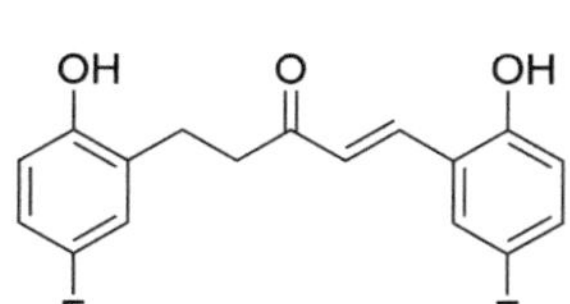

92

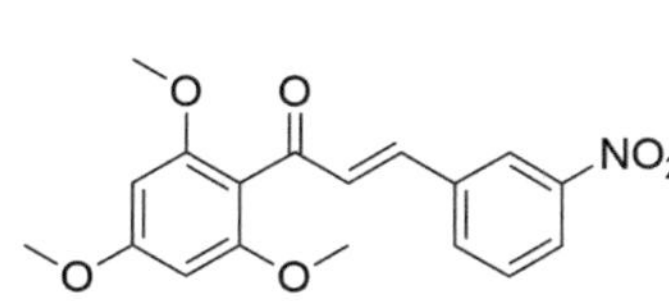

93

Figure 23.
Chemical structures of selected chalcones known as TrxR inhibitors [21].

selective inhibition of TrxR, and induction of cell apoptosis. Mechanistically, the U498C mutation of TrxR was performed to support the covalent mechanism. As a result, this compound could significantly decrease the cellular thiol level and induce the expression of reactive oxygen species (ROS) [98].

2.7 Targeting CYPs

The parent analogue, ANF (**94**), has long been recognized as displaying a broad range of pharmacological activities. Of particular note is its effects on CYP1. It has been shown that ANF (**94**) is capable of reversing CYP1B1-mediated drug resistance, increasing the efficacy of cytotoxic drugs. Simple ring opening of the flavone moiety releases a hydroxynaphthyl chalcone (**95**). Modification of the pendant phenyl ring was shown to impart modest CYP inhibition relative to ANF (**Table 3**). The parent phenyl (**96**) displays a CYP1B1 IC_{50} of 157.7 nM (c.f. ANF IC_{50} 5.9 nM). Introduction of ring substituents enhances activity with the 4-F (**97**; 48 nM),

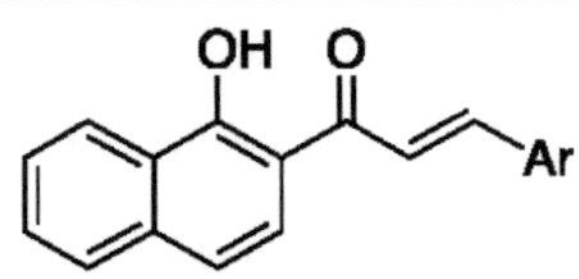

Ar	**CYP IC_{50} values (nM)**			**IC_{50} ratio**	
	1B1	**1A1**	**1A2**	**1A1/1B1**	**1A2/1B1**
ANF **94**	5.9 ± 1.3	80.3 ± 3.6	18.0 ± 3.6	13.6	3.1
Ph **95**	157.7 ± 18.5	>1000	>1000	>6.3	>6.3
4-FPh **96**	48.3 ± 8.2	>1000	>1000	>20.7	>20.7
2-OCH3Ph **97**	37.8 ± 5.8	556.6 ± 28.7	>1000	14.7	>26.5
3-Pyridyl **98**	16.7 ± 3.7	117.1 ± 18.9	227.0 ± 25.2	7.0	13.6
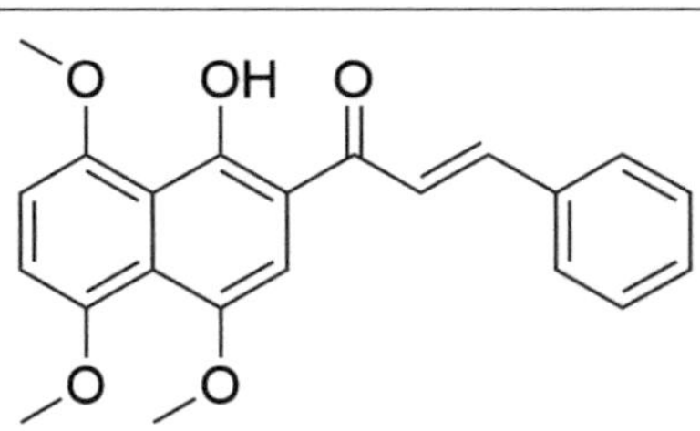					
99	4.9 ± 0.6	161.3 ± 17.4	734.7 ± 31.2	32.9	149.9
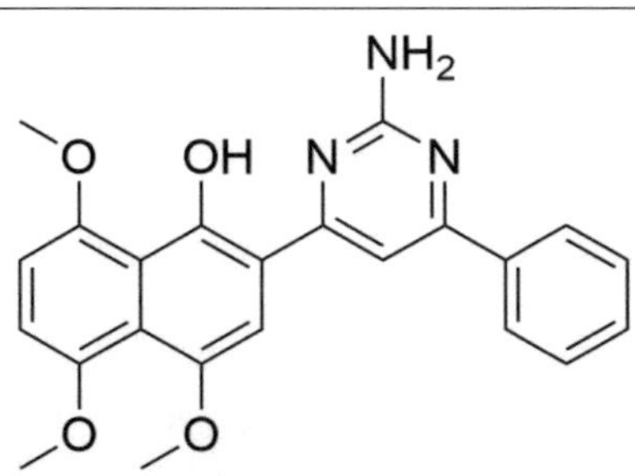					
100	4.8 ± 0.5	51.8 ± 9.7	>1000	10.8	>208.3

Table 3.
Inhibitor potency of modified chalcones against CYP1 enzymes.

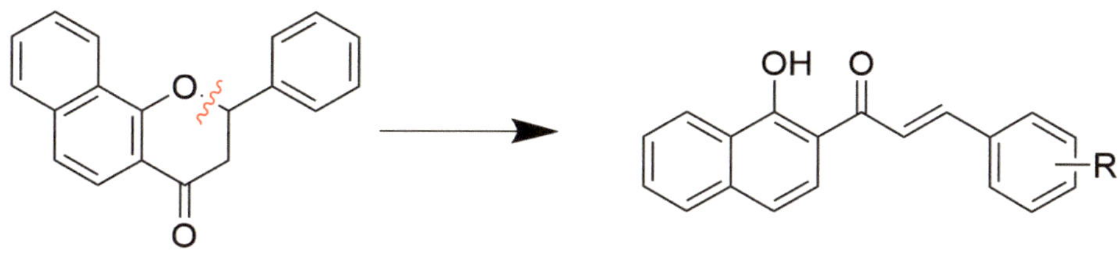

94 **95-100**

Figure 24.
Structural modification of ANF leading to a family of CYP1B1 inhibitors displaying high levels of cytotoxicity, see **Table 3** *for details of "R" [99].*

	IC_{50} values (μM)			
Compound	**MCF-7**	**MDA-MB-231**	**LCC6/P-gp**	**MCF-7/1B1**
ANF (**94**)	80.7 ± 7.6	>100	82.3 ± 8.5	>100
95	25.9 ± 3.2	46.2 ± 5.3	>100	32.3 ± 4.5
96	48.1 ± 3.7	79.6 ± 4.9	48.6 ± 2.9	>100
97	43.4 ± 1.6	75.3 ± 6.8	43.9 ± 4.4	>100
98	7.6 ± 0.7	19.8 ± 2.8	8.0 ± 2.3	12.7 ± 1.7
99	6.3 ± 1.4	15.8 ± 2.2	9.6 ± 1.3	15.1 ± 1.8
100	46.8 ± 4.7	48.9 ± 4.1	>100	20.4 ± 3.3

Table 4.
Cytotoxic activities of benzochalcones against MCF-7, MDA-MB-231, LCC6/P-GP, and MCF-7 cell lines.

2-OCH_3 (**98**; 37.7 nM), and 3-pyridyl (**99**; 16.7 nM), also with improved CYP1A2/B1 selectivity. Increasing the hydrophobicity of the phenyl moiety was detrimental to potency, but the introduction of a tetrasubstituted naphthyl moiety proved to be highly efficacious [99] (**Figure 24**).

Of the modified ANF analogues reported, **100** and **101** displayed CYP1B1 inhibition level equivalent to ANF but with significantly enhanced selectivities of 150- and >200-fold (ANF, CYP1A2/B1 = 3.1) (**Table 3**).

Examination of these analogues against MCF-7, MDA-MB-231, LCC6/P-gp, and MCF-7/1B1 revealed the 2-pyridyl chalcone analogue to be broad-spectrum active in both the wild type (MCF-7 and MDA-MB-231 cells) and also in the drug-resistant cells (LCC6/P-gp and MCF-7/1B1) (**Table 3**). Replacement of the phenyl moiety with a tetramethoxynaphthalene resulted in a drop in CYP1B1 activity ($IC_{50} > 1000$ nM), but the MCF-7 and LCC6/P-gp cytotoxicity increased. This presumably is a consequence of increased cellular uptake [99] (**Table 4**).

3. Conclusions

The medicinal chemistry landscape is a mobile one. Approaches that were viewed as unviable mere 5- to 10-years ago are now gaining traction. The introduction of PAINS filters has stymied some areas of medicinal chemistry development, correctly; but in other areas, the changing paradigms may necessitate a reexamination of the type of screening filters applied. This is especially relevant to the potential development of chalcones in the anticancer drug space. It has been consistently shown that not only do these agents possess high levels of antiproliferative activity as single agents, they synergise well across a significant number of clinically used anticancer drugs.

As this field progresses, careful reevaluation of off-target effects, compound specificity, and promiscuity will remain key, but there is significant potential for transformation of chalcones into true clinical compounds. It is worth noting that it is the role of the medicinal chemist to modulate the unfavorable effects of lead compounds in the development of clinical candidates. This, perhaps though is best left in an academic environment until "compound cleaning" to a true development candidate can be achieved.

Acknowledgements

AM is the recipient of NH&MRC project funding targeting the development of novel anticancer agents. CCR and AM are recipients of funding from the University of Newcastle Priority Research Centre for Drug Development.

Conflicts of interest

The authors declare no conflicts of interest.

Author details

Adam McCluskey and Cecilia Russell*
Chemistry, The University of Newcastle, University Drive, Callaghan, NSW, Australia

*Address all correspondence to: cecilia.russell@newcastle.edu.au

References

[1] Ferlay J, Colombet M, Soerjomataram I, Mathers C, Parkin DM, Piñeros M, et al. Estimating the global cancer incidence and mortality in 2018: GLOBOCAN sources and methods. International Journal of Cancer. 2019;**144**:1941-1953

[2] Reichardt P. The story of imatinib in GIST—A journey through the development of a targeted therapy. Oncology Research and Treatment. 2018;**41**:472-477

[3] Kannaiyan R, Mahadevan D. A comprehensive review of protein kinase inhibitors for cancer therapy. Expert Review of Anticancer Therapy. 2018;**18**: 1249-1270

[4] Lu RM, Hwang YC, Liu IJ, Lee CC, Tsai HZ, Li HJ, et al. Development of therapeutic antibodies for the treatment of diseases. Journal of Biomedical Science. 2020;**27**:1. DOI: 10.1186/s12929-019-0592-z

[5] Sun J, Russell C, Scarlett CJ, McCluskey A. Small molecule inhibitors in the treatment of pancreatic cancer. RSC Medicinal Chemistry. 2020;**11**: 164-183. DOI: 10.1039/c9md00447e

[6] Alphandéry E. Glioblastoma Treatments: An account of recent industrial developments. Frontiers in Pharmacology. 2018;**9**:1-31. DOI: 10.3389/fphar.2018.00879

[7] GBD 2016 Brain and Other CNS Cancer Collaborators. Global, regional, and national burden of brain and other CNS cancer, 1990–2016: A systematic analysis for the Global Burden of Disease Study 2016. Lancet Neurology. 2019;**18**:376-393

[8] Zhou B, Xing C. Diverse molecular targets for chalcones with varied bioactivities. Medicinal Chemistry. 2015;**5**:388-404

[9] Zhuang C, Zhang W, Sheng C, Zhang W, Chengguo Xing C, Miao Z. Chalcone: A privileged structure in medicinal chemistry. Chemical Reviews. 2017;**117**:7762-7810

[10] Gomes MN, Muratov EN, Pereira M, Peixoto JC, Rosseto LP, Cravo PVL, et al. Chalcone derivatives: Promising starting points for drug design. Molecules. 2017;**22**:1210

[11] Baell JB, Holloway GA. New substructure filters for removal of pan assay interference compounds (PAINS) from screening libraries and for their exclusion in bioassays. Journal of Medicinal Chemistry. 2010;**53**: 2719-2740

[12] Capuzzi SJ, Muratov EN, Tropsha A. Phantom PAINS: Problems with the utility of alerts for pan—Assay interference compounds. Journal of Chemical Information and Modeling. 2017;**57**:417-427

[13] Lagorce D, Oliveira N, Miteva MA, Villoutreix BO. Pan-assay interference compounds (PAINS) that may not be too painful for chemical biology projects. Drug Discovery Today. 2017; **22**:1131-1133. DOI: j.drudis.2017.05.017

[14] Newman DJ. Natural products as leads to potential drugs: An old process or the new hope for drug discovery? Journal of Medicinal Chemistry. 2008; **51**:2589-2599

[15] Batovska DI, Todorova IT. Trends in utilization of the pharmacological potential of chalcones. Current Clinical Pharmacology. 2010;**5**:1-29

[16] Sahu NK, Balbhadra SS, Choudhary J, Kohli DV. Exploring pharmacological significance of chalcone scaffold: A review. Current Medicinal Chemistry. 2012;**19**:209-225

[17] Singh P, Anand A, Kumar V. Recent developments in biological activities of chalcones: A mini review. European Journal of Medicinal Chemistry. 2014; **85**:758-777

[18] Karthikeyan C, Moorthy NS, Ramasamy S, Vanam U, Manivannan E, Karunagaran D, et al. Advances in chalcones with anticancer activities. Recent Patents on Anti-Cancer Drug Discovery. 2015;**10**:97-115

[19] Dinkova-Kostova AT, Massiah MA, Bozak RE, Hicks RJ, Talalay P. Potency of Michael reaction acceptors as inducers of enzymes that protect against carcinogenesis depends on their reactivity with sulfhydryl groups. Proceedings of the National Academy of Sciences of the United States of America. 2001;**98**:3404-3409

[20] Dinkova-Kostova AT, Cheah J, Samouilov A, Zweier JL, Bozak RE, Hicks RJ, et al. Phenolic Michael reaction acceptors: Combined direct and indirect antioxidant defenses against electrophiles and oxidants. Medicinal Chemistry. 2007;**3**:261-268

[21] Gan FF, Kaminska KK, Yang H, Liew CY, Leow PC, So CL, et al. Identification of Michael acceptor-centric pharmacophores with substituents that yield strong thioredoxin reductase inhibitory character correlated to antiproliferative activity. Antioxidants & Redox Signaling. 2013;**19**:1149-1165

[22] Dinkova-Kostova AT, Abeygunawardana C, Talalay P. Chemoprotective properties of phenylpropenoids, bis(benzylidene)-cycloalkanones, and related Michael reaction acceptors: Correlation of potencies as phase 2 enzyme inducers and radical scavengers. Journal of Medicinal Chemistry. 1998;**41**:5287-5296

[23] Srinivasan B, Johnson TE, Lad R, Xing C. Structure activity relationship studies of chalcone leading to 3-hydroxy-4,3′,4′,5′-tetramethoxychalcone and its analogues as potent nuclear factor kappaB inhibitors and their anticancer activities. Journal of Medicinal Chemistry. 2009; **52**:7228-7235

[24] Jackson PA, Widen JC, Harki DA, Brummond KM. Covalent modifiers: A chemical perspective on the reactivity of α,β-unsaturated carbonyls with thiols via hetero-Michael addition reactions. Journal of Medicinal Chemistry. 2016; **60**:839-885

[25] He W, Wang Q, Srinivasan B, Xu J, Padilla MT, Li Z, et al. A JNK-mediated autophagy pathway that triggers c-IAP degradation and necroptosis for anticancer chemotherapy. Oncogene. 2014;**33**:3004-3013

[26] Xu J, Xu X, Shi S, Wang Q, Saxton B, He W, et al. Autophagy-mediated degradation of IAPs and c-FLIP potentiates apoptosis induced by combination of TRAIL and Chal-24. Journal of Cellular Biochemistry. 2016; **117**:1136-1144

[27] Shi S, Wang Q, Xu J, Jang JH, Padilla MT, Nyunoya T, et al. Synergistic anticancer effect of cisplatin and Chal-24 combination through IAP and c-FLIPL degradation, Ripoptosome formation and autophagy-mediated apoptosis. Oncotarget. 2015;**6**:1640-1651

[28] Zhang Y, Wu J, Ying S, Chen G, Wu B, Xu T, et al. Discovery of new MD2 inhibitor from chalcone derivatives with anti-inflammatory effects in LPS induced acute lung injury. Scientific Reports. 2016;**6**:25130

[29] Senger MR, Fraga CAM, Dantas RF, Silva-Júnior FP. Filtering promiscuous compounds in early drug discovery: Is it a good idea? Drug Discovery Today. 2016;**21**:868-872

[30] Burmaoglu S, Algul O, Aktas D, Gobek A, Gulbol G. Synthesis and

anti-proliferative activity of fluoro-substituted chalcones. Bioorganic & Medicinal Chemistry Letters. 2016;**26**: 3172-3176

[31] Romagnoli R, Baraldi PG, Carrion MD, Cara CL, Cruz-Lopez O, Preti D, et al. Design, synthesis, and biological evaluation of thiophene analogues of chalcones. Bioorganic & Medicinal Chemistry. 2008;**16**:5367-5376

[32] Mao Z, Zheng X, Qi Y, Zhang M, Huang Y, Wan C, et al. Synthesis and biological evaluation of novel hybrid compounds between chalcone and piperazine as potential antitumor agents. RSC Advances. 2016;**6**:7723-7727

[33] Koziel R, Szczepanowska J, Magalska A, Piwocka K, Duszynski J, Zablocki K. Ciprofloxacin inhibits proliferation and promotes generation of aneuploidy in Jurkat cells. Journal of Physiology and Pharmacology. 2010;**61**: 233-239

[34] Aranha O, Grignon R, Fernandes N, McDonnell TJ, Wood DP, Sarkar FH. Suppression of human prostate cancer cell growth by ciprofloxacin is associated with cell cycle arrest and apoptosis. International Journal of Oncology. 2003;**22**:787-794

[35] Miclau T, Edin ML, Lester GE, Lindsey RW, Dahners LE. Effect of ciprofloxacin on the proliferation of osteoblast-like MG-63 human osteosarcoma cells in vitro. Journal of Orthopaedic Research. 1998;**16**:509-512

[36] Somekh E, Douer D, Shaked N, Rubinstein E. In vitro effects of ciprofloxacin and pefloxacin on growth of normal human hematopoietic progenitor cells and on leukemic cell lines. The Journal of Pharmacology and Experimental Therapeutics. 1989;**248**: 415-418

[37] Lawrence NJ, McGown AT, Ducki S, Hadfield JA. The interaction of chalcones with tubulin. Anti-Cancer Drug Design. 2000;**15**:135-141

[38] Ducki S. Antimitotic chalcones and related compounds as inhibitors of tubulin assembly. Anti-Cancer Agents in Medicinal Chemistry. 2009;**9**:336-347

[39] Romagnoli R, Baraldi PG, Carrion MD, Cruz-Lopez O, Cara CL, Balzarini J, et al. Hybrid alpha-bromoacryloylamido chalcones. Design, synthesis and biological evaluation. Bioorganic & Medicinal Chemistry Letters. 2009;**19**:2022-2028

[40] Fu DJ, Zhang SY, Liu YC, Zhang L, Liu JJ, Song J, et al. Design, synthesis and antiproliferative activity studies of novel dithiocarbamate-chalcone derivates. Bioorganic & Medicinal Chemistry Letters. 2016;**26**:3918-3922

[41] Yang Y, Hahne H, Kuster B, Verhelst SH. A simple and effective cleavable linker for chemical proteomics applications. Molecular & Cellular Proteomics. 2013;**12**:237-244

[42] Austin MB, Noel JP. The chalcone synthase superfamily of type III polyketide synthases. Natural Product Reports. 2003;**20**:79-110

[43] Dong X, Du L, Pan Z, Liu T, Yang B, Hu Y. Synthesis and biological evaluation of novel hybrid chalcone derivatives as vasorelaxant agents. European Journal of Medicinal Chemistry. 2010;**45**:3986-3992

[44] Kamal A, Shankaraiah N, Prabhakar S, Reddy CR, Markandeya N, Reddy KL, et al. Solid-phase synthesis of new pyrrolobenzodiazepine-chalcone conjugates: DNA-binding affinity and anticancer activity. Bioorganic & Medicinal Chemistry Letters. 2008;**18**: 2434-2439

[45] Kamal A, Prabhakar S, Janaki Ramaiah M, Venkat Reddy P, Ratna Reddy C, Mallareddy A, et al. Synthesis

and anticancer activity of chalcone-pyrrolobenzodiazepine conjugates linked via 1,2,3-triazole ring side-armed with alkane spacers. European Journal of Medicinal Chemistry. 2011;**46**: 3820-3831

[46] Gaur R, Pathania AS, Malik FA, Bhakuni RS, Verma RK. Synthesis of a series of novel dihydroartemisinin monomers and dimers containing chalcone as a linker and their anticancer activity. European Journal of Medicinal Chemistry. 2016;**122**:232-246

[47] Kamal A, Mallareddy A, Suresh P, Shaik TB, Lakshma Nayak V, Kishor C, et al. Synthesis of chalcone-amidobenzothiazole conjugates as antimitotic and apoptotic inducing agents. Bioorganic & Medicinal Chemistry. 2012;**20**:3480-3492

[48] Schobert R, Biersack B, Dietrich A, Knauer S, Zoldakova M, Fruehauf A, et al. Pt(II) complexes of a combretastatin A-4 analogous chalcone: Effects of conjugation on cytotoxicity, tumor specificity, and long-term tumor growth suppression. Journal of Medicinal Chemistry. 2009;**52**:241-246

[49] Pingaew R, Saekee A, Mandi P, Nantasenamat C, Prachayasittikul S, Ruchirawat S, et al. Synthesis, biological evaluation and molecular docking of novel chalcone coumarin hybrids as anticancer and antimalarial agents. European Journal of Medicinal Chemistry. 2014;**85**:65-76

[50] Zhao L, Mao L, Hong G, Yang X, Liu T. Design, synthesis and anticancer activity of matrine-1H-1,2,3-triazole-chalcone conjugates. Bioorganic & Medicinal Chemistry Letters. 2015;**25**: 2540-2544

[51] O'Boyle NM, Carr M, Greene LM, Bergin O, Nathwani SM, McCabe T, et al. Synthesis and evaluation of azetidinone analogues of combretastatin A-4 as tubulin targeting agents. Journal of Medicinal Chemistry. 2010;**53**: 8569-8584

[52] Singh P, Raj R, Kumar V, Mahajan MP, Bedi PM, Kaur T, et al. 1,2,3-Triazole tethered beta-lactam-chalcone bifunctional hybrids: Synthesis and anticancer evaluation. European Journal of Medicinal Chemistry. 2012; **47**:594-600

[53] Loch-Neckel G, Bicca MA, Leal PC, Mascarello A, Siqueira JM, Calixto JB. In vitro and in vivo anti-glioma activity of a chalcone-quinoxaline hybrid. European Journal of Medicinal Chemistry. 2015;**90**:93-100

[54] Shankaraiah N, Siraj KP, Nekkanti S, Srinivasulu V, Sharma P, Senwar KR, et al. DNA-binding affinity and anticancer activity of beta-carboline-chalcone conjugates as potential DNA intercalators: Molecular modelling and synthesis. Bioorganic Chemistry. 2015;**59**:130-139

[55] Kamal A, Balakrishna M, Nayak VL, Shaik TB, Faazil S, Nimbarte VD. Design and synthesis of imidazo[2,1-b] thiazolechalcone conjugates: Microtubule-destabilizing agents. ChemMedChem. 2014;**9**:2766-2780

[56] Kamal A, Kashi Reddy M, Viswanath A. The design and development of imidazothiazole-chalcone derivatives as potential anticancer drugs. Expert Opinion on Drug Discovery. 2013;**8**:289-304

[57] Kamal A, Dastagiri D, Ramaiah MJ, Reddy JS, Bharathi EV, Srinivas C, et al. Synthesis of imidazothiazole-chalcone derivatives as anticancer and apoptosis inducing agents. ChemMedChem. 2010; **5**:1937-1947

[58] Kolundzija B, Markovic V, Stanojkovic T, Joksovic L, Matic I, Todorovic N, et al. Novel anthraquinone based chalcone analogues containing an imine fragment: Synthesis, cytotoxicity

and anti-angiogenic activity. Bioorganic & Medicinal Chemistry Letters. 2014; **24**:65-71

[59] Lemstrova R, Melichar B, Mohelnikova-Duchonova B. Therapeutic potential of taxanes in the treatment of metastatic pancreatic cancer. Cancer Chemotherapy and Pharmacology. 2016;**78**:1101-1111

[60] Martino E, Casamassima G, Castiglione S, Cellupica E, Pantalone S, Papagni F, et al. Vinca alkaloids and analogues as anti-cancer agents: Looking back, peering ahead. Bioorganic & Medicinal Chemistry Letters. 2018;**28**: 2816-2826

[61] Jordan MA, Wilson L. Microtubules as a target for anticancer drugs. Nature Reviews. Cancer. 2004;**4**:253-265

[62] Dumontet C. Mechanisms of action and resistance to tubulin-binding agents. Expert Opinion on Investigational Drugs. 2000;**9**:779-788

[63] Niu M, Qin J, Tian C, Yan X, Dong F, Cheng Z, et al. Tubulin inhibitors: Pharmacophore modeling, virtual screening and molecular docking. Acta Pharmacologica Sinica. 2014;**35**:967-979

[64] Pettit GR, Cragg GM, Herald DL, Schmidt JM, Lohavanijaya P. Antineoplastic agents. Part 84. Isolation and structure of combretastatin. Canadian Journal of Chemistry. 1982; **60**:1374-1376

[65] Kamal A, Ramakrishna G, Raju P, Viswanath A, Ramaiah MJ, Balakishan G, et al. Synthesis and anti-cancer activity of chalcone linked imidazolones. Bioorganic & Medicinal Chemistry Letters. 2010;**20**:4865-4869

[66] Markovic V, Debeljak N, Stanojkovic T, Kolundzija B, Sladic D, Vujcic M, et al. Anthraquinone-chalcone hybrids: Synthesis, preliminary antiproliferative evaluation and DNA-interaction studies. European Journal of Medicinal Chemistry. 2015;**89**:401-410

[67] Wani ZA, Guru SK, Rao AV, Sharma S, Mahajan G, Behl A, et al. A novel quinazolinone chalcone derivative induces mitochondrial dependent apoptosis and inhibits PI3K/Akt/mTOR signaling pathway in human colon cancer HCT-116 cells. Food and Chemical Toxicology. 2016;**87**:1-11

[68] Canela M-D, Noppen S, Bueno O, Prota AE, Bargsten K, Sáez-Calvo G, et al. Antivascular and antitumor properties of the tubulin-binding chalcone TUB091. Oncotarget. 2017;**8**: 14325-14342

[69] Wu W, Ye H, Wan L, Han X, Wang G, Hu J, et al. Millepachine, a novel chalcone, induces G2/M arrest by inhibiting CDK1 activity and causing apoptosis via ROS-mitochondrial apoptotic pathway in human hepatocarcinoma cells in vitro and in vivo. Carcinogenesis. 2013;**34**: 1636-1643

[70] Yang Z, Wu W, Wang J, Liu L, Li L, Yang J, et al. Synthesis and biological evaluation of novel millepachine derivatives as a new class of tubulin polymerization inhibitors. Journal of Medicinal Chemistry. 2014;**57**: 7977-7989

[71] Wang G, Peng F, Cao D, Yang Z, Han X, Liu J, et al. Design, synthesis and biological evaluation of millepachine derivatives as a new class of tubulin polymerization inhibitors. Bioorganic & Medicinal Chemistry. 2013;**21**: 6844-6854

[72] Wang G, Li C, He L, Lei K, Wang F, Pu Y, et al. Design, synthesis and biological evaluation of a series of pyrano chalcone derivatives containing indole moiety as novel anti-tubulin agents. Bioorganic & Medicinal Chemistry. 2014;**22**:2060-2079

[73] Zhu C, Zuo Y, Wang R, Liang B, Yue X, Wen G, et al. Discovery of potent cytotoxic ortho-aryl chalcones as new scaffold targeting tubulin and mitosis with affinity-based fluorescence. Journal of Medicinal Chemistry. 2014;**57**:6364-6382

[74] Shen KH, Chang JK, Hsu YL, Kuo PL. Chalcone arrests cell cycle progression and induces apoptosis through induction of mitochondrial pathway and inhibition of nuclear factor kappa B signalling in human bladder cancer cells. Basic & Clinical Pharmacology & Toxicology. 2007;**101**: 254-261

[75] Martel-Frachet V, Keramidas M, Nurisso A, DeBonis S, Rome C, Coll JL, et al. IPP51, a chalcone acting as a microtubule inhibitor with in vivo antitumor activity against bladder carcinoma. Oncotarget. 2015;**6**: 14669-14686

[76] Qiao Z, Wang Q, Zhang F, Wang Z, Bowling T, Nare B, et al. Chalconebenzoxaborole hybrid molecules as potent antitrypanosomal agents. Journal of Medicinal Chemistry. 2012;**55**:3553-3557

[77] DiCesare N, Lakowicz JR. Chalcone-analogue fluorescent probes for saccharides signaling using the boronic acid group. Tetrahedron Letters. 2002; **43**:2615-2618

[78] Kumar SK, Hager E, Pettit C, Gurulingappa H, Davidson NE, Khan SR. Design, synthesis, and evaluation of novel boronic-chalcone derivatives as antitumor agents. Journal of Medicinal Chemistry. 2003;**46**: 2813-2815

[79] Sasayama T, Tanaka K, Mizukawa K, Kawamura A, Kondoh T, Hosoda K, et al. Trans-4-Iodo,4′-boranylchalcone induces antitumor activity against malignant glioma cell lines in vitro and in vivo. Journal of Neuro-Oncology. 2007;**85**:123-132

[80] Achanta G, Modzelewska A, Feng L, Khan SR, Huang P. A boronic-chalcone derivative exhibits potent anticancer activity through inhibition of the proteasome. Molecular Pharmacology. 2006;**70**:426-433

[81] Ducki S, Mackenzie G, Lawrence NJ, Snyder JP. Quantitative structure-activity relationship (5D-QSAR) study of combretastatin-like analogues as inhibitors of tubulin assembly. Journal of Medicinal Chemistry. 2005;**48**:457-465

[82] Ducki S, Rennison D, Woo M, Kendall A, Chabert JF, McGown AT, et al. Combretastatin-like chalcones as inhibitors of microtubule polymerization. Part 1: Synthesis and biological evaluation of antivascular activity. Bioorganic & Medicinal Chemistry. 2009;**17**:7698-7710

[83] Edwards ML, Stemerick DM, Sunkara PS. Chalcones: A new class of antimitotic agents. Journal of Medicinal Chemistry. 1990;**33**:1948-1954

[84] Peyrot V, Leynadier D, Sarrazin M, Briand C, Menendez M, Laynez J, et al. Mechanism of binding of the new antimitotic drug MDL 27048 to the colchicine site of tubulin: Equilibrium studies. Biochemistry. 1992;**31**: 11125-11132

[85] Kim DY, Kim KH, Kim ND, Lee KY, Han CK, Yoon JH, et al. Design and biological evaluation of novel tubulin inhibitors as antimitotic agents using a pharmacophore binding model with tubulin. Journal of Medicinal Chemistry. 2006;**49**:5664-5670

[86] Zhang H, Liu JJ, Sun J, Yang XH, Zhao TT, Lu X, et al. Design, synthesis and biological evaluation of novel chalcone derivatives as antitubulin agents. Bioorganic & Medicinal Chemistry. 2012;**20**:3212-3218

[87] Ruan BF, Lu X, Tang JF, Wei Y, Wang XL, Zhang YB, et al. Synthesis,

biological evaluation, and molecular docking studies of resveratrol derivatives possessing chalcone moiety as potential antitubulin agents. Bioorganic & Medicinal Chemistry. 2011;**19**:2688-2695

[88] Kamal A, Kumar GB, Vishnuvardhan MV, Shaik AB, Reddy VS, Mahesh R, et al. Synthesis of phenstatin/isocombretastatin-chalcone conjugates as potent tubulin polymerization inhibitors and mitochondrial apoptotic inducers. Organic & Biomolecular Chemistry. 2015;**13**:3963-3981

[89] Konieczny MT, Bulakowska A, Pirska D, Konieczny W, Skladanowski A, Sabisz M, et al. Structural factors affecting affinity of cytotoxic oxathiole-fused chalcones toward tubulin. European Journal of Medicinal Chemistry. 2015;**89**: 733-742

[90] Konieczny MT, Bulakowska A, Polak J, Pirska D, Konieczny W, Gryn P, et al. Structural factors affecting cytotoxic activity of (E)-1-(Benzo[d][1,3]oxathiol-6-yl)-3-phenylprop-2-en-1-one derivatives. Chemical Biology & Drug Design. 2014;**84**:86-91

[91] Pommier Y, Leo E, Zhang H, Marchand C. DNA topoisomerases and their poisoning by anticancer and antibacterial drugs. Chemistry & Biology. 2010;**17**:421-433

[92] Kim SH, Lee E, Baek KH, Kwon HB, Woo H, et al. Chalcones, inhibitors for topoisomerase I and cathepsin B and L, as potential anti-cancer agents. Bioorganic & Medicinal Chemistry Letters. 2013;**23**:3320-3324

[93] Akihisa T, Kikuchi T, Nagai H, Ishii K, Tabata K, et al. 4-Hydroxyderricin from Angelica keiskei roots induces caspase-dependent apoptotic cell death in HL60 human leukemia cells. Journal of Oleo Science. 2011;**60**:71-77

[94] Na Y, Nam JM. Synthesis and topoisomerase II inhibitory and cytotoxic activity of oxiranylmethoxy- and thiiranylmethoxy-chalcone derivatives. Bioorganic & Medicinal Chemistry Letters. 2011;**21**:211-214

[95] Paterni I, Bertini S, Granchi C, Macchia M, Minutolo F. Estrogen receptor ligands: A patent review update. Expert Opinion on Therapeutic Patents. 2013;**23**:1247-1271

[96] Hajirahimkhan A, Simmler C, Yuan Y, Anderson JR, Chen SN, et al. Evaluation of estrogenic activity of licorice species in comparison with hops used in botanicals for menopausal symptoms. PLoS ONE. 2013;**8**:e67947

[97] Hegazy ME, El-Hamd H, Mohamed A, El-Halawany AM, Djemgou PC, Shahat AA, et al. Estrogenic activity of chemical constituents from *Tephrosia candida*. Journal of Natural Products. 2011;**74**: 937-942

[98] Zhang B, Duan D, Ge C, Yao J, Liu Y, Li X, et al. Synthesis of xanthohumol analogues and discovery of potent thioredoxin reductase inhibitor as potential anticancer agent. Journal of Medicinal Chemistry. 2015; **58**:1795-1805

[99] Dong J, Huang G, Zhang Q, Wang Z, Cui J, Wu Y, et al. Development of benzochalcone derivatives as selective CYP1B1 inhibitors and anticancer agents. MedChemComm. 2019;**10**:1606-1614

Chapter 6

New Screening for the Development of Radioprotectors: Radioprotection and Anti-Cancer Effect of β-Glucan (*Enterococcus faecalis*)

Yeun-Hwa Gu

Abstract

In this study, β-glucan was orally administered and irradiated with whole body 2 Gy. It was then confirmed that the mortality of mice and tumor growth of mice with tumors were significantly reduced. Since the number of leukocytes and lymphocytes increased with a single dose of β-glucan, the crystal was encountered where the radioprotective effect of β-glucan was probably increased by the hematopoietic action of irradiated mice. In previous studies, β-(1–3)-D-glucan extract has a radioprotective effect and an antitumor effect, and regarding the mechanism of action, the immune activity and antioxidant were elucidated. In this study, we investigated the antitumor effects of β-glucan on radiation, protection of immune disorders, and antioxidant effects. After intraperitoneal inoculation of about 2×10^6 sarcoma 180, ICR mice were administered 200 mg/kg β-glucan every other day every two weeks. We irradiated 2 Gy radiation 3 times and counted the number of white blood cells and lymphocytes. In addition, body weight and tumor size were measured 2 weeks after cancer cells were seeded. Antioxidant activity was measured using the AAPH (2,2-azobis (2-amidinopropane) dihydrochloride) method. There was a clear decrease in tumor size in the radiation and glucan groups compared to the group receiving only cancer cells that increased tumor size over time. Almost all mice inoculated with only cancer cells died two weeks after radiation, but two-thirds of radiation and the glucan group were alive. Regardless of radiation exposure, the number of leukocytes and lymphocytes increased when β-glucan was administered. Antioxidant activity has been demonstrated in both groups of glucans. These results may indicate that administration of β-glucan increases immune activity, prevents side effects during cancer radiotherapy, and provides a supplemental tool for the treatment of cancer.

Keywords: lymphocyte, CD4 + , CD8 + , β-(1–3)-D-glucan, radioprotection, radiotherapy

1. Introduction

Recent studies have demonstrated the immunomodulatory effects of heat-killed lactic acid bacteria. The aim of this study was to evaluate the protective effect of heat-killed *Enterococcus faecalis EF-2001* (EF-2001) on a radiation protective and immunopotentiating Effect.

Drugs that suppress the radiosensitizer that enhances the biological action of ionizing radiation are collectively called radioprotector. Drugs that show protective effects by radical scavenging or hypoxic action, such as WR-2721, need to be administered before exposure [1]. Interleukins and the like are also effective with prior administration. Drugs that enhance *in vivo* production of hematopoietic cell growth factors, such as hematopoietic cell growth factors such as G-CSF and immunostimulants such as 432OK, are effective even after administration [2]. Chelating agents and iodine agents that prevent radionuclides from being absorbed from the skin and gastrointestinal tract and deposited in tissues and promote excretion are broadly considered protective agents [3].

Protective agents for radical scavengers have been studied as an adjunct to cancer radiotherapy, and WR-2721 (S-2-(3-Aminopropylamino) ethylphosphorothioic acid) is the most promising among many compounds. It is thought to show a protective action by eliminating radicals caused by indirect action of radiation, hydrogenation, reduction of oxygen effect, etc. A drug that can reduce radiation damage when administered immediately before radiation exposure is called a radioprotective drug. Typical examples are aminothiol derivatives such as cysteamine (mercaptoethylamine) and WR-2721. At the time of tumor radiotherapy, clinical application has been considered for protecting normal tissues around the tumor, but it has not been put into practical use. In addition, there is a possibility that these radiation prevention drugs may be used to protect rescue workers and decontamination workers in the event of a nuclear facility accident, but all currently known drugs are stamina, judgment, agility. Side effects such as decreased sex and vomiting are strong and have not been put to practical use [4].

Mn, Zn, and Cd ions, as activators of biological defense mechanisms, induce protective effects by inducing biosynthesis of metallothionein with radical scavenging ability in cells. In addition, gelen, interleukin 1 (IL-1), lipopolysaccharide (lipopolysaccharide, LPS), muramyl dipeptide (MDP) derivatives, ginseng extract, etc. Effective when administered prior to exposure. Leucons and innocities are nucleic acid precursors that are approved as drugs for leukopenia and have radiation protection but are not strong [5].

G-CSF (granulocyte colony-stimulating factor), a hematopoietic cell growth factor, is a growth factor for leukocyte progenitor cells such as neutrophils. Prevents infection and bleeding and provides lifesaving effect. GM-CSF (granulocyte/macrophage colony-stimulating factor) and interleukin 6 (IL-6) have similar effects, but G-CSF is most expected in terms of fewer side effects. These proteins are natural substances collectively called cytokines, but can be produced as recombinants by genetic engineering techniques. In addition, picibanil (OK-432), glucan, lactic acid bacteria preparations, etc. are said to enhance in vivo production of hematopoietic cell growth factor and are effective when administered after exposure. Hematopoietic hormones, such as GM-CSF, are actually post-accidents in Brazil and San Salvador used for exposed people [6].

New Protective Agents Stable nitroxide radicals have SOD activity and protect animal cells from oxidative stress caused by superoxide and hydrogen peroxide. Tempol, one of the stable nitroxide radicals, has been shown to exhibit radioprotective effects on C3H mice both in vitro and in vivo. It has also been shown to prevent radiation-induced bone marrow damage and appears promising as a protective agent in cancer radiotherapy [7].

Chelating agents and iodine agents that prevent radionuclides from being absorbed from the skin and gastrointestinal tract, or deposited in tissues, or promote excretion as agents for preventing absorption and deposition of radionuclides in the body and promoting elimination these are protective agents in a broad sense. Prussian blue is used to prevent absorption of ^{137}Cs. To promote ^{90}Sr excretion, calcium citrate and sodium alginate are recommended. In addition, sodium citrate and a low phosphorus diet are effective. Geralmine (aluminum hydroxide gel) has the same effect as a low phosphorus diet because it inhibits the absorption of phosphoric acid. Zn-DTPA or Ca-DTPA is used to promote plutonium excretion. An iodine agent (potassium iodide agent) is effective for preventing radioactive iodine from collecting in the thyroid gland [8–10].

β-glucan is an edible mushroom, belonging to the β-glucan, and named β-glucan. It particularly resembles *L.shimeji* Hongo in its taste and touch. It is a stump mushroom, which grows in forest, having a grayish brown-shaped umbrella about 4–9 cm in diameter [11]. Glucan (β-*glucan decastes* Sing) was called the β-glucan aggregate and has highly been valued for a long time, and its artificial cultivation was difficult till now. Recently, there has been artificial cultivation using bacterial strains as seedlings [12]. Now you can see it with general partial exposure. The authors studied glucan for antitumor, angiotensin converting enzyme inhibition, and serum cholesterol-lowering activity [13]. Glucan was found to have higher activity than the same class of shiitake Enteroccous Faecalis in anti-tumor activity, β-1,6 D-glucan and β-1,3D-glucan, and their active β-1, 6 D-glucan contains β-1,3D-glucan [14]. Here, we report the effect of glucan extract on radiation therapy in mice with cancer.

2. Materials and methods

2.1 β-Glucan

EF-2001 is a commercially available probiotic that was originally isolated from healthy human infant feces. Nihon BRM Co. Ltd. (Tokyo, Japan) supplied it as a heat-killed, dried powder. One gram of dried EF-2001 is equivalent to over 7.5×10^{12} colony-forming units prior to being heat-killed. *Nihon BRM Co. Ltd. (Tokyo, Japan) supplied Enteroccous Faecalis 2001®, a glucan product, composed of yeast extract, dextrin and gelatin*.

Dry Enterococcus faecalis contains 35–45 g of β-glycan per 100 g. *Enteroccous Faecalis* was orally administered using a zoned for 2 weeks before the start of the experiment.

2.2 Animal

The experimental animals used in this study are ICR / Slc mice. ICR/Slc mice (5 weeks old, male) were obtained from SLC, Japan. Once received, the mice were pre-bred for a week and only healthy mice were used for testing. Mice were fed with commercial feed (CA-1, CLEA Japan) and water ad libitum, with a 12-hour light cycle (8:00 lights, 20:00 lights off). The room humidity and temperature were 60–65% and 22 ± 2° C, respectively.

2.3 Experimental groups

The experimental groups were divided into control group, tumor seeding group, tumor seeding +2 Gy exposure group, β-glucan treatment group, β-glucan + tumor seeding group, β-glucan + tumor seeding +2 Gy exposure by 6 groups.

2.4 Irradiation device

The X-ray generator used was Philips MG226/4.5. For the pipe voltage, a dose of 200 kV was applied at a rate of 0.35 Gy/min. The total amount of X-rays exposed was 2 Gy. The exposed place of the mouse was fixed to the position of the front part of the left foot (place where cancer cells were seeded) with a holder, and the place not irradiated was covered with a lead container. X-rays were irradiated on the 1 and 3 days.

The specific radiation irradiation method in each experimental group is shown below. For changes in blood cells, single irradiation with 2 Gy was performed. However, in the radiation tumor effect experiment, 2 Gy was divided into 3 divided doses.

2.5 Tumor inoculation

In order to obtain reproducible experimental data, mice were inoculated on the 15th day after breeding for more than 1 month. Approximately 2 x 10^6 sarcoma 180 cancer cells were inoculated into the muscle of the left foot of an ICR male mouse.

2.6 Administration method of β-glucan

Dissolve the extract in physiological saline, and for the control group, tumor-seeding group, β-glucan administration group, β-glucan + tumor seeding group, extract the water extract (200 mg/kg) every other day for several weeks. Administered. In the control group, tumor seeding +2 Gy-exposed group and β-glucan + tumor seeding +2 Gy-exposed group, only saline was injected. After 2 weeks of cancer cell seeding, the tumor size was measured weekly. We also measured body weight on exactly the same schedule as tumor size measurements.

Each group consisted of 10 mice. Tumor size was measured using.

Formula:

$$\text{Tumor size}\left(\text{cm}^3\right) = 3/4\,\pi\,\text{A2B}/2$$

A; Minor axis (cm);

B; Longer axis (cm)

At 14 (just before the first X-ray exposure), 1, 3, 5, 7, 9 and 11 days after tumor dissemination, each mouse is fixed with a holder and the caudal vein is covered with an extended female to get about 20 ul of dripping blood. Blood was collected in a blood collection container (Dolamond Co. Ltd.) and diluted with diluent (Nihon Kohden Co. Ltd.). White blood cell counts, including lymphocyte counts and granulocyte counts, were measured using an automated blood cell analyzer (Nihon Kohden Co. Ltd., Celltac-α-MEK-6318). The results obtained were expressed as mean ± standard deviation (S.D.). Student's t-test was applied and results above 0.05 were considered significant.

3. Results

3.1 Number of peripheral blood cells: leukocytes

Figure 1 shows the changes over time of leukocytes in the 4 groups.

Compared with the control group, the β-glucan group showed a significant increase in the number of white blood cells. The rate of significant increase throughout the treatment period was 5/8 (β-glucan group). These results suggest that β-glucan decisively increases white blood cell count.

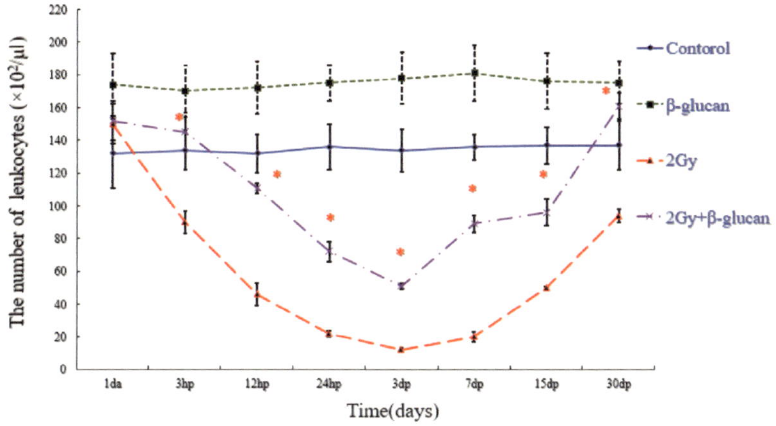

Figure 1.
β-glucan on blood leukocyte counts in mice. There were 10 animals in each experimental group. Data are mean ± standard deviation values. Statistically significantly different (P < 0.05) from the control group. Statistically significantly different (* P < 0.05) from the 2 Gy group. Administration of β-glucan was administered for 2 weeks and then treated with radiation. da; days after, hp.; hours post, dp; days post.*

In the irradiated group, white blood cell counts began to decrease in all experimental groups immediately after irradiation and tended to recover after 3 days. Compared to the 2 Gy group over time, the white blood cell count was always higher in the β-glucan +2 Gy group. When observed in each period, the white blood cell count in the β-glucan +2 Gy group was significantly higher than the 2 Gy single group the day before irradiation ($P < 0.05$). This suggests that an increase in white blood cell count is shown in the un-irradiated state. A significant ratio was observed in the β-glucan +2 Gy group. These results suggest a decrease in 2 Gy-induced decrease in white blood cell count in the β-glucan +2 Gy group.

3.2 Number of lymphocytes

Figure 2 shows the time course of lymphocyte counts by β-glucan administration in each non-irradiated and 2 Gy whole body irradiated groups.

In the non-irradiated group, all treatment groups showed higher lymphocyte counts compared to the control group. Specifically, there was a significant ratio in the β-glucan

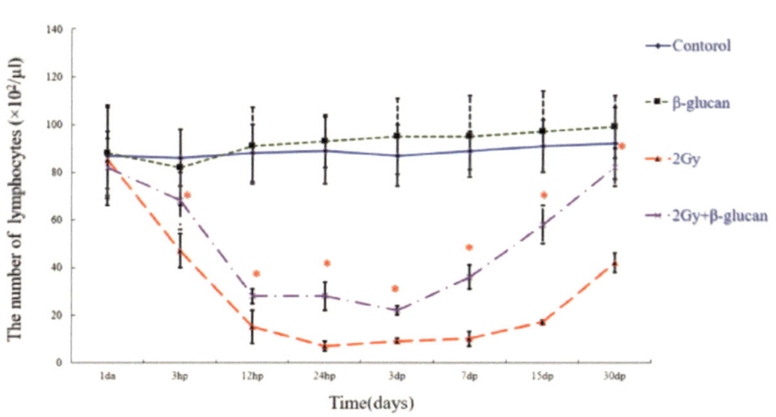

Figure 2.
β-Glucan on blood lymphocyte counts in mice. There were 10 animals in each experimental group. Data are mean ± standard deviation values. Statistically significantly different (P < 0.05) from the control group. Statistically significantly different (* P < 0.05) from the 2 Gy group. Administration of β-glucan was administered for 2 weeks and then treated with radiation. da; days after, hp.; hours post, dp; days post.*

group (4/8), and statistically significant differences were observed over many periods ($P < 0.05$). Overall, lymphocytes tended to increase compared to the control group.

This is the same trend seen in the non-irradiated group. Time-dependent changes after irradiation, all experimental groups showed a decrease, and subsequent recovery was observed 3 days after irradiation. The β-glucan +2 Gy group also showed higher lymphocyte counts than the X group. A significant ratio was observed in the β-glucan +2 Gy group ($P < 0.05$). These treatments have been shown to be particularly effective with a recovery period of 3 days after irradiation.

3.3 CD4 + and CD8 +

Figures 3 and **4** show the changes in CD4 + and CD8 + after β-glucan administration compared to the control group.

Figures 3 and **4** shows the increase frequency of CD4 + or CD8 + by β-glucan administration in each non-irradiated and 2 Gy whole body irradiation groups.

The β-glucan +2 Gy group showed a higher increase in CD4 + or CD8 + than the X group.

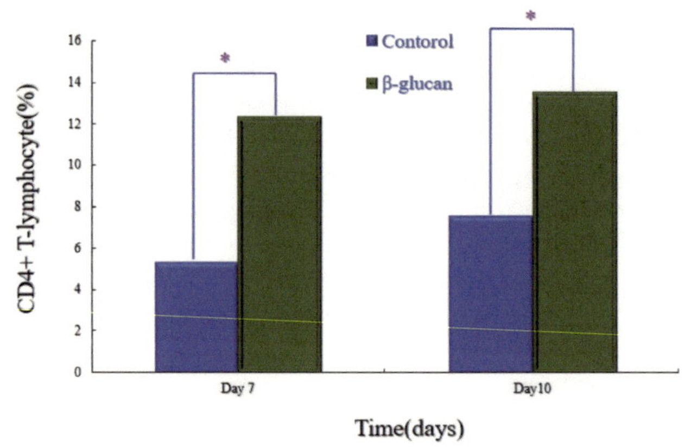

Figure 3.
Lymphocytes were analyzed for CD4+ in C3H mic. The change of CD4+ cells after control and β-glucan administration group. The change of CD4+ cells control and β-glucan administration group. Statistically significantly different (P < 0.05) from the control group.*

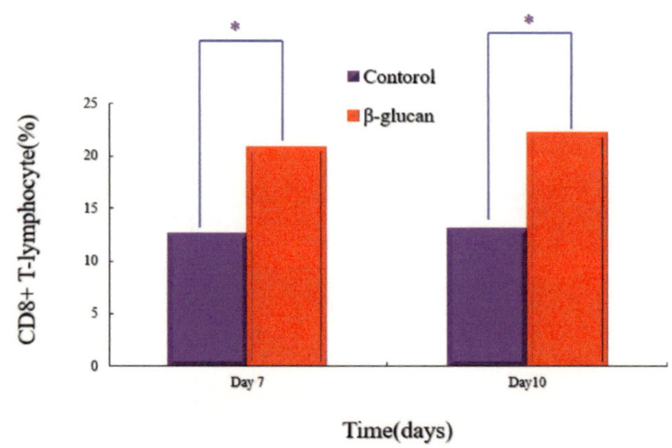

Figure 4.
Lymphocytes were analyzed for CD8+ in C3H mic. The change of CD8+ cells after control and β-glucan administration group. The change of CD8+ cells control and β-glucan administration group. Statistically significantly different (P < 0.05) from the control group.*

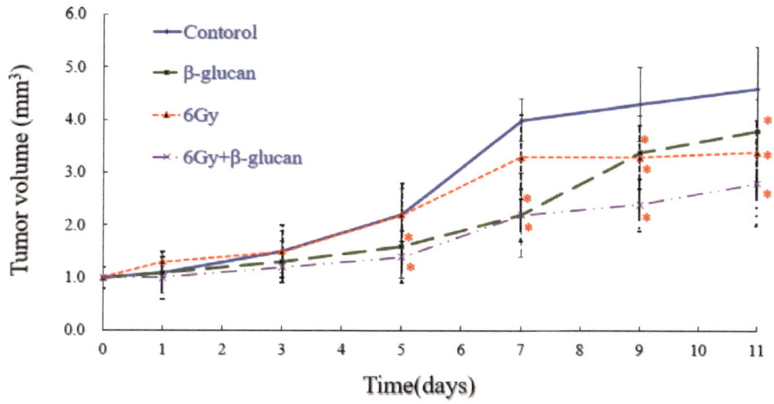

Figure 5.
*Effect of β-glucan on the tumor growth in mice inoculated with 4 T1 (high grade) of mouse cancer cell line. Groups of ten mice each were subjected to each treatment. Results represent means ± S.D. * Statistically significant ($P < 0.05$) from the control.*

3.4 Effect of antioxidant activity (AOA_{AAPH})

Although an effect was observed in the β-glucan administration group, there was no statistically significant difference. The antioxidant activity against peroxy radicals after treatment was subtle.

3.5 Anti-tumor effects

Figure 5 shows the measurement of tumor growth rate by β-glucan administration. The doubling time of the non-irradiated group was not different from the doubling time of the control group with respect to the number of days required to double the tumor size and the ratio of the control group to the 6 Gy group. In the local irradiation group (treatment group), the doubling time of the β-glucan +6 Gy group was 1.4 times longer than that of the control group. The doubling time of the β-glucan +6 Gy group did not exceed the doubling time of the 6 Gy group and tended to be slightly shorter. Compared to the 6 Gy group, it was confirmed that tumor growth was suppressed.

4. Discussion

White blood cells consisting of lymphocytes, granulocytes, and monocytes are deeply involved in immunity. Lymphocytes are roughly classified into T cells and B cells. T cells are associated with cellular immunity, while B cells are associated with humoral immunity through the production of antibodies. T cells are further classified into helper T cells and suppressor T cells, helper T cells play a role in directing and activating B cells, NK cells, killer T cells, cytotoxic T cells, and granulocytes are mediated by blood Phagocytoses vascular walls, bacteria and foreign bodies. Monocytes are transformed into macrophages through morphological changes after moving to tissues, and transmit antigen information to T lymphocytes. In addition, macrophages activate NK and LAK cells. Thus, in white blood cells, lymphocytes distinguish between self and non-self, give instructions, and play a central role in the immune response [15–19]. In this study, in the non-irradiated group, the β-glucan group showed an increase in the number of lymphocytes, suggesting an increase in the overall white blood cell count.

β-Glucan is a mushroom that contains abundant β-(1–3)-D-glucan and β-(1–6)-D-glucan. It has been reported that the number of granulocytes increases in response to Petrchenko et al. B-(1–3)-D-glucan. Treatment with β-(1–6)-D-glucan has also been reported to cause macrophage activation, increased T cells, and increased TNF-α and IL-release 8 macrophage activation [16–18]. However, intra-peritoneal administration of these polysaccharides has also been reported to induce inflammation in the peritoneal cavity due to difficulty in intestinal absorption [20]. Furthermore, β-(1–6)-D-glucan has been reported to accumulate in the liver and spleen after peritoneal and oral administration [21].

This study and previous reports strongly suggest the involvement of β-(1–3)-D-glucan and β-(1–6)-D-glucan. Polysaccharide polysaccharides such as β-(1–3)-D-glucan are difficult to absorb these substances in the peritoneal cavity and intestine and may stimulate intestinal immunity with a slight inflammatory condition. Intestinal mucosal epithelial T lymphocytes are located between intestinal mucosal epithelial cells, and Peyer's patch and lymphoid tissue are located around the digestive tract. The intestine is considered the largest immune system because 70–80% of B lymphocytes are present in the intestinal lymphoid tissue [22–24]. However, with the exception of β-(1–3)-D-glucan, there are few reports that food is directly related to the immune system, regardless of how difficult it is to absorb.

Therefore, this is thought to be due to slight differences in physicochemical structures such as the side chain of β-(1–3)-D-glucan. In addition, β-(1–6)-D-glucan is degraded by beneficial intestinal bacteria and is relatively well absorbed, so it is necessary to consider the relationship with intestinal bacteria [25]. It is therefore speculated that macrophages are activated by the intestinal immune system. IL-8 and TNF-α are released from macrophages, activate helper T cells, and activate the systemic immune system consisting of macrophages, cytotoxic T cells, killer T cells, NK cells, and B cells.

However, there is no good basis for connecting these series of mechanisms and further experimentation is required. Cell damage is the most important side effect of radiation, and lymphocytes are the most sensitive cells [22]. Radiation causes interphase death in the short term [23]. Therefore, the control of radiation effects on lymphocytes essential to the immune system is very important, and the effects on lymphocytes can be viewed as an indicator of radiation-induced cell damage. When the body is exposed to radiation, free radicals such as H •, OH •, and O^2- (superoxide anion) are generated by the decomposition of water molecules by radiation. DNA free radical damage is called an indirect effect. Administration of the redox agent reduced the cytotoxicity induced by O^2 produced by ionizing radiation [25].

It has been suggested that the administration of α-glucan, which has a radio-protective effect, does not inhibit the suppression of tumor growth by radiation, but inhibits tumor growth independently [26]. This may be due to low blood flow in hypoxic cells such as tumor cells and low radical scavenger factors in plasma. Therefore, the antitumor components and tumor suppressors of these substances act by activating immune cells [27–30].

In this study, we examined tumor growth of sarcoma 180 alone, but in the future, we will need to explore different types of tumors and adopt more accurate experimental systems.

Figure 6 shows mechanisms of cell repair in radiation protection.

Figure 7 shows radiation protection and radical scavenger processes.

Figure 8 shows the free radical removal mechanism of β-glucan by radiation.

Enterococcus faecalis is a gram-positive bacterium that belongs to the LAB family. Its cell walls are reported to induce B-cell activation along with stimulation of IgA

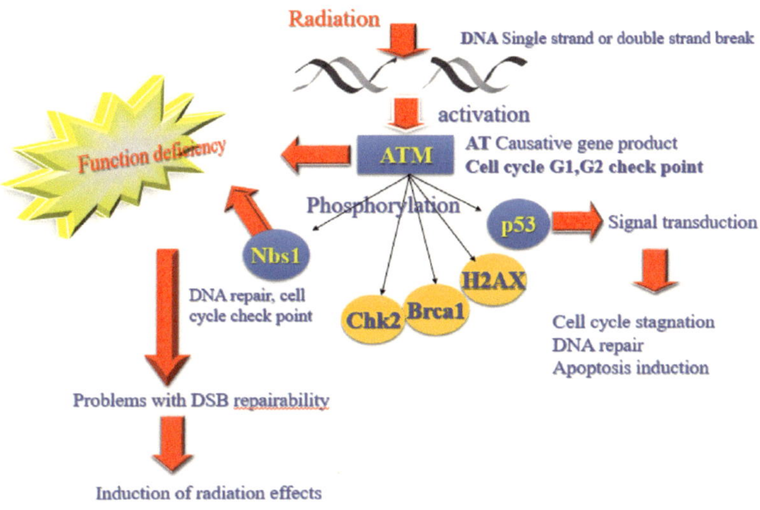

Figure 6.
Mechanisms of cell repair in radiation protection.

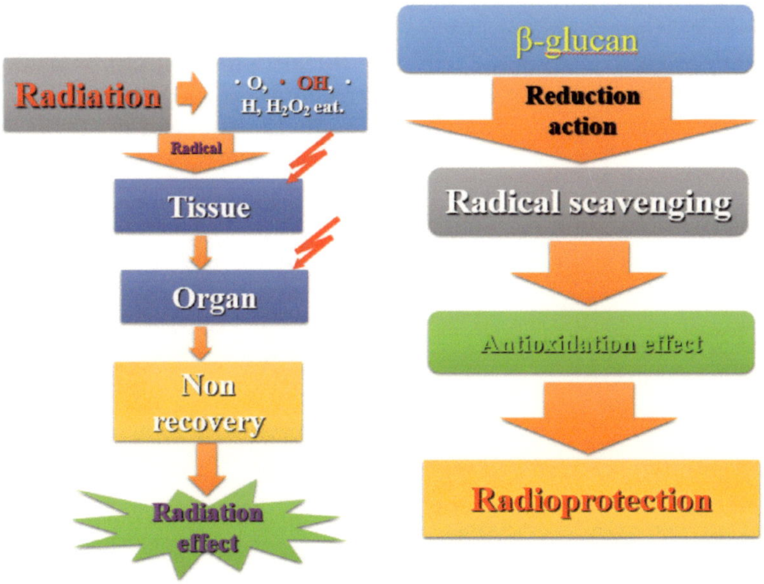

Figure 7.
Radiation protection and radical scavenger processes.

secretion in the intestine [31], which could remove pathogens from the intestine [32]. To date, several functions of EC-12 have been reported [33, 34]. However, the preventive effects of heat-killed EC-12 on intestinal carcinogenesis have not yet been elucidated. In this study, we demonstrated that administration of heat-killed EC-12 weakly decreased intestinal tumorigenesis in Min mice, Apc-mutant mice that develop many intestinal polyps through activation of β-catenin signaling. Moreover, were vealer that heat-killed EC-12 possesses suppressive function of β-catenin signaling in vitro by measuring T-cell factor/lymphoid enhancer factor (TCF/LEF) transcriptional activity.

High IFN-γ production as part of the Th1 immune response has been associated with colitis in mice [33]. Furthermore, Ito et al. reported that IFN-γ plays a

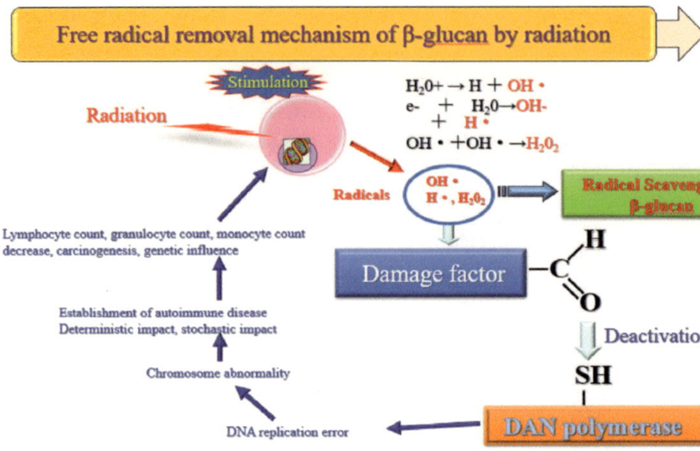

Figure 8.
The free radical removal mechanism of β-glucan by radiation.

fundamental role in the development of colitis in mice [34]. In addition, IFN-γ activates downstream effector cells to produce inflammatory cytokines such as IL-1β. Therefore, suppression of IFN-γ and IL-1β induction may explain the anti-inflammatory properties observed with EF-2001. In addition, Th1 or humoral responses are important for resistance to extracellular pathogens and these cells produce certain IL family cytokines, including IL-1β, IL-6, and IL-10 [35–37].

Author details

Yeun-Hwa Gu
Department of Radiological Science, Faculty of Health Science, Junshin Gakuen University, 1-1-1 chikushigaoka, Minami-ku, Fukuoka 815-8510, Japan

*Address all correspondence to: gu.y@junshin-u.ac.jp

References

[1] Gu YH, Yamashita T, Yamamoto H, Matsuo T, Washino N, Song JH and Kang KM. Plant Enzymes Decrease Prostate Cancer Cell Numbers and Increase TNF-α In Vivo: A Possible Role in Immunostimulatory Activity. *International Journal of Food Science*. Hindawi, Article ID 8103480, 1-7, doi:10.1155/2019/8103480. 2019.

[2] Yamashita T, Kato T, Isogai T, Gu YH, Ma N. Protective Effects of Taurine on the Radiation Exposure Induced Cellular Damages in the Mouse Intestine. *Adv. Exp. Med. Biol.*, **1115**, 443-450. 2019.

[3] Ma N, Kato T, Isogai T, Gu Y, Yamashita T. The Potential Effects of Taurine in Mitigation of Radiation Nephropathy. *Adv. Exp. Med. Biol.*, **1115**,497-505. 2019

[4] Gu YH, Yamasita T, Inoue T, Song JH and Kang KM. Cellular and Molecular Level Mechanisms against Electrochemical Cancer Therapy. *Journal of Pathogens.*Hindawi, 1-11 pages. Article ID 3431674,doi:10.1155/2019/3431674. 2019.

[5] Gu YH, Yamasita T, Choi DJ, Yamamoto H, Matsuo T, Washino N, Song JH and K. M. Kang KM. The anticancer effect of plant enzymes on mouse breast cancer model. Adv. Medi. Plant Res., **6**(4), 70-77, 2018.

[6] Gu YH, Yamasita T, Kang KM. Subchronic oral dose toxicity study of *Enterococcus faecalis* 2001(EF 2001) in mice. *Toxi. Res.*,**34**(1).55-63. 2018.

[7] Gu YH, Choi HJ, Yamashita T, Kang KM, Iwasa M, Lee MJ, Lee KH and Kim CH. Pharmaceutical Production of Anti-tumorand Immune-potentiating *Enterococcus faecalis*-2001 β-glucans: EnhancedActivity of Macrophage and Lymphocytes in Tumor-implanted Mice. *Current Pharmaceutical Biotechnology*,**18**(8),653-661.2017.

[8] Yamashita T, Kato T, Tunekawa M, Gu YH, Wang S, Ma N. Effect of Radiation on the Expression of Taurine Transporter in the Intestine of Mouse. *Adv. Exp. Med. Biol.*, **975**,729-740. 2017.

[9] Gu YH, Huang CS, Inoue T, Yamashita T, Ishida T, Kang KM, Nakao A. Drinking hydrogenwater ameliorated cognitive impairment in senescence-accelerated mice. *J Clin Biochem Nutr.* **46**(3):269-276., 2010.

[10] Gu YH, Takeo T, Kim HG, Suzuki I, Mori T, Yamamoto Y. Study of the radioprotective effects of TMG on teratogenic malformations in irradiated mice. Nihon *Igaku Hoshasen Gakkai Zasshi*, **60**, 845-55. 2000.

[11] Gu YH, Kai M, Kusama T. The embryonic and fetal effects in ICR mice irradiated in the various stages of the preimplantation period. *Radi. Res.* **147**,735-740. 1997.

[12] Gu YH, Choi HJ, Yamashita T, Kang KM, Iwasa M, Lee MJ, Lee KH, Kim CH.: Pharmaceutical production of anti-tumor and immune-potentiating *Enterococcus faecalis*-2001 β-glucans: enhanced activity of macrophage and lymphocytes in tumor-implanted mice. *Current Pharmaceutical Biotechnology*,**18(8)**,653-661.2017.

[13] Gu YH, Fujimiya Y, Itokwa Y, Oshima M, J Choi JS, Miura T, Ishida T.: Tumoricidal effects of beta-glucans: mechanisms include both antioxidant activity plus enhanced systemic and topical immunity. *Nutr Cancer*, **60(5)**, 685-691, 2008.

[14] Gu YH, Takagi Y, Nakamura T, Hasegawa T, Suzuki I, Oshima M, Tawaraya H, NiwanoY.: Enhancement of radioprotection and anti-tumor

immunity by yeast-derived β-glucan in Mice. *J Med Food*, **8(2)**, 154-158, 2005.

[15] Nakamura T, Itokawa Y, Tajima M, Ukawa Y, Cho KH, Choi JS, Ishida T, Gu YH.: Radioprotectve effect of β-glucan decastes and the effect on immunological functions in irradiated mice. *J Tradi Chi Med.* **27(1)**, 70-75. 2007.

[16] Gu YH, Park SR, Hasegawa T, Koike M.: Antihypertensive effect of B-glucan decastes Sing in spontaneously hypertensive rats. *Int J Med Mus.*, **3(1)**,103-110. 2001.

[17] Gu YH, Hasegawa T, Suzuki I, Hayashi I, Ahn KS, Twaraya H.: A study of the radioprotection effect of macro-glucan(β-1-3 glucan) on fetuses of ICR mice. *J Ori Med.*, **5(1)**, 63-70. 2000.

[18] Gu YH, Yamasita T, Kang KM.: Subchronic oral dose toxicity study of *Enterococcus faecalis* 2001(EF 2001) in mice. *Toxi Res.*,**34(1)**.55-63. 2018.

[19] Yamashita T, Kato T, Tunekawa M, Gu YH, Wang S, Ma N.: Effect of radiation on the expression of Taurine transporter in the intestine of mouse. *Adv Exp Med Biol.*, **975**.729-740, 2017.

[20] Gu YH, Maenaka T, Saito K, Yamashita T, Choi IS, Terai K, Ahn KS. Antioxidant and immuno-enhancing effects of *Echinacea purpurea* (American herb) in vivo. *Ori. Pharm. Exp. Med.* **5**, 48-56. 2005.

[21] Liu J, Edamatsu R, Hamada H, Mori A. Scavenging effect of Guilingji on free radicals. *Neurosciences,* **16**, 623-630. 1990.

[22] Kim JH, Park MY, Lee JY, Okuda H, Kim S, Hwang WI. Antioxidant and antitumor effects of manda. *Biochem. Arch.* **14**, 211-219. 1998.

[23] Gu YH, Takebe M. Immunological enhancement effect and radiation protection effect of *Fuscoporia oblique*. *Med. Bio.* **153**, 165-175. 2009.

[24] Gu YH, Iwasa M, Iwasa H, Kobayashi K, Itokawa Y, Ishida T. Radiation protection effect for *EF 2001 (Enterococcus faecalis 2001). Med. Bio.* **151,** 289-295. 2007.

[25] Gu YH, Itokawa Y, Maenaka T, Yamashita T, Oshima M, Nakamura T, Young-nam Kang, Takeo Hasegawa, Ikukatsu Suzuki, Insuk Choi, Tano Kaori, Torao Ishida: The Blood Estradiol-17β, Testosterone and Progesterone of Male and Female Mice Change by *Lepidium meyenii Walp (MAX-180)* and *Muira Puama*. *Med Bio*, **150(4)**, 159-168, 2006.

[26] Kang YN, Maenaka T, Itokawa Y, Yamashita T, Nakamura T, Oshima M, Hasegawa T, Suzuki I, Tano K, Ishida T, Gu YH: Embryonic Death Effects of Hyperthermia Induced by RF (Radiofrequency) Waves *Med Bio*, **150(3)**, 97-103, 2006.

[27] Gu YH, Yamashita T, Maenaka T, Itokawa Y, Nakamura T, Choi IS, Tano K, Ryu MS, Hasegawa T, Oshima M. Anti-tumor Immunity and Radioprotection effect of *Fuscoporia oblique*.; *Med Bio*, *149(9)*, 304-318, 2005.

[28] Choi IS, Gu YH. Anti-cancer and Radioprotection Effects of Hatakeshimeji (*B-glucan decastes*).; *Med. Bio.*, **149(7)**, 256-262, 2005.

[29] Gu YH, Yamashita T, Oshima M, Takagi Y. The blood estradiol-17β, Testosterone and progesterone of male and female mice change by *Lepidium meyenii Walp* (MAX-180); *Med Bio*, **148(1)**, 14-73, 2004.

[30] Gu YH, Yamashita T, Oshima M, Takagi Y. Immunological enhancement effect in *PASSION FRUIT (MARACUJYA)*; *Med Bio*, Vol.**148(1)**, 20-25, 2004.

[31] Vacheron F, Guenounou M, Nauciel C. Induction of interleukin 1 secretion by adjuvant-active peptidoglycans. *Infect Immun,* **42**, 1049-1054, 1983.

[32] Humphrey BD, Huang N, Klasing KC. Rice expressing lactoferrin and lysozyme has antibiotic-like properties when fed to chicks. *J Nutr,* **132**, 1214-1418, 2002.

[33] Nishibayashi R, Inoue R, Harada Y, Watanabe T, Makioka Y, Ushida K. RNA of *Enterococcus faecalis* strain EC-12 is a major component inducing interleukin-12 production from human monocytic cells. *PLoS ONE,* **10**, e0129806, 2015.

[34] Inoue R, Tsukahara T, Matsukawa N, Watanabe T, Bukawa W, Nakayama K, Ushida K. Rapid induction of an immune response in rat Peyer's patch after oral administration of *Enterococcus faecalis* strain EC-12. *Biosci Biotechno. Bioche,.* **77**, 863-866, 2013.

[35] Tsukahara T, Inoue R, Nakanishi N, Nakayama K, Matsubara N, Ushida K. Evaluation of the low dose level of a heat-killed and dried cell preparation of *Enterococcus faecalis* to prevent porcine edema disease using experimental infection model with enterotoxcemic *Escherichia coli* in weaning pigs. *J Vet Med Sci,* **69**, 103-109, 2007.

[36] Singer II, Kawka DW, Scott S, Weidner JR, Mumford RA, Riehl TE, Stenson WF. Expression of inducible nitric oxide synthase and nitrotyrosine in colonic epithelium in inflammatory bowel disease. *Gastroenterology,* **111**, 871-885, 1996.

[37] Debnath T, Kim DH, Lim BO. Natural products as a source of anti-inflammatory agents associated with inflammatory bowel disease. *Molecules*, **18**, 7253-7270, 2013.

Chapter 7

Evaluation by Monte Carlo Simulation of Doses Distribution in Tumors with Hypoxia

Mirko Salomón Alva-Sánchez and Thatiane Alves Pianoschi

Abstract

Radiotherapy is one of the most useful modalities applied for tumor treatments, which use ionization radiation to eradicate the tumor, in major cases. Cells with normal oxygenation are more sensitive to the effects of ionizing radiation than those with hypoxic conditions, because O_2 molecules react rapidly with free radicals, produced by irradiation, originating highly reactive radicals. Thus, the different concentrations of hypoxia in tumors can modulate the response of the irradiation through the radioresistance they present and consequently the success of the treatment. This chapter deals with the dose distributions in cranial tumors with different concentrations of hypoxia through a code based on Monte Carlo simulation.

Keywords: radiotherapy, tumor hypoxia, dose distribution, Monte Carlo simulations

1. Introduction

The modality of treatment with ionization radiation, specifically, for cancer can be considered routinely in several hospital centers, which must have human and technological resources capable of conforming the radiation dose into the target volumes and trying to avoid high toxicity in the adjuvant tissues. Although all these resources exist, the treatment planning is based on prior knowledge of the structures of the patient that can be obtained through any kind of medical images. Once the tumor has been diagnosed, appropriate treatment is indicated without, often, considering some factors that may influence treatment success, due the limitation of the medical images. Factors known as repair of sublethal DNA damage, cell repopulation, redistribution of cells, and reoxygenation are not considered [1].

Experimental data showed that oxygen is the most component that modified the radiation sensitivity and hypoxic cells that can be 2–3 times more resistant to ionizing radiation, which would imply administering doses higher than doses to achieve the same effect in oxygenated cells under normal conditions [2–4].

An important concept in clinical radiobiology is that the tumor may have subpopulations in hypoxic areas, thus leading to success of radiotherapy. Still, there are concepts related to acute or chronic hypoxic cells that may also alter treatment outcomes [5]. The low concentration of oxygen or hypoxia in the tumor tissues is a radiobiological phenomenon that has been observed since the beginning of the twentieth century [6].

The dependence of oxygen in tissue is related with the generation of free radicals, which came from interacting between the radiation energy and tissues. The quantity that measures the likelihood of this interacting is the cross section, which decreases when the beam energy increases [7]. Thus, few radicals will interact with the DNA of the tumor cell and consequently decreasing the chain reaction. This dependence is known as the oxygen effect that is ignored in the accuracy of ionization radiation treatments [8, 9], which is why hypoxia characterizes a tissue as radioresistant. Therefore, hypoxia and radiosensitivity are related to lower oxygen concentration rate; there will be higher survival cell rate, in postirradiation. On the other hand, there is an optimal oxygenation value wherewith the radiosensitivity increases [10]. Concentrations of oxygen in some tumors can be found in different regions in the same tumor complex. In this case, the tumor hypoxia may occur in a chronic or acute form. A form of oxygen concentration is due to the accelerated growth of the tumor in the most central parts, which are usually originated by the lack of adequate blood supply. In this way, in an axial section of one tumor, have concentric circles of regions of different oxygenation, whose central areas are necrotic [4]. One way to express the decreased radiosensibilty of cell, due to hypoxia, is through the parameter oxygen enhancement ratio (OER), which is defined as the amount of dose reduction required for cell of a given oxygenation level compared to cell with no oxygen to obtain the same effect [11].

One way to study the oxygen effect in tumors is through computational modeling. Thus, different modeling of oxygen effect has been proposed such as a voxel-based multiscale tumor response model [12]. The model used in this work was written in C++ simulating a virtual tumor with considering biological parameters as vascular fraction that is related to the oxygenation of the tumor.

Laura Antonovic and co-authors [13] used a treatment planning system TRiP [14] to simulated spherical tumors in silico based on a biological model of oxygen diffusion [15]. The beam used was carbon ion.

Another publication showed the use of a computational model for trans-vascular oxygen transport and blood vessel networks in tumors [16, 17].

The paper title *Dose prescription and optimisation based on tumor hypoxia* [18] proposed a method to prescribe dose distributions in radioresistant tumors.

The Monte Carlo HYP-RT model was used to simulate tumors considering the repopulation and reoxygenation for hypoxic head and neck tumors [19].

A 4D cellular model was applied to simulate head and neck cancer with oxygenation varying with vascularity and blood oxygenation [20].

An algorithm implemented on Geant4-DNA (codes based on Monte Carlo) was developed to show the effect of oxygen on DNA [21].

The Monte Carlo simulation, specifically the codes based on this method, can also be an effective dosimetric tool for the study of dose deposited. The dose–response from the codes shows an advantage of providing detailed studies in different conditions that involve procedures which are lengthy, complex, and expensive. The most commonly used Monte Carlo simulation codes in radiotherapy simulations are EGS, MCNP, and PENELOPE [22–28]. The quality of the results provided by the different codes is directly related to the accuracy of the implemented transport model and its data libraries associated with the cross section of the transported particles. Thus, the mixed charged particle transport algorithm, implemented by the penetration and energy loss of positron and electrons (PENELOPE) code [29], led to its intense use in radiotherapy [30–35].

This chapter presents a study of dose distribution in simulated cranial tumor with different concentrations of oxygen [18, 36–39] through the PENELOPE simulation code, which is based on the Monte Carlo method [40, 41]. The tumor with different concentrations of oxygen will be compared with one under normal oxygen conditions.

1.1 PENELOPE-Monte Carlo code

PENELOPE is a code used to simulate the transport of electrons, positrons, and photons considering interactions of photons and charged particles (such as the photoelectric effect, Rayleigh scattering, Compton scattering, production and annihilation of pairs, elastic and inelastic collisions), which are simulated in complex geometries and arbitrary materials.

In the PENELOPE package, there are subroutines written in FORTRAN distributed in various (open) source codes, applications, a database with characteristics of various materials, as well as application examples. The FORTRAN subroutines are organized into four basic files: PENELOPE.f, PENGEOM.f, PENVARED.f, and TIMER.f.

PENELOPE.f contains the simulated particle scattering and absorption subroutines, primary and secondary particle generation and storage, and particle transport management and simulation as a whole.

PENGEOM.f defines the structures, or geometries, to be simulated, which may consist of several homogeneous bodies, defined by a specified material and also by their limits in space. The bounding surfaces of the geometry bodies are described by quadratic functions. Through these functions surfaces such as planes, plane pairs, spheres, cylinders, cones, ellipsoids, parables, and hyperboloids can be defined.

For each body defined in the geometry file of a given simulation, a material index must be defined, corresponding to the material that will be a constituent of the body, having an agreement between the geometry file and the material file. In the material archive, the interaction data of the radiation with the material being used are shown in tables, as interaction coefficients for electrons and photons in energies from 1 eV to 1GeV. A material file is created using the subroutines of the MATERIAL.f and PENELOPE.f source codes. One of the advantages of PENELOPE is that it uses a recent database with the characteristics of various materials of interest in radiological physics [42] and current cross section libraries and other quantities required for particle transport [43].

The PENVARED.f source code contains subroutines that perform the variational reduction methods of the code, without increasing simulation time and neither the statistical uncertainty of the simulated results.

Finally, source code TIMER.f manages the simulation time.

The simulation algorithm is based on a model that combines numerical and analytical cross section data for the different types of interaction and is applied for initial energies from 1 keV to 1 GeV. Photons transport are simulated by the conventional or detailed, and for electron and positron are simulated using a mixed algorithm. Thus, for electrons and positrons, the PENELOPE code differs from other simulation codes by using a mixed algorithm that implements two simulation models: the detailed, for strong events, defined from angular deflection (scattering angle) or energy loss above a set value, and the condensate for weak interactions with angular deflection or energy loss less than the preset values. Condensed interactions are described by a multiple-scatter approximation consisting of transforming a given number of weak interactions into a single artificial event [44]. To develop a simulation with PENELOPE, the user must edit a FORTRAN file, user.f, with calls from the subroutines PENELOPE.f, PENGEOM.f, PENVARED.fe, and TIMER.f, providing overall simulation management and creating with these five FORTRAN files a user.exe file.

The simulation is started by running the user.exe file that reaches the user-supplied input information through the input.in file, geometry information through the geometry.geo file, and cross section information for the materials involved in the simulation through the material.mat file.

Another executable program comes together with PENELOPE package, the GEOVIEW.exe, which allows the visualization of the defined bodies and the materials that constitute a simulation geometry.

1.2 Simulation of the dose distribution in tumors with hypoxia through PENELOPE code

As some tumors have concentric circles of regions of low concentration of oxygenation, which are deprived of adequate blood supply, the evaluation of those regions becomes essential to guarantee the success of radiotherapy treatments [4]. The study evaluated the hypoxia effect in the dose distribution for simulated cranial tumor with different concentrations of oxygen [18, 36–39] through the PENELOPE simulation code. The code allows the "construction" of tumors through the compound's chemical composition, mass density, mean excitation energy, and energy and oscillator strength [45, 46]. The tumor with different concentrations of oxygen will be compared with one under normal oxygen conditions. The parameter OER was applied to express the decreased radiosensibilty of the tumor with hypoxia. The simulation of the dose distribution in tumors with hypoxia through PENELOPE code is based on the published by Alva-Sánchez [47].

2. Material and methods

The Monte Carlo code, PENELOPE®, version 2008 was used to achieve the main objective to simulate tumors with hypoxia. Since the code allows the "construction" of materials by the compound's chemical composition, the soft tissue material from the code, number 262, was modified by adding different concentrations tumors with hypoxia, from knowledge that chemical compounds of the normal tissue are approximately equal to the tumor. The geometry of simulation used was a parallelepiped of $8 \times 15 \times 21$ cm^3 containing six identical spherical tumors of 1.2 cm radius, as shown in **Figure 1** [47]. In that work 2×10^9 primary particles and 0.1mm^2 pixel size and photon spectra at 6 MV [48], which was applied in the input file of the code, were used. The tumors were located before the buildup region for the

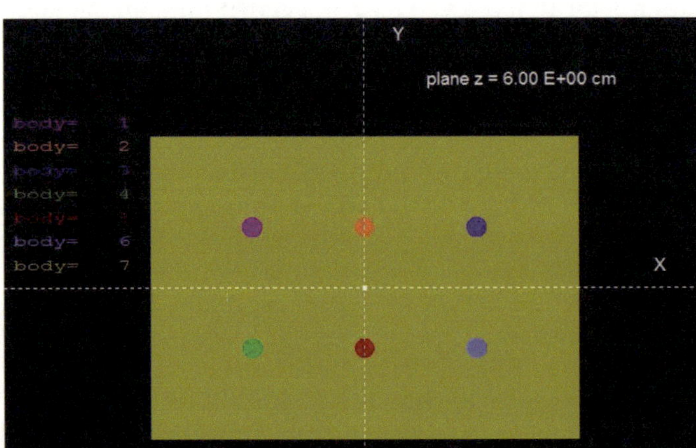

Figure 1.
Geometric representation through of the PENELOPE code, for the simulation of six tumors (spheres) spaced within the parallelepiped, in the XY plane.

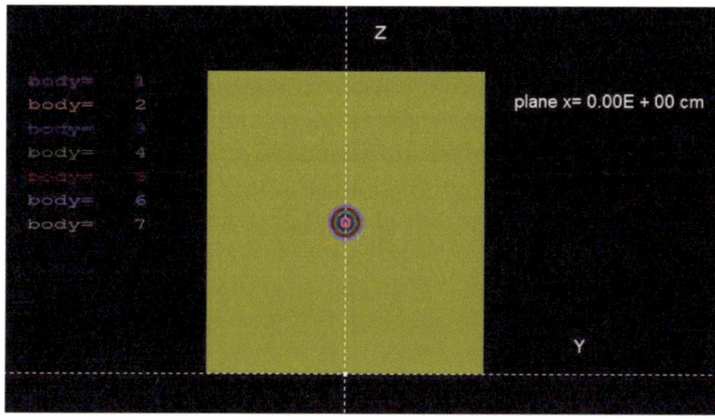

Figure 2.
Geometric representation of the PENELOPE code, for the simulation of a tumor (sphere) centralized in the center of the brain (cylinder), in the ZY plane.

6 MV beam at 10 cm from the top of the phantom. The simulated material of the parallelepiped was a soft tissue, available in the code, while the tumors had different pressures of oxygen, from 5 to 70 mmHg. Simulation responses were obtained through the values average in the whole target or spherical tumors.

This geometry used to simulate the radiation conditions was 22 × 22 cm^2 radiation field, 100 cm source-tumor distance, with a 6 MV energy beam. The obtained results from the simulation were analyzed in terms of deposited energy and values of OER relative to the pressure O_2 in terms of mmHg, following the OER equation proposed for [55].

$$OER = 1 + 0.81 \left(pO_2{}^{0.616}\right) / \left(1 + pO_2{}^{0.616}\right) \tag{1}$$

The second part of that work published [47] analyzed the oxygen effect in the dose distributions in simulated cranial tumors: one with different oxygen concentrations and the other with normal oxygenation [18, 36–39]. A cylinder with 18 cm in diameter and 20 cm in height was simulated to represent the head of an adult, containing concentric spheres of radii of 0.5–1.2 cm that can represent the dimensions of a glioblastoma tumor. Due the characteristics of localization of this kind of tumor, the simulation tumors were centralized at 10 cm height, beyond the equilibrium range to charged particle for the energy used in this study. The bean incident was simulated in the direction to the phantom, parallel to the Z axis. In **Figure 2** the geometry for radiation for a simulated tumor with different concentrations of oxygen from minor (radius sphere 0.5 cm) to greater is shown (radius sphere 1.2 cm).

The simulated material of the tumors and brain structures was soft tissue due to similar chemical compounds present. This material is available in the simulation code. In the spheres (tumors) these materials were modified with different concentrations of oxygen. The radiation conditions used were 1.2 × 1.2 cm radiation field, source-tumor distance of 100 cm, and photon spectra at 6 MV.

3. Results

From the results obtained to the six spheres inserted in the parallelepiped (**Figure 1**), the deposited energy was plotted for each spherical tumor containing different pressures of oxygen as shown in **Figure 3**. Values of the OER were obtained through Eq. (1) and plotted for each pressure of oxygen, as shown in **Figure 4**.

The *penmain* file of the code generates an output file with generic information, such as number of simulated primary showers, secondary-particle generation probabilities, average deposited energies, and statistical error, etc. Each simulation was written in a separate file. The program computes and delivers the statistical uncertainties (3σ) of all evaluated quantities and distributions. Thus, for all obtained results, an error at least 3.58% was reported by the code used.

Figure 5a shows the dose distributions for a simulated tumor of 1.2 cm radius with different pressures of O_2, and **Figure 5b** shows the same tumor of **Figure 5a** with normal oxygenation.

These distributions were compared through a dose profile, as shown in **Figure 6**, along the center of the dose maps.

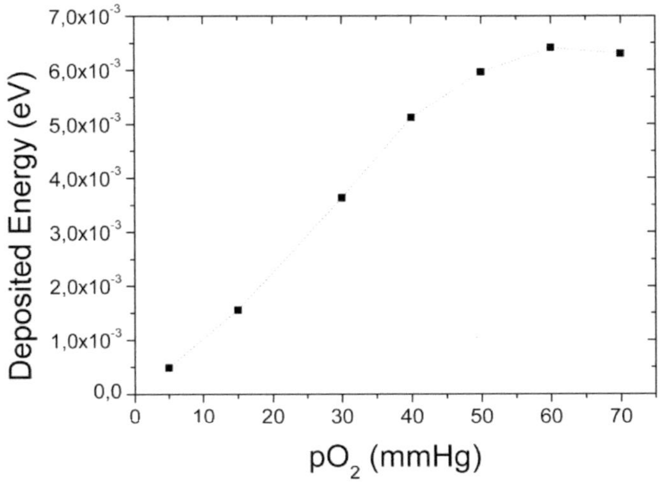

Figure 3.
Behavior and deposited energy for six identical spheres with different pressures of O_2.

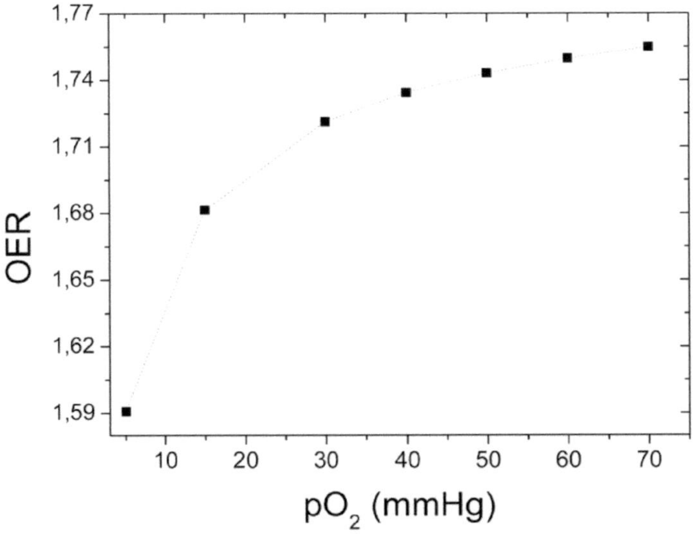

Figure 4.
OER values relative to each of the six identical spheres with different pressures of O_2.

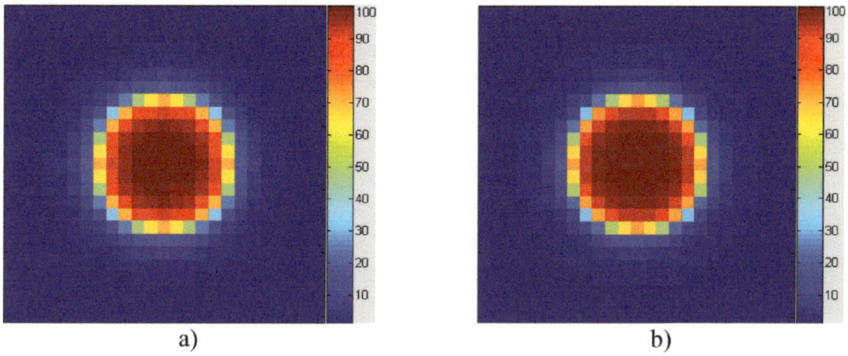

Figure 5.
Dose distribution of the tumor of 7.24 cm³: (a) tumor 1, with different pressures O_2, and (b) tumor 2, normal oxygenation.

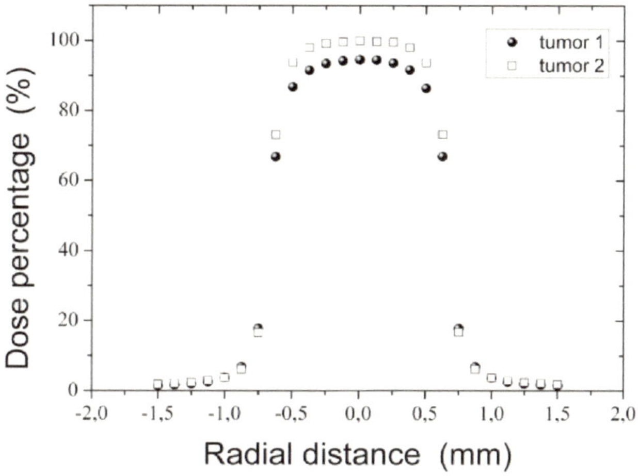

Figure 6.
Dose relative profile of tumor 1 (with different pressures of O_2) and tumor 2 (with normal oxygenation).

4. Discussions and conclusions

Statistical uncertainties at least 3.58% was reported by the code for all simulations. From the results shown in **Figure 3**, we can observe that the deposited energy have an approximately linear behavior with the increases in pressure until 50 mmHg of O_2; from this pressure the deposited energy shows a constant trend for higher pressures than 60 mmHg of O_2. This behavior was also equivalent to those presented in the literature [36, 49].

The obtained values of the OER relative to pressure of O_2 shown in **Figure 4** have a behavior similar to an increasing logarithm function as found in literature [50–54]. After the 60 mmHg of pressure of O_2, the OER values have a trend to value constant. **Figures 3** and **4** confirm the increasing of the deposited energy for tumors with a high concentration of oxygen, because of the oxygen effect that is disregarded in accuracy of the ionization radiation treatment [53, 55].

The dose distributions shown in **Figure 5** visually show almost the same distribution, but in the field profile of both distributions, shown in **Figure 6**, a difference of 7.29% was found at a radial distance of 0.6 mm of the tumor. The code allowed evaluated the influences of effect of oxygen for tumors with hypoxia that is related with the outcome of treatment with radiotherapy. However, the hypoxic tumor cells are resistant to radiation [8]. From the comparisons of the dose distribution in the central plane of the phantom, it was observed that there are regions where the concentration of oxygen was lower (that of sphere of less radius), thus, the energy deposited was lower, unlike the spheres with higher oxygen concentrations.

Despite the fact that the code cannot simulate the physiological factor, which it can modulate a variety of normal developmental and metabolic processes that cause injury to the tumor cell, the present study of tumors with hypoxia plays an important role in dose distribution that can compromise the treatment outcomes and individual prognosis.

5. Considerations

There are a number of simulation and numerical methods and codes that demonstrate the importance of the low concentration oxygen effect in response to ionizing radiation treatments. This chapter shows the work *Study of the distribution of doses in tumors with hypoxia through the PENELOPE code* which showed physical parameters with results similar to the literature through the PENELOPE-Monte Carlo code.

Acknowledgements

The authors thank professor Ph.D. Patricia Nicolucci for her orientation and suggestions for all the works, which are part of our doctorate work.

Author details

Mirko Salomón Alva-Sánchez* and Thatiane Alves Pianoschi
Department of Exact Science and Applied Social, Federal University of Health Sciences of Porto Alegre, Porto Alegre, Rio Grande do Sul, Brazil

*Address all correspondence to: mirko@ufcspa.edu.br

References

[1] Lind BK, Brahme A. The radiation response of heterogeneous tumors. Physica Medica. 2007;**23**:919

[2] Schwarz G. Ueber Desensibilisierung gegen Roentgen und Radium Strahlen. Muenchner Medizinische Wochenschrift. 1909;**24**:1-2

[3] Thomlinson RH, Gray LH. The histological structure of some human lung cancers and the possible implications for radiotherapy. British Journal of Cancer. 1955;**9**:539-549

[4] Hall EJ, Giaccia AJ. Radiobiology for the Radiologist. 6th ed. Philadelphia: Lippincott Williams & Wilkins; 2006

[5] Bristow RG, Hill RP. Hypoxia and metabolism. Hypoxia, DNA repair and genetic instability. Nature Reviews. Cancer. 2008;**8**(3):180-192

[6] De olveira R, Alves R. Agentes antineoplásicos biorredutiveis: uma nova alternativa para o tratamento de tumores sólidos. Quimica Nova. 2002;**25**(6):976-984

[7] Itikawa Y. Cross sections for electron collisions with oxygen molecules. The Journal of Physical Chemistry. 2009;**38**:1

[8] Wenzl and Wilkins. Theoretical analysis of the dose dependence of the oxygen enhancement ratio and its relevance for clinical applications. Radiation Oncology. 2011;**6**:171

[9] Yamashitaa S, Katsumurab Y, Linc M, Muroyad Y, Miyazakia T, Murakamie T. Water radiolysis with heavy ions of energies up to 28 GeV. 1. Measurements of primary g values as track segment yields. Radiation Physics and Chemistry. 2008;**77**:439-446

[10] Nias A. An Introduction to Radiobiology. 2nd ed. Chichester: Wiley; 2000

[11] Anon. Quantitative Concepts and Dosimetry in Radiobiology. International Commission on Radiation Units and Measurements. ICRU Report 30. Bathesda, MD; 1979

[12] Espinoza I, Peschke P, Karger CP. A voxel-based multiscale model to simulate the radiation response of hypoxic tumors. Medical Physics. 2015;**42**:90-102. DOI: 10.1118/1.4903298

[13] Antonovic L, Lindblom E, Daşu A, Bassler N, Furusawa Y, Toma-DAşu I. Clinical oxygen enhancement ratio of tumors in carbon ion radiotherapy: The influence of local oxygenation changes. Journal of Radiation Research. 2014;**55**:902-911

[14] Krämer M, Scholz M. Treatment planning for heavy-ion radiotherapy: Calculation and optimization of biologically effective dose. Physics in Medicine and Biology. 2000;**45**:3319-3330

[15] Daşu A, Toma-Daşu I, Karlsson M. Theoretical simulation of tumour oxygenation and results from acute and chronic hypoxia. Physics in Medicine & Biology. 2003;**48**:2829-2842

[16] Welter M, Fredrich T, Rinneberg H, Rieger H. Computational model for tumor oxygenation applied to clinical data on breast tumor hemoglobin concentrations suggests vascular dilatation and compression. PLoS One. 2016;**11**(8):e0161267. DOI: 10.1371/journal.pone.0161267

[17] Gödde R, Kurz H. Structural and biophysical simulation of angiogenesis and vascular remodeling. Developmental Dynamics. 2001;**220**(4):387-401

[18] Toma-Daşu I, Daşu A, Brahme A. Dose prescription and optimisation based on tumour hypoxia. Acta Oncologica;**48**:2009, 11811192

[19] Harriss-Phillips WM, Bezak E, Yeoh EK. Monte Carlo radiotherapy simulations of accelerated repopulation and reoxygenation for hypoxic head and neck cancer. The British Journal of Radiology. 2011;**84**(1006):903-918. DOI: 10.1259/bjr/25012212

[20] Forster JC, MJJ D, Harriss-Phillips WM, Bezak E. Simulation of head and neck cancer oxygenation and doubling time in a 4D cellular model with angiogenesis. Scientific Reports. 2017;7(1):11037. DOI: 10.1038/s41598-017-11444-1

[21] Forster JC, MJJ D, Phillips WM, Bezak E. Monte Carlo simulation of the oxygen effect in dna damage induction by ionizing radiation. Radiation Research;**190**(3):248-261

[22] De Vlamynck K et al. Dose measurements compared with Monte Carlo simulations of narrow 6 MV multifead collimator shaped photon beams. Medical Physics. 1999;**26**:1874-1882

[23] Pooter JA et al. Computer optimization of nocoplanar beam setups improves stereotactic treatment of liver tumors. International Journal of Radiation Oncology Biology Physics. 2006;**66**:913-922

[24] Yamamoto T et al. An integrated Monte Carlo dosimetric verification system for radiotherapy treatment planning. Physics in Medicine and Biology. 2008;**52**:1991

[25] Ghassoun J, Senhou N, Jehouani A. Neutron and photon doses in high energy radiotherapy facilities and evaluation of shielding performance by Monte Carlo method. Annals of Nuclear Energy. 2011;**38**(10):2163-2167

[26] Kim JH, Hill R, Kuncic Z. An evaluation of calculation parameters in the EGSnrc/BEAMnrc Monte Carlo codes and their effect on surface dose calculation. Physics in Medicine and Biology. 2012;**57**(4):N267-N278

[27] Rodriguez M, Sempau J, Brualla L. Combined approach of variance reduction techniques for the efficient Monte Carlo simulation of linacs. Physics in Medicine & Biology. 2012;**57**(10)

[28] Martinez-Rovira I, Sempau J, Prezado Y. Monte Carlo-based treatment planning system calculation engine for microbeam radiation therapy. Medical Physics. 2012;**39**(5):2829-2838

[29] Sempau J et al. A PENELOPE-based system for the automated Monte Carlo simulation of clinacs and a voxelized geometries—Application to far-from-axis fields. Medical Physics. 2011;**38**(11):5887-5895

[30] Koivunoro H et al. Accuracy of the electron transport in MCNP5 and its suitability for ionization chamber response simulations: A comparison with the EGSNRC and PENELOPE codes. Medical Physics. 2012;**39**(3):1335-1344

[31] Ramirez VJ et al. Dosimetry of small radiation field in inhomogeneous medium using alanine/EPR minidosimeters and PENELOPE Monte Carlo simulation. Radiation Measurements. 2011;**46**:941-944

[32] Carvajal MA et al. Monte Carlo simulation using the PENELOPE code with ant colony algorithm to study MOSFET detectors. Physics in Medicine and Biology. 2009;**54**:6263-6276

[33] Górka B et al. Optimization of a tissue-equivalent CVD-diamond dosimeter for radiotherapy using the Monte Carlo code PENELOPE. Nuclear Instruments and Methods in Physics Research Section A. 2008;**59**(3):578-587

[34] Badal A et al. Monte Carlo simulation of a realistic anatomical

phantom described by triangle meshes: Application to prostate brachytherapy imaging. Radiotherapy and Oncology. 2008;**86**:99-103

[35] Brualla L et al. Comparison between PENELOPE and electron Monte Carlo simulations of electron fields used in the treatment of conjunctival lymphoma. Physical Biology. 2009;**54**:5469-5481

[36] Tuckwell W, Bezak E, Yeoh E, Marcu L. Efficient Monte Carlo modelling of individual tumor cell propagation for hypoxic head and neck cáncer. Physics in Medicine and Biology. 2008;**53**:4489-4507

[37] Diabira S, Morandi X. Gliomagenesis and neural stem cells: Key role of hypoxia and concept of tumor "neo-niche". Medical Hypotheses. 2008;**70**:96-104

[38] Evans S, Judy K, Dunphy I. Comparative measurements of hypoxia in human brain tumor using needle electrodes and EF5 binding. Cancer Research. 2004;**64**:1886-1892

[39] Wang J, Klem J, Wyrick J. Detection of hypoxia in human brain tumor xenografts using a modified comment assay. Neoplasia. 2003;**4**:288-296

[40] Salvat F, Fernández-Varea J, Sempau J. PENELOPE-2008: A Code System for Monte Carlo Simulation of Electron and Photon Transport, Nuclear Energy Agency OECD/NEA, Issy-les-Moulineaux, France. 2008. Available from: http://www.nea.fr

[41] Sempau J, Acosta E, Baró J, et al. An algorithm for Monte Carlo simulation of coupled electron-photon transport. Nuclear Instruments and Methods in Physics Research Section B. 1997;**1997**(132):377-390

[42] International Commission on Radiation Units and Measurements. Tissue substitutes in radiation dosimetry and measurement. ICRU report 44. Bethesda: EUA; 1989

[43] Salvat F, Fernández-Varea JM, Sempau J. A Code System for Monte-Carlo Simulation of Electron and Photon Transport, September, France. 2005

[44] Sempau J, Andreo P. Configuration of the electron transport algorithm of PENELOPE to simulate íon chambers. Physics in Medicine & Biology. 2006;**51**:3533-3548

[45] Alva M, Pianoschi1 T, Marques T, Santanna M, Baffa O, Nicolucci P. Monte Carlo simulation of MAGIC-f gel for radiotherapy using PENELOPE. Journal of Physics: Conference Series. 2010;**250**(1)

[46] Sánchez A, Salomón M. Verificação 3D da distribuição da dose em radiocirurgia estereotáxica através de simulação Monte Carlo e dosimetria por ressonância magnética nuclear. 2012. Tese (Doutorado em Física Aplicada à Medicina e Biologia) - Faculdade de Filosofia, Ciências e Letras de Ribeirão Preto, Universidade de São Paulo, Ribeirão Preto. 2012. DOI: 10.11606/T.59.2012.tde-15052013-193530. Acesso em: 2020-03-31

[47] Alva-Sánchez MS, Pianoschi TA. Study of the distribution of doses in tumors with hypoxia through the PENELOPE code. Radiation Physics and Chemistry. 2019;**167**:108428

[48] Sheik-Bagheri D, Rogers DWO. Monte Carlo calculation of nine megavoltage photon beam spectra using the BEAM code. Medical Physics. 2002;**29**:391-402

[49] Grimes DR, Warren DR, Warren S. Hypoxia imaging and radiotherapy: Bridging the resolution gap. The British Journal of Radiology. 2017 Aug;**90**(1076):20160939. DOI: 10.1259/bjr.20160939. [Epub May 25, 2017]

[50] Kirkpatrick J, Cárdenas-Navia LI, Dewhirst MW. Predicting the effect of temporal variations in PO_2 on tumor radiosensitivity. International Journal of Radiation Oncology Biology Physics. 2004;**59**(3):822-833

[51] Taha E, Djouider F, Banoqitah E. Monte Carlo simulations for dose enhancement in cancer treatment using bismuth oxide nanoparticles implanted in brain soft tissue. Australasian Physical & Engineering Sciences in Medicine. 2018;**41**:363-370

[52] Grimes R, Partridge M. A mechanistic investigation of the oxygen fixation hypothesis and oxygen enhancement ratio. Biomedical Physics & Engineering Express. 2015, 2015;**1**:045209

[53] Grimes R, Fletcher A, Partridge M. Oxygen consumption dynamics in steady-state tumor models. Royal Society Open Science. 2014;**1**:140080

[54] Alper T, Howard-Flanders P. Role of oxygen in modifying the radiosensitivity of *E. coli* B. Nature. 1956;**178**:978-979

[55] Ye SJ. Monte Carlo based protocol for cell survival and tumour control probability in BNCT. Physics in Medicine & Biology. 1999;**44**:447-461

Chapter 8

Bozepinib: A Promising Selective Derivative Targeting Breast Cancer Stem Cells

Joaquín M. Campos, Ana Conejo-García and Olga Cruz-López

Abstract

Bozepinib is a potent antitumour compound that shows an IC_{50} of 0.166 μM against MDA-MB-231 human breast cancer cell line. It is also a very selective drug that presents a therapeutic index (TI) of 11.0 against MDA-MB-231 in relation to the normal MCF-10A. It is important to identify new cancer stem-like cells (CSCs) anticancer drugs to struggle against the resistance and the high risk of relapse in patients. In the present chapter, we show how bozepinib demonstrated selectivity on cancer cells and showed an inhibitory effect over kinases involved in carcinogenesis, proliferation and angiogenesis. Bozepinib inhibits HER-2 signaling pathway and JNK and ERK kinases. In addition, it has an inhibitory effect on AKT and VEGF together with anti-angiogenic and anti-migratory activities. Interestingly, bozepinib suppresses the formation of both mammo- and colonospheres and eliminated ALDH+ CSC subpopulations at a low micromolar range similar to salinomycin. It also induces the downregulation of SOX2, c-MYC and β-CATENIN and upregulation of the GLI-3 Hedgehog signaling repressor. Finally, bozepinib shows in vivo antitumor and anti-metastatic efficacy in xenotransplanted nude mice without presenting subacute toxicity. However, further studies in cancer patients are needed to confirm the therapeutic potential of bozepinib.

Keywords: benzoxazepine, bozepinib, cancer stem-like cells, MDA-MB-231, MCF-7, MCF-10A, protein kinases, seven-membered ring

1. Introduction

Expansion of cancer keeps going on as an important health problem in the developed, undeveloped and developing countries. Although major advances have been made in the chemotherapeutic management of some patients, the continued commitment to the laborious task of discovering new anticancer agents remains critically important, in the course of identifying various chemical substances, which may serve as leads for designing novel antitumor agents.

1.1 Cancer stem cells

Currently, one of the most interesting concepts being explored in cancer research is the theory of cancer stem cells. CSCs can be defined as the subpopulations of cells within tumors that possess the ability to self-renew and differentiate into the different lines of cancer cells that make up the tumor. This type of cell is proposed as the promoter of resistance against antitumor therapies, being able to maintain benign and malignant tumors, as well as causing relapses [1]. Compared to normal stem cells, CSCs are thought to have no control over their proliferation. These CSCs, present in tumors in small numbers, are characterized by their ability to remain quiescent for long periods of time, capacity for self-renewal, maintenance of growth and heterogeneity of the tumor, affinity for environment resistance to chemotherapy and development of metastases [2].

CSCs are characterized by their ability to form spherical colonies when cultivated in suspension [3]. Al-Hajj et al. managed to demonstrate that the injection of 200 tumoural cells expressing characteristic markers of CSCs was more effective in generating tumors in immunodepressed mice than the injection of 50,000 tumor cells with differentiated cell markers of the same histological lineage [4]. It has been found that multiple molecules related to the characteristic properties of stem cells such as self-renewal and pluripotency and certain enzymatic activities are largely expressed in CSCs, including c-MYC, β-CATENIN [5], SOX-2 [6] and aldehyde dehydrogenase activity (ALDH1) [7]. New strategies for selective and effective cancer therapy can be provided by selectively acting on overregulated pathways or molecules in differentiated cancer cells and/or in CSC populations, but not in normal cells.

1.2 Therapies targeted against cancer stem cells

Cancer treatment currently targets its proliferation potential, and therefore most treatments target rapidly dividing cells. The presence of CSCs may explain the failure of treatments to eradicate the disease or the recurrence of cancer [1]. CSCs have to remain in a state of quiescence, a state in which the cell does not divide staying in the G0 phase of the cell cycle [8] allows them to survive most anticancer treatments. This characteristic makes relapses possible, even decades after initial treatment, such as in colon or breast cancers [1, 9]. Although current treatments may reduce the tumor size, these effects are transient and generally do not improve patients' survival. For tumors in which CSCs play a role, there are three possibilities. First, the mutation of normal stem cells or CSC progenitor cells can lead to the development of the primary tumor. Second, during chemotherapy, most cells in the primary tumor can be destroyed, but if CSCs are not eradicated, they become refractory CSCs and can lead to the recurrence of the tumor [10]. Third, CSCs can migrate to distant sites of the primary tumor and cause metastasis [11–13]. Theoretically, the identification of CSCs can allow the development of treatment modalities that target these cells rather than rapidly dividing cells [14].

One of the therapeutic approaches currently being studied to combat CSCs is related to the signaling pathways involved in the processes of their self-renewal, proliferation and differentiation. This is because the loss of regulation of pathways such as Hedgehog (Hh), Notch and Wnt/β-catenin results in the key processes involved in the characteristics of CSCs. Currently, the therapy directed against these routes represents one of the most promising mechanisms of action against these initiation cells of the tumor [15, 16].

Herein we will discuss the search and biological activity of small synthetic derivatives: racemate **2**, named as bozepinib (isomer of **1**), was selected for anti-CSC studies (**Figure 1**). The information presented in this chapter should be of interest to medicinal chemists and represents an effort to summarize the experimental research and advances in the field of CSCs [17, 18].

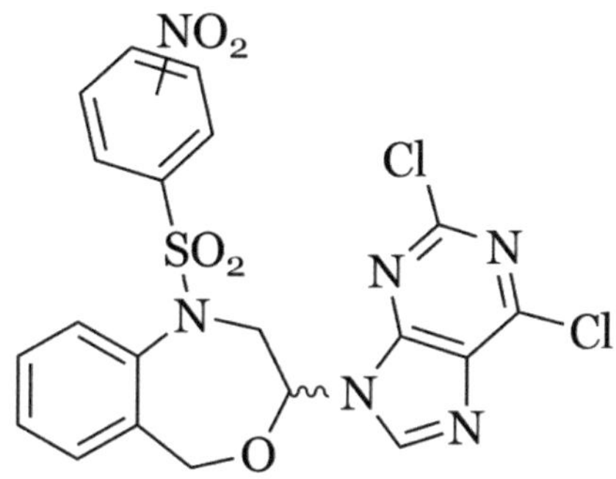

1: o-NO_2 isomer
2: *p*-NO_2 isomer (bozepinib)

Figure 1.
*Chemical structures of bezoxazepine derivatives **1** and **2**.*

A better understanding of the molecular mechanisms responsible for CSC formation probably lead to the design and synthesis of new anticancer drugs which will be able to eliminate CSC or to halt tumor growth by interfering with important intracellular signaling pathways related with CSC stemness or CSC differentiation or both.

2. (*RS*)-2,6-Dichloro-9-[1-(*o*- or *p*-nitrobenzenesulfonyl)-1,2,3,5-tetrahydro-4,1-benzoxazepine-3-yl]-9*H*-purines 1 and 2

2.1 Synthesis of tetrahydrobenzoxazepine *O*,*O*-acetals with electron withdrawing groups on the nitrogen atom

As part of an Anticancer Drug Programme, we were interested in the preparation of the heterocycles **3a-b** (**Figure 2**) that could be useful intermediates for the synthesis of novel bioactive compounds. **Figure 2** shows the synthesis of derivatives **3a-b** [19]. The Mitsunobu reaction is a versatile method for the transformation of aliphatic alcohols into alkylating agents in situ and under mild conditions [20]. A successful Mitsunobu displacement depends on the pK_a associated with the N—H bond [21]. Thus, a powerful electron withdrawing group for the amino moiety was needed such as the *p*- or *o*-nitrobenzenesulfonyl fragment.

The synthesis of compounds **3a-b** begins with the protection of the hydroxyl group of anthranilic alcohol by the *tert*-butyldimethylsilanyl group to give **4**; the synthesis of sulfonamides **5a** and **5b** was accomplished under the conditions of Fukuyama et al. [22]. Compound **6a** was obtained in a 70% yield under Mitsunobu conditions from **5a** and glycolaldehyde dimethyl acetal. The yield of this reaction depends greatly on the temperature: at rt., it is 19%, increasing up to 70% at 30°C and falling to 40% when the temperature is 40°C (**Figure 2**). When the optimized temperature conditions were applied to **5b**, **6b** was obtained in an 80% yield. After deprotection of the silanyl group of **6a** (and **6b**) with tetra-*n*-butylammonium fluoride (TBAF) in tetrahydrofuran (THF), **7a** was obtained in an 83% yield (and **7b** in 100% yield). Compounds **7a** and **7b** quantitatively afforded the benzo-fused seven-membered *O*,*O*-acetals **3a** and **3b**, respectively, using boron trifluoride diethyl etherate as previously reported [23].

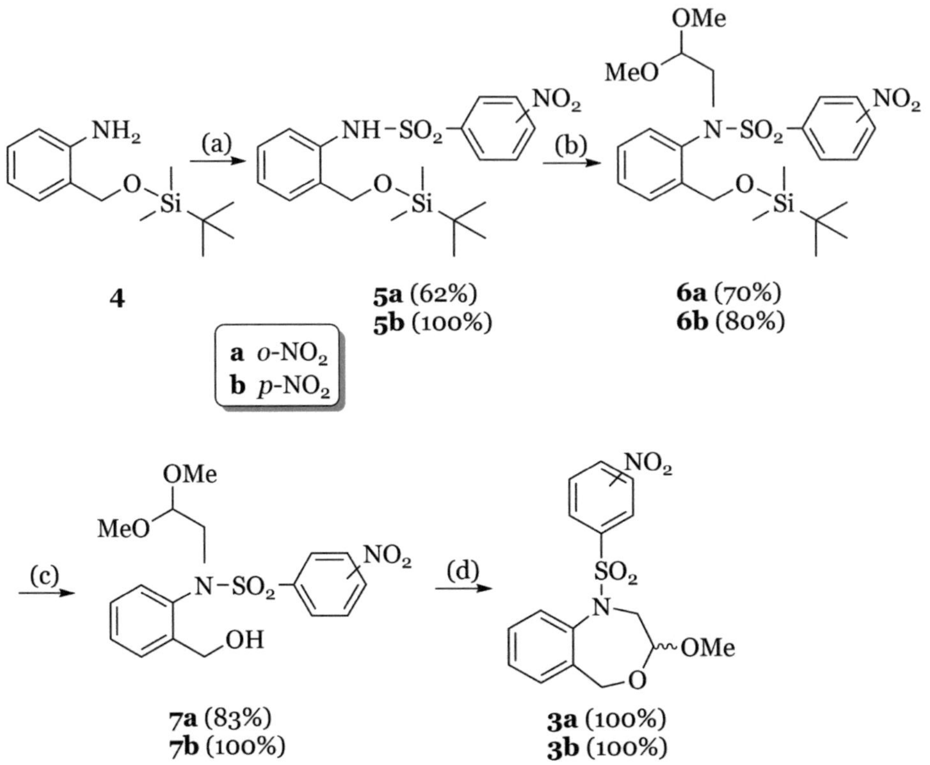

Figure 2.
*Reagents and conditions: (a) o-O_2N-C_6H_4-SO_2Cl (1.1 equiv), TEA (1.5 equiv), CH_2Cl_2, reflux, 24 h, for **5a**; p-O_2N-C_6H_4-SO_2Cl (0.5 equiv), CH_2Cl_2, rt., 3 h, for **5b**; (b) $HOCH_2CH(OMe)_2$ (1 equiv), diisopropyl azodicarboxylate (DIAD, 1.1 equiv), PPh_3 (1.2 equiv), anhydrous THF, 21 h; (c) TBAF (1 equiv), THF, rt., 1 h; (d) $BF_3{\cdot}OEt_2$ (2 equiv), anhydrous Et_2O, rt., 7 days for **3a**; when these conditions were used to obtain **3b**, the yield was 67%; p-H_3C-C_6H_4-SO_3H (0.03 equiv), anhydrous toluene, 110°C, 2 h under argon for **3a** and **3b** [19].*

Until compounds **3a** and **3b** were obtained under the optimal conditions described above, other conditions were studied giving rise to unwanted products. Product **5b** was obtained using a twofold excess of the *o*-aminobenzyl silanyl ether **4**, and these conditions were most important for the preparation of this compound (**5b, Figure 2**). Actually, the derivative **8** was isolated when the reaction was carried out using triethylamine (TEA) as a hydrochloride acid scavenger and 1.1 equiv. of the sulfonyl chloride was added (**Figure 3**) [19].

A reasonable explanation implied the previous ionization of the sulfonamide hydrogen atom of **5b** to give a $^{-}NSO_2$ anion which reacts more rapidly than the starting amine to give **8**. Disulfonimides have been stated [24] to be by-products in reactions of sulfonyl halides with primary amines and ammonia. The *o*-nitro group might sterically hinder the $^{-}NSO_2$ anion, and therefore the analogous side product was not isolated.

We also investigated other conditions to synthesize **6b** (**Figure 4**) [19]. The isopropyl alkylated derivative **9** (38%) was obtained together with the expected acetal **6b** (31%) when an excess of glycolaldehyde dimethyl acetal (4.3 equiv) was added. Such a compound could be interpreted by the transesterification reaction of glycolaldehyde dimethyl acetal and diisopropyl azodicarboxylate (DIAD), with the concomitant leaving of isopropanol. A similar process was previously reported for diethyl azodicarboxylate (DEAD) but not when DIAD was used [25].

The *O,O*-acetals **3a** and **3b** were formed after treatment of the *p*-toluenesulfonic acid-mediated cyclization from the acyclic acetals **7a** and **7b**, using anhydrous toluene as solvent. When neutral and mild conditions using triphenylphosphine/carbon tetrachloride were employed, the substitution of the hydroxyl group by the chlorine took place, and compounds **10a** and **10b** were obtained instead of the cyclic derivatives **7a** and **7b** (**Figure 5**) [26]. Compounds **7a** and **7b** present bulky groups that limit their conformational motions, making them rigid structures. The oxygen atoms of the acetalic groups cannot act as nucleophiles against the benzylic position (with the triphenylphosphine ether) due to steric hindering. Hydrogen atoms of the methylene groups of both compounds (**7a** and **7b**) are diastereotopic protons (J_{gem} = 12.6–14.1 Hz) [19].

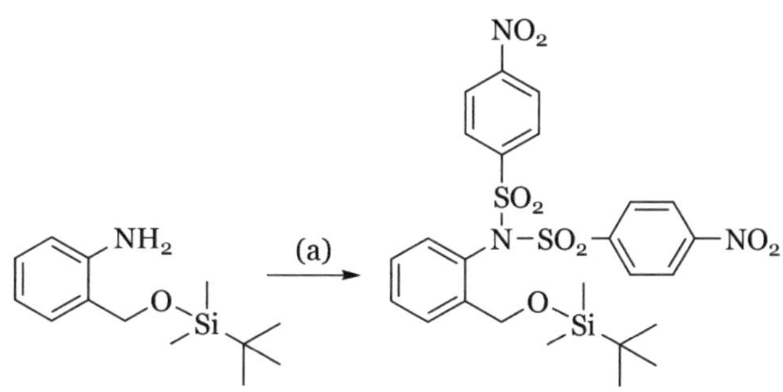

4 **8** (100%)

Figure 3.
Reagents and conditions: (a) p-O_2N-C_6H_4-SO_2Cl (1.1 equiv), TEA (1.5 equiv) and anhydrous CH_2Cl_2, rt., 5 h when 0.5 equiv. of p-O_2N-C_6H_4-SO_2Cl was used, see **Figure 2** *(conversion* **4** → **5b***) [19].*

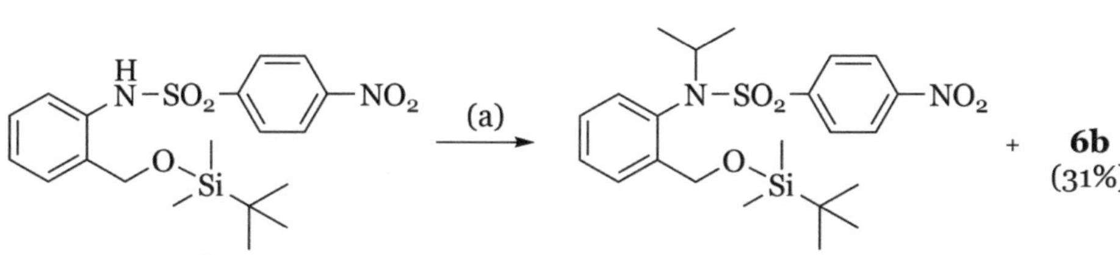

5b **9** (38%)

Figure 4.
Reagents and conditions: (a) $HOCH_2CH(OMe)_2$ (4.3 equiv), DIAD (1.2 equiv), PPh_3 (1.2 equiv) and anhydrous THF, rt., 18; h; when 1.2 equiv. of $HOCH_2CH(OMe)_2$ were used, see **Figure 2** *(conversion* **5b** → **6b***) [19].*

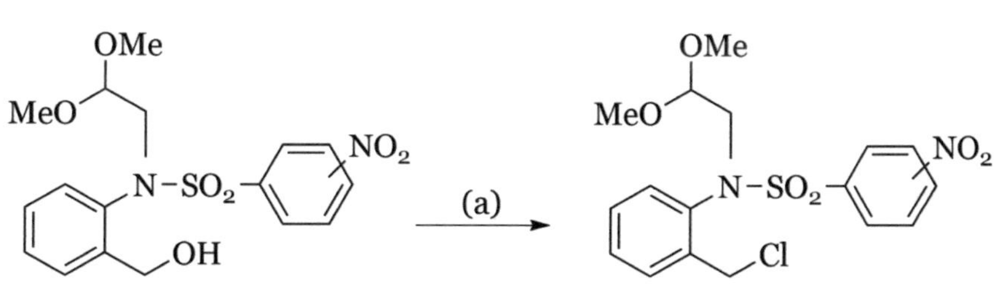

7a (83%)
7b (100%)

10a (40%)
10b (100%)

Figure 5.
Reagents and conditions: (a) Ph3P (1 equiv), CCl_4, 110°C, 30 min [19].

2.2 Synthesis of tetrahydrobenzoxazepine 2,6-dichloropurine *O,N*-acetals with nitrosulfonyl groups on the nitrogen atom

The preparation of the *O,N*-acetals **1** and **2** was achieved by the microwave-assisted Vorbrüggen one-pot condensation of the cyclic acetals **3a** and **3b** [27] and the commercially available purine base 2,6-dichloropurine, using trimethylsilyl chloride (TMSCl), 1,1,1,3,3,3-hexamethyldisilazane (HMDS) and tin(IV) chloride as the Lewis acid in anhydrous acetonitrile. The reaction mixture was microwave-irradiated at a temperature of 140°C for 5 min (**Figure 6**).

Compounds **11** and **12** were obtained along with the cyclic 2,6-dichloropurine *O,N*-acetals (**1** and **2**, bozepinib) and the acyclic one **13** (when starting from **3b**) in the reaction of purines with **3a** and **3b**, respectively. The mechanism of the reaction of these compounds is important as none of them were previously isolated in the

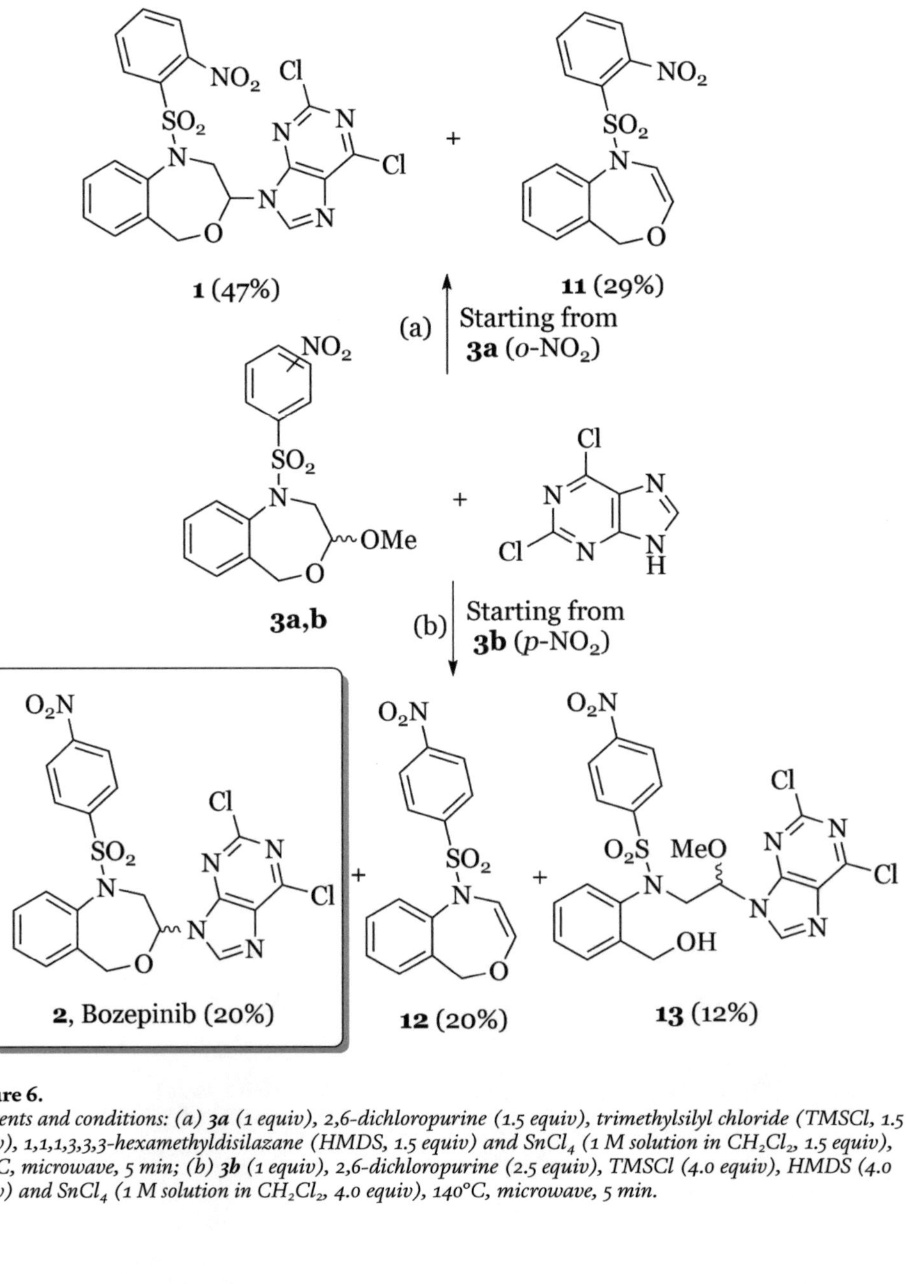

Figure 6.
Reagents and conditions: (a) ***3a*** *(1 equiv), 2,6-dichloropurine (1.5 equiv), trimethylsilyl chloride (TMSCl, 1.5 equiv), 1,1,1,3,3,3-hexamethyldisilazane (HMDS, 1.5 equiv) and* $SnCl_4$ *(1 M solution in* CH_2Cl_2*, 1.5 equiv), 140°C, microwave, 5 min; (b)* ***3b*** *(1 equiv), 2,6-dichloropurine (2.5 equiv), TMSCl (4.0 equiv), HMDS (4.0 equiv) and* $SnCl_4$ *(1 M solution in* CH_2Cl_2*, 4.0 equiv), 140°C, microwave, 5 min.*

corresponding reactions with uracil or 5-FU [27]. We have previously explained the mechanism of the reaction leading to the benzo-fused derivatives **1**, **2**, **11** and **12** [28].

2.3 Homochiral drugs

A better understanding of the molecular recognition of the therapeutic targets in many diseases highlights the issue of drug in the design and development of new drugs. The separation of racemates, chiral pool and asymmetric synthesis are the three most used methods for the production of a chiral drug. Since the 1980s there has been a significant increase in the development of chiral pharmaceutical drugs. When patents of racemic drugs expire, pharmaceutical companies can extend patents by developing the synthesis of enantiomers that exhibit the desired biological activity [29].

Compound **2** was resolved into its two enantiomers: [(*R*)-**2**: $[\alpha]^{25}_{D} = -43.6$ (c = 0.22, THF) and (*S*)-**2**: $[\alpha]^{25}_{D} = +41.0$ (c = 0.23, THF)]; using a semipreparative column CHIRALPAK® and a mixture of hexane/*t*-BuOMe/*i*PrOH as eluant [28]. From this moment on, the racemic **2** [(*RS*)-**2**] will be named only as bozepinib.

2.4 Biological studies

Table 1 shows the anti-proliferative activity (IC_{50} values) for **1**, bozepinib and 5-fluorouracil (5-FU) as a reference drug. Compounds were first assayed as anti-proliferative agents against the human breast adenocarcinoma cell line MCF-7 (p53 wild type and ras mutated). Compounds **1** and bozepinib were further assayed against the human breast cancer cell line MDA-MB-231 which presents high levels of mutant p53 [28, 30]. The IC_{50} = 0.166 μM for bozepinib against the human cancerous cell line MDA-MB-231 stands out.

In order to determine the in vitro therapeutic index of the compounds, they were assayed against the non-cancerous human mammary epithelial cell line MCF-10A. The TI of a drug is defined as the ratio of the toxic dose to the therapeutic dose (in vitro TI = IC_{50} non-tumor cell line/IC_{50} tumor cell line) [28]. Bozepinib is more selective against both human breast adenocarcinoma MCF-7 and MDA-MB-231 cancer cell lines (TIs = 5.14 and 11.0, respectively) in relation to the normal one (**Table 2**).

As bozepinib is more active and more selective and more active than its isomer **1**, we decided to carry out the separation of bozepinib into their component enantiomers (resolution). (*S*)-**2** shows higher anti-proliferative effect that of (*R*)-**2** in the MCF-7 cell line. However no differences against the MDA-MB-231 cell line were observed (**Table 3**). The enantioselective cytotoxicity indicates that the

Compound	IC_{50} MCF-7 (μM)	IC_{50} MDA-MB-231 (μM)	IC_{50} MCF-10A (μM)
1	0.383 ± 0.027	0.280 ± 0.006	1.530 ± 0.198
Bozepinib	0.355 ± 0.011	0.166 ± 0.063	1.825 ± 0.503
5-FU[c]	4.32 ± 0.020	N.D.[b]	N.D.[b]

[a]*All experiments were conducted in duplicate and gave similar results. Data are means ± SEM of three independent determinations. The treatment time was 48 h.*
[b]*N.D. = not determined.*
[c]*Taken from Ref. [31].*

Table 1.
Anti-proliferative activities[a] for compounds 1 and bozepinib against the cancerous cell lines MCF-7 and MDA-MB-231 and the non-cancerous cell line MCF-10A.

Compound	Therapeutic index (TI)	
	MCF-7	MDA-MB-231
1	4.00	5.50
Bozepinib	5.14	11.0

Table 2.
*Therapeutic indexes for **1** and bozepinib.*

Compound	MCF-7 (μM)[a]	MDA-MB-231 (μM)[a]
Bozepinib	0.355 ± 0.011	0.166 ± 0.063
(*R*)-2	0.19 ± 0.001	0.11 ± 0.001
(*S*)-2	0.10 ± 0.001	0.11 ± 0.001

[a]*All experiments were conducted in duplicate and gave similar results. The data are means ± SEM of three independent determinations.*

Table 3.
Anti-proliferative activities of bozepinib and its enantiomers against the cancerous cell lines MCF-7 and MDA-MB-231.

enantiomers of some chiral drugs may differ both quantitatively and qualitatively in their biological activity [32, 33]. Moreover, enantiomers can show minimal in vitro but a dramatic in vivo chiral dependency in their antitumor activities [34, 35].

2.4.1 Effect of bozepinib against CSC subpopulations

The cytotoxic effect of bozepinib was determined on SKBR-3 and MDA-MB 468 breast and HCT-116 colon CSC-enriched subpopulations by growing them into low attachment plates with sphere-forming medium for 72 h. Salinomycin is a selective and potent drug used in the treatment of CSCs, but its use is limited in humans due to considerable toxicity [36]. Thus, we decided to include salinomycin in our studies as reference drug. Bozepinib displayed IC50 values in a similar range to salinomycin in SKBR-3 and MDA-MB 468 cells [30].

CSCs were separated using ALDH activity by FACS. IC_{50} values were determined in both ALDH positive cells (called ALDH+), ALDH negative cells (called ALDH−) and cells growing in sphere-forming medium without sorter enrichment process [30]. Since there is controversy about the efficacy of sphere-forming cultures to select CSCs [37, 38], we used ALDH activity to enrich cell cultures with clonal ability and stem-like properties. Bozepinib substantially diminished the number and size of spheres at 5 μM and abolished the formation of spheres at 20 μM [30] in subpopulations isolated by ALDH activity. High ALDH activity is associated with metastasis, resistance to chemotherapies and poor prognosis in human cancers, and it has been identified as one of the most specific markers of human CSCs [39].

Apoptosis is also an important factor in the onset of a tumor. It has been reported than CSCs are resistant to apoptosis to ensure succeeding generation [40] and may be on the causes to chemo- or radiotherapy survival. Reactivating death programmes in CSCs may increase efficacy of the treatment. Bozepinib induced a significant level of cell death by apoptosis in the resistant ALDH+ subpopulations from both SKBR-3 and HCT-116 cell lines. Higher levels of apoptosis were detected in the ALDH− subpopulations.

Bozepinib induced the downregulation of important genes involved in Notch and Wnt signaling. These genes contribute to the CSC phenotype when they are deregulated [41]. A downregulation was detected of the co-activator

Mastermind-like MAML-2 protein, which decreases Notch signaling, reducing the primary tumor sphere formation and side population in MCF-7 cell line, contributing to the decrease in the number of CSC subpopulations [42]. We also found an evident downregulation of the *NOTCH 3* gene, which has recently been involved in the proliferation of both HER2 positive and negative breast cancer cells, suggesting that targeted suppression of this signaling pathway may be a promising strategy for the treatment of determined HER2-related breast cancers [43, 44].

The modification of proteins related to the CSC phenotype such as β-catenin, GLI-3, c-MYC and SOX-2 was additionally analysed. This study was carried out in both ALDH+ and ALDH− SKBR-3 breast and HCT-116 colon cancer subpopulations.

β-Catenin is a key mediator of the Wnt signaling which has a crucial role in CSCs [45]. β-Catenin expression was detected in ALDH+ SKBR-3 but not in ALDH− SKBR-3 cells. A high level of expression in HCT-116 cell lines with an ALDH+ subpopulations in comparison with the ALDH− in HCT-116 subpopulations was also detected. After bozepinib treatment, β-catenin expression was reduced in ALDH+ HCT-116 subpopulation. Its inhibition in ALDH− HCT-116 cells was also observed.

GLI-3, a described target gene transcription repressor of Hedgehog signaling pathway [16], was detected in ALDH− HCT-116 isolated cells and was not present in the ALDH+ cells, denoting that the Hedgehog signaling pathway is involved in the CSC phenotype as previously reported [16]. Bozepinib greatly induced the expression of GLI-3 in both ALDH+ and ALDH− HCT-116 cells. However, no changes at protein level were observed in ALDH+/− subpopulations isolated from the SKBR-3 cell line. Furthermore, the activation of GLI-3 protein corresponded with an inactivation of β-catenin expression in CSC subpopulations after bozepinib treatment in accordance with the previous published studies [46]. Considering that GLI-3 overexpression decreased tumor cell proliferation and induced apoptosis in colon CSCs [47], the GLI-3 induction by bozepinib could be one of the mechanisms by which this drug exerts its antitumor activity in colon CSCs. This hypothesis will be deeply study the future.

The c-MYC oncoprotein was observed in SKBR-3 and HCT-116 cell lines with a high level of expression in ALDH+ subpopulations in comparison with the ALDH− subpopulations. Bozepinib induced a significant decrease of c-MYC level in ALDH+ HCT-116 cells and inhibited its expression in ALDH+ SKBR-3-treated cells. It also inhibited ALDH− subpopulations of both HCT-116 and SKBR-3 cells [30]. In accordance with the high level of stem signaling proteins described for CSCs, higher levels of these proteins in the ALDH+ subpopulations in comparison with ALDH- cells were detected. The downregulation of c-MYC activates the inhibition of cancer cell proliferation, invasion and migration [48].

The transcription factor SOX2 was detected in HCT-116 ALDH+ subpopulation. However SOX2 was not observed in breast cancer cells, and the expression of SOX2 was very weak in HCT-116 ALDH− subpopulation [30]. Its expression practically disappeared after treatment with bozepinib. SOX2 is involved in the induction and maintenance of pluripotent stem cells and has also been associated with metastases and poor prognosis in colon cancer [49].

2.4.2 *In vivo studies of bozepinib*

The acute toxicity profile of bozepinib was determined in BALB/c mice. After 2 weeks, bozepinib was nontoxic to BALB/c mice even at the highest intraperitoneal bolus dose of 200 mg/kg and orally bolus dose of 50 mg/kg. Control mice were treated with vehicle alone. All 50 bozepinib-treated mice remained healthy and gained weight throughout the 15-day observation period, with no evidence of morbidity [28].

We then evaluated the subacute toxicity after 29 days of intraperitoneal treatment with 100 mg/kg twice a week. Bozepinib-treated mice presented no weight loss or unusual behaviour, and the histopathologic examination did not find any detectable toxicity in the liver or kidneys. These data indicate that, at the concentration used, bozepinib did not cause any systemic damage [30].

3. Conclusion

Although we show promising data proving the efficacy of bozepinib over CSCs, the mechanism by which bozepinib inhibits the CSC growth requires further detailed investigation. Moreover, the in vivo antitumor and anti-metastatic effect and the non-systemic toxicity of bozepinib encourage further studies on the therapeutic potential of this synthetic compound in breast and colon cancer patients.

The detection of CSCs in multiple solid tumors over the past years represents a paradigm shift in oncology and will probably change our understanding of the tumourigenic process. The impressive number of publications that have appeared in this field in recent years bears testimony to its enormous current interest.

We expect this chapter to stimulate fresh activity within the medicinal chemistry community and to result in the enlargement of chemical structures active against CSCs.

Abbreviations

ALDH	aldehyde dehydrogenase activity
CSCs	cancer stem cells
DEAD	diethyl azodicarboxylate
DIAD	diisopropyl azodicarboxylate
FACS	fluorescence-activated cell sorter
5-FU	5-fluorouracil
Hh	Hedgehog
HMDS	1,1,1,3,3,3-hexamethyldisilazane
PKR	protein kinase R
TBAF	tetra-*n*-butylammonium fluoride
TEA	triethylamine
THF	tetrahydrofuran
TI	therapeutic index
TMSCl	trimethylsilyl chloride
VEGF	vascular endothelial growth factor

Author details

Joaquín M. Campos[1,2]*, Ana Conejo-García[1,2] and Olga Cruz-López[1,2]

1 Department of Pharmaceutical and Organic Chemistry, Faculty of Pharmacy, University of Granada, Granada, Spain

2 Granada Biosanitary Institute (ibs. GRANADA), Andalusian Health Service, University of Granada, Granada, Spain

*Address all correspondence to: jmcampos@ugr.es

References

[1] Reya T, Morrison SJ, Clarke MF, Weissman IL. Stem cells, cancer, and cancer stem cells. Nature. 2001;**414**:105-111. DOI: 10.1038/35102167

[2] Tirino V, Desiderio V, Paino F, De Rosa A, Papaccio F, La Noce M, et al. Cancer stem cells in solid Tumours: An overview and new approaches for their isolation and characterization. The FASEB Journal. 2013;**27**:13-24. DOI: 10.1096/fj.12-218222

[3] Dontu G, Abdallah WM, Foley JM, Jackson KW, Clarke MF, Kawamura MJ, et al. In vitro propagation and transcriptional profiling of human mammary stem/progenitor cells. Genes & Development. 2003;**17**:1253-1270. DOI: 10.1101/gad.1061803

[4] Al-Hajj M, Wicha MS, Benito-Hernández A, Morrison SJ, Clarke MF. Prospective identification of tumourigenic breast cancer cells. Proceedings of the National Academy of Sciences of the United States of America. 2003;**100**:3983-3988. DOI: 10.1073/pnas.0530291100

[5] Moumen M, Chiche A, Decraene C, Petit V, Gandarillas A, Deugnier MA, et al. Myc is required for β-catenin-mediated mammary stem cell amplification and tumourigenesis. Molecular Cancer. 2013;**12**:132-140. DOI: 10.1186/1476-4598-12-132

[6] Leis O, Eguiara A, López-Arribillaga E, Alberdi MJ, Hernández-García S, Elorriaga K, et al. Sox2 expression in breast tumours and activation in breast cancer stem cells. Oncogene. 2012;**31**:1354-1365. DOI: 10.1038/onc.2011.338

[7] Deng S, Yang X, Lassus H, Liang S, Kaur S, Ye Q, et al. Distinct expression levels and patterns of stem cell marker, aldehyde dehydrogenase isoform 1 (ALDH1), in human epithelial cancers. PLoS One. 2010;**5**:e10277. DOI: 10.1371/journal.pone.0010277

[8] Arai F, Hirao A, Ohmura M, Sato H, Matsuoka S, Takubo K, et al. Tie2/angiopoietin-1 signalling regulates hematopoietic stem cell quiescence in the bone marrow niche. Cell. 2004;**118**:149-161. DOI: 10.1016/j.cell.2004.07.004

[9] Dick JE. Stem cell concepts renew cancer research. Blood. 2008;**112**:4793-4807. DOI: 10.1182/blood-2008-08-077941

[10] Stockler M, Wilcken N, Ghersi D, Simes RJ. Systematic reviews of chemotherapy and endocrine therapy in metastatic breast cancer. Cancer Treatment Reviews. 2000;**26**:151-168. DOI: 10.1053/ctrv.1999.0161

[11] Jordan CT, Guzman ML. Mechanisms controlling pathogenesis and survival of leukemic stem cells. Oncogene. 2004;**23**:7178-7187. DOI: 10.1038/sj.onc.1207935

[12] Jordan CT, Guzman ML, Noble M. Cancer stem cells. New England Journal of Medicine. 2006;**355**:1253-1261. DOI: 10.1056/NEJMra061808

[13] Liu HG, Chen C, Yang H, Pan YF, Zhang XH. Cancer stem cell subsets and their relationships. Journal of Translational Medicine. 2011;**9**:50-58. DOI: 10.1186/1479-5876-9-50

[14] Sagar J, Chaib B, Sales K, Winslet M, Seifalian A. Role of stem cells in cancer therapy and cancer stem cells: A review. Cancer Cell International. 2007;7:9-14. DOI: 10.1186/1475-2867-7-9

[15] Maugeri-Saccà M, Zeuner A, De Maria R. Therapeutic targeting of cancer stem cells. Frontiers in Oncology. 2011;**1**:10. DOI: 10.3389/fonc.2011.00010

[16] Takebe N, Harris PJ, Warren RQ, Ivy SP. Targeting cancer stem cells by inhibiting Wnt, Notch, and Hedgehog pathways. Nature Reviews. Clinical Oncology. 2011;**8**:97-106. DOI: 10.1038/nrclinonc.2010.196

[17] Oreste P, García-Rubiño ME, Franchini C, Campos J. Cancer stem cells: The new objective for the eradication of tumours. In: Watanabe HS, editor. Horizons in Cancer Research. Vol. 56. 2015. pp. 41-81. ISSN: 2159-1326. ISBN: 978-1-63482-248-0 (eBook)

[18] García-Rubiño ME, Lozano-López C, Campos JM. Inhibitors of cancer stem cells. Anti-Cancer Agents in Medicinal Chemistry. 2016;**16**:1230-1239. DOI: 10.2174/1871520616666160330104715

[19] Díaz-Gavilán M, Rodríguez-Serrano F, Gómez-Vidal JA, Marchal JA, Aránega A, Gallo MA, et al. Synthesis of tetrahydrobenzoxazepine acetals with electron-withdrawing groups on the nitrogen atom. Novel scaffolds endowed with anticancer activity against breast cancer cells. Tetrahedron. 2004;**60**:11547-11557. DOI: 10.1016/j.tet.2004.09.072

[20] Fletcher S. The Mitsunobu reaction in the 21st century. Organic Chemistry Frontiers. 2015;**2**:739-752. DOI: 10.1039/C5QO00016E

[21] Koppel I, Kippel J, Degerbeck F, Grehn L, Ragnarsson V. Acidity of imidodicarbonates and tosylcarbamates in dimethyl sulfoxide. Correlation with yields in the Mitsunobu reaction. The Journal of Organic Chemistry. 1991;**56**:7172-7174. DOI: 10.1021/jo00025a041

[22] Fukuyama T, Jow CK, Cheung M. 2,4-Dinitrobenzenesulfonamides: A simple and practical method for the preparation of a variety of secondary amines and diamine. Tetrahedron Letters. 1995;**36**:6373-6374. DOI: 10.1016/S0040-4039(97)01334-8

[23] Campos J, Pineda MJ, Gómez JA, Entrena A, Trujillo MA, Gallo MA, et al. 5-fluorouracil derivatives. 1. Acyclonucleosides through a Tin (IV) chloride-mediated regiospecific ring opening of alkoxy-1,4-diheteroepanes. Tetrahedron. 1996;**52**:8907-8924. DOI: 10.1016/0040-4020(96)00439-5

[24] Andersen KK, Jones DN, editors. Comprehensive Organic Chemistry. Vol. 3. Pergamon: Oxford; 1979. pp. 339-341. https://doi.org/10.1002/jps.2600690651

[25] Rew Y, Goodman M. Solid-phase synthesis of amine-bridged cyclic enkephalin analogues via on-resin cyclization utilizing the Fukuyama–Mitsunobu reaction. The Journal of Organic Chemistry. 2002;**67**:8820-8826. https://doi.org/10.1021/jo020447l

[26] Espinosa A, Gallo MA, Campos J, Gómez JA. Diastereoselective intramolecular cyclization through the triphenylphosphine/carbon tetrachloride system: Synthesis of saturated 1,4-dihetero seven-membered Cycloacetals. Synlett. 1995;**11**:1119-1120. DOI: 10.1055/s-1995-5207

[27] Díaz-Gavilán M, Gómez-Vidal JA, Entrena A, Gallo MA, Espinosa A, Campos JM. Study of the factors that control the ratio of the products between 5-fluorouracil, uracil, and tetrahydrobenzoxazepine *O,O*-acetals bearing electron-withdrawing groups on the nitrogen atom. The Journal of Organic Chemistry. 2006;**71**:1043-1054. DOI: 10.1021/jo052167m Ref. 12 del EJMC 2011

[28] López-Cara LC, Conejo-García A, Marchal JA, Macchione G, Cruz-López O, Boulaiz H, et al. New (*RS*)-benzoxazepin-purines with antitumour activity: The chiral switch from (*RS*)-2,6-dichloro-9-[1-(*p*-nitrobenzenesulfonyl)-1,2,3,5-tetrahydro-4,1-benzoxazepin-3-yl]-9*H*-purine. European Journal of Medicinal Chemistry. 2011;**46**:249-258. DOI: 10.1016/j.ejmech.2010.11.011

[29] Núñez MC, García-Rubiño ME, Conejo-García A, Cruz-López O, Kimatrai M, Gallo MA, et al. Homochiral drugs: A demanding tendency of the pharmaceutical industry. Current Medicinal Chemistry. 2009;**16**:2064-2074. DOI: 10.2174/092986709788682173

[30] Ramírez A, Boulaiz H, Morata-Tarifa C, Perán M, Jiménez G, Picón-Ruiz M, et al. HER2-signalling pathway, JNK and ERKs kinases, and cancer stem-like cells are targets of bozepinib. Oncotarget. 2014;**5**:3590-3606. DOI: 10.18632/oncotarget.1962

[31] Núñez MC, Díaz-Gavilán M, Conejo-García A, Cruz-López O, Gallo MA, Espinosa A, et al. Design, synthesis and anticancer activity against the MCF-7 cell line of benzo-fused 1,4-dihetero seven- and six-membered tethered pyrimidines and purines. Current Medicinal Chemistry. 2008;**15**:2614-2631. DOI: 10.2174/092986708785909021

[32] Liu H, Xu L, Zhao M, Liu W, Zhang C, Zhou S. Enantiomer-specific, bifenthrin-induced apoptosis mediated by MAPK signalling pathway in Hep G2 cells. Toxicology. 2009;**261**:119-125. DOI: 10.1016/j.tox.2009.05.002

[33] Shelley MD, Hartley L, Fish RG, Groundwater P, Morgan JJG, Mort D, et al. Stereo-specific cytotoxic effects of gossypol enantiomers and gossypolone in tumour cell lines. Cancer Letters. 1999;**135**:171-180. DOI: 10.1016/S0304-3835(98)00302-4

[34] Lai JC, Brown BD, Voskresenskiy AM, Vonhoff S, Klussman S, Tan W, et al. Comparison of D-G3139 and its enantiomer L-G3139 in melanoma cells demonstrates minimal in vitro but dramatic in vivo chiral dependency. Molecular Therapy. 2007;**15**:270-278. DOI: 10.1038/sj.mt.6300037

[35] Brown NM, Belles CA, Lindley SL, Zimmer-Nechemias LD, Zhao X, Witte DP, et al. The chemopreventive action of equol enantiomers in a chemically induced animal model of breast cancer. Carcinogenesis. 2010;**31**:886-893. DOI: 10.1093/carcin/bgq025

[36] Naujokat C, Steinhart R. Salinomycin as a drug for targeting human cancer stem cells. Journal of Biomedicine & Biotechnology. 2012;**2012**:950658. DOI: 10.1155/2012/950658

[37] Smart CE, Morrison BJ, Saunus JM, Vargas AC, Keith P, Reid L, et al. In vitro analysis of breast cancer cell line tumourspheres and primary human breast epithelia mammospheres demonstrates inter- and intrasphere heterogeneity. PLoS One. 2013;**8**:e64388. DOI: 10.1371/journal.pone.0064388

[38] Ma L, Lai D, Liu T, Cheng W, Guo L. Cancer stemlike cells can be isolated with drug selection in human ovarian cancer cell line SKOV3. Acta Biochimica et Biophysica Sinica. 2010;**42**(9):593-602. DOI: 10.1093/abbs/gmq067

[39] Charafe-Jauffret E, Ginestier C, Iovino F, Tarpin C, Diebel M, Esterni B, et al. Aldehyde dehydrogenase 1-positive cancer stem cells mediate metastasis and poor clinical outcome in inflammatory breast cancer. Clinical Cancer Research. 2010;**16**:45-55. DOI: 10.1158/1078-0432.CCR-09-1630

[40] Kruyt FA, Schuringa JJ. Apoptosis and cancer stem cells: Implications for apoptosis targeted therapy. Biochemical Pharmacology. 2010;**80**:423-430. DOI: 10.1016/j.bcp.2010.04.010

[41] Dontu G, Jackson KW, McNicholas E, Kawamura MJ, Abdallah WM, Wicha MS. Role of Notch signalling in cell-fate

determination of human mammary stem/progenitor cells. Breast Cancer Research. 2004;**6**:R605-R615. DOI: 10.1186/bcr920

[42] Wong NK, Fuller M, Sung S, Wong F, Karsan A. Heterogeneity of breast cancer stem cells as evidenced with Notch-dependent and Notch-independent populations. Cancer Medicine. 2012;**1**:105-113. DOI: 10.1002/cam4.18

[43] Pradeep CR, Kostler WJ, Lauriola M, Granit RZ, Zhang F, Jacob-Hirsch J, et al. Modeling ductal carcinoma in situ: A HER2-Notch3 collaboration enables luminal filling. Oncogene. 2012;**31**:907-917. DOI: 10.1038/onc.2011.279

[44] Yamaguchi N, Oyama T, Ito E, Satoh H, Azuma S, Hayashi M, et al. NOTCH3 signalling pathway plays crucial roles in the proliferation of ErbB2-negative human breast cancer cells. Cancer Research. 2008;**68**:1881-1888. DOI: 10.1158/0008-5472.CAN-07-1597

[45] Reya T, Clevers H. Wnt signalling in stem cells and cancer. Nature. 2005;**434**(7035):843-850. DOI: 10.1038/nature03319

[46] Ulloa F, Itasaki N, Briscoe J. Inhibitory Gli3 activity negatively regulates Wnt/beta-catenin signalling. Current Biology. 2007;**17**:545-550. DOI: 10.1016/j.cub.2007.01.062

[47] Merchant AA, Matsui W. Targeting Hedgehog—A cancer stem cell pathway. Clinical Cancer Research. 2010;**16**:3130-3140. DOI: 10.1158/1078-0432.CCR-09-2846

[48] Zhao Y, Jian W, Gao W, Zheng YX, Wang YK, Zhou ZQ, et al. RNAi silencing of c-Myc inhibits cell migration, invasion, and proliferation in HepG2 human hepatocellular carcinoma cell line: c-Myc silencing in hepatocellular carcinoma cell. Cancer Cell International. 2013;**13**:23. DOI: 10.1186/1475-2867-13-23

[49] Neumann J, Bahr F, Horst D, Kriegl L, Engel J, Luque RM, et al. SOX2 expression correlates with lymph-node metastases and distant spread in right-sided colon cancer. BMC Cancer. 2011;**11**:518. DOI: 10.1186/1471-2407-11-518

Chapter 9

NQO1-Bioactivatable Therapeutics as Radiosensitizers for Cancer Treatment

Naveen Singh, Edward A. Motea, Xiumei Huang, Colton L. Starcher, Jayne Silver, I-Ju Yeh, S. Louise Pay, Xiaolin Su, Kristen A. Russ, David A. Boothman and Erik A. Bey

Abstract

Developing cancer therapeutics that radiosensitize in a tumor-selective manner remains an ideal. We developed a novel means of radiosensitization, exploiting NAD(P)H:Quinone Oxidoreductase 1 (NQO1) overexpression, and lowered catalase expression in solid human tumors using NQO1-bioactivatable drugs. Non-small cell lung (NSCLC), pancreatic (PDAC), prostate, and breast cancers overexpress NQO1. Ionizing radiation (IR) creates a spectrum of DNA lesions, including lethal DNA double-strand breaks (DSBs), and mutagenic but rarely lethal altered DNA bases and DNA single-strand breaks (SSBs). NQO1-bioactivatable drugs (e.g., β-lapachone and deoxynyboquiones) also promote abasic DNA lesions and SSBs. These hyperactivate poly (ADP-ribose) polymerase 1 (PARP1) and dramatically increase calcium release from the endoplasm reticulum (ER). Exposure of human cancer cells overexpressing NQO1 to NQO1-bioactivatable drugs immediately following IR, therefore, hyperactivates PARP1 synergistically, which in turn depletes NAD+ and ATP, inhibiting DSB repair. Ultimately, this leads to cell death. Combining IR with NQO1-bioactivatable drugs allows for a reduction in drug dose. Similarly, a lower IR dose can be used in combination with the drug, reducing the effects of IR on normal tissue. The combination treatment is effective in preclinical animal models with NSCLC, prostate, and head and neck xenografts, indicating that clinical trials are warranted.

Keywords: NQO1 expression, PARP hyperactivation, abasic site synergy, NAD+/ATP losses, DSB repair inhibition, programmed necrosis

1. Introduction

For decades, radiobiologists and physician-scientists have collaborated to develop effective combination therapies with ionizing radiation and radiosensitizing agents to reduce the overall dose of radiation required in cancer therapy. This minimizes adverse side-effects observed in normal tissues and increases the efficacy of radiation in reducing tumor burden. Here, we discuss the pros and cons of radiosensitizing agents used in the clinic in comparison with NAD(P)H quinone oxidoreductase-1 (NQO1)-bioactivatable drugs. β-Lapachone (β-Lap) is a clinical chemotherapeutic agent discovered to be a potent DNA repair inhibitor in the late 1980s. It has since been shown to be bioactivated by NQO1, an enzyme elevated more than 20-fold in most solid human cancers, e.g., non-small cell lung, pancreas, prostate, head and neck, and breast cancers, and shows promise as a potent radiosensitizer.

2. Radiotherapy as a single agent

2.1 Initial use of ionizing radiation

The late 19th-century discovery of the X-ray by Wilhelm Roentgen led to diagnostic tools and therapies for diseases such as blood disorders and benign and malignant growths [1, 2]. Initially, radiation was delivered using unfocused beams, causing skin and blood malignancies in both patients and radiologists [1, 2]. Today, patients benefit from vast technological improvements, allowing for focused radiation beams, which markedly increased patient survival. Current approaches include conformal radiation therapy, proton beam radiation therapy, stereotactic radiation therapy (using linear accelerators or gamma knife devices), and intraoperative therapy [3]. Despite improvements in targeting tumors and reducing normal tissue damage, high doses of radiation are still required for a curative effect. Some tumors can also be resistant to radiotherapy, including hypoxic tumors and dormant cancer cells that regrow when the optimal tumor microenvironment presents itself. Thus, methods to improve the safety and efficacy of ionizing radiation were initiated, including combination with chemotherapeutics or radiosensitizers.

2.2 Enhancing radiation therapy with radiosensitizers

Radiosensitizing agents are molecules that enhance the dose of ionizing radiation delivered to a patient's tumor. The optimal clinical radiosensitizer (a) lowers the required dose of ionizing radiation, (b) increases its antitumor effect, and

Radiosensitizer	Tumor type	Mechanism
Hyperbaric oxygen	Brain tumors	Oxygenation
Nicotinamide	Glioblastoma	Oxygenation
Metronidazole	Cervical cancer	Oxygenation
Mitomycin-C	Breast cancer	Kills hypoxic cells
5-fluorouracil (5FU)	Gastrointestinal	S-phase check points
Bromodeoxyuridine (BrDU)	Breast	Repair inhibition
Topo-inhibitors	Breast, cervical	DNA damage
NBTXR3	Solid tumors	Direct
Nimoral	Head and neck	Modifies hypoxia
Trans sodium crocetinate	Glioblastoma	Oxygenation
NVX108	Glioblastoma	Oxygenation

*List of commonly used radiosensitizing methods/agents for combination with radiotherapy in various tumor types. The last four are **emboldened** to denote their current use in ongoing clinical trials.*

Table 1.
Clinical radiosensitizers.

(c) synergistically kills cancer cells. To date, no radiosensitizer has met these demands. Many radiosensitizers have been used clinically (**Table 1**, normal text) with limited success, or are currently in clinical trial (**Table 1**, bold text). These include suppressors of radioprotectors (e.g., thiol) [4], molecules releasing cytotoxic substances when radiolyzed [5], thymine/cytidine analogs [6], oxygen mimic sensitizers [7], and DNA repair inhibitors [8].

3. β-Lapachone, a DNA repair inhibitor

3.1 Initial discovery of β-lapachone's effect on DNA repair

In the late 1980s, our laboratory began searching for DNA repair modulators that synergize with ionizing radiation to kill cancer cells more effectively. The goal was to thwart cancer cells' ability to repair IR damage, to avoid the survival of IR-resistant malignant cells that have undergone potentially lethal damage repair (PLDR). One of those compounds was (3,4-dihydro-2,2-dimethyl-2H-naphthol[1,2-b]pyran-5,6-dione), also known as β-lapachone [9].

We found that just four micromolar β-lapachone inhibited single-strand DNA break repair in cancer cells exposed to DNA-damaging agent methyl methane sulfonate [9, 10], killing 99% of cells at an exposure time 90–120 min [11]. Additionally, we found that combining β-lapachone with ionizing radiation in Hep2 cells increased double-strand breaks and dramatically lowered the dose of radiation required for cell death, highlighting β-lapachone as a potent radiosensitizer [12].

In the 1990s and early 2000s, we conducted subtraction-hybridization screening to isolate X-ray inducible genes to investigate ionizing radiation resistance and found Xip3, also known as NQO1 [13]. Dicoumarol, an NQO1 inhibitor, specifically blocked β-lapachone's toxicity, indicating that the radiosensitizer may be bioactivated by this enzyme. As NQO1 is specifically expressed in tumor cells, this indicated a promising use of β-lapachone as a cancer therapeutic with or without ionizing radiation.

4. Mechanism of action for NQO1-bioactivatable therapies

4.1 NQO1 vs. catalase ratio and specificity

NQO1 is a Phase II detoxification enzyme that reduces ROS levels in cancer cells. NQO1 converts quinones into stable intermediate hydroquinones that are exported out of the cell by conjugation [10]. Most solid cancers, including non-small cell lung and pancreatic cancers (>85%), prostate, colon, and breast cancers (60%) and head and neck cancers (40%) overexpress NQO1 5- to 200- fold above normal tissue. Corresponding levels of catalase in these cancers were strikingly reduced, impacting the ability of cancer cells to eliminate ROS [14]. Overexpression of NQO1 appears to stabilize HIF-1alpha and promotes metastasis [15].

Though NQO1 detoxifies most quinones through two-electron oxidoreduction, a few quinones undergo a rapid futile redox cycle response, generating an unstable intermediate hydroquinone that spontaneously reverts back to its original form using two oxygenation steps and creating two superoxides. Deoxynyboquiones (DNQ), KP372 agents, and β-lapachone are three classes of NQO1-bioactivatable drugs currently known [16]. Recently, Napabucasin, an orphan drug in clinical trials for pancreatic and cervical cancer, has also been reported to be bioactivated by NQO1 [17]. Though mitomycin C and streptonigrin are metabolized by NQO1, these agents can also be activated by other drug metabolizing enzymes [18]. Human cancer cells overexpressing NQO1 have been shown to be sensitive to NQO1-bioactivatable drugs alone and in combination with PARP inhibitors, cisplatin, radiation, and NAMPT inhibitors both in cell culture and xenograft models [14, 19].

4.2 NQO1-dependent ROS formation and PARP hyperactivation

Cancer cells overexpressing NQO1 and exposed to NQO1-bioactivatable drugs, such as β-lapachone, DNQ or IB-DNQ, acquire extensive DNA lesions as evidenced by alkaline comet assays [11]. The unstable hydroquinone form of these NQO1 bioactivatable drugs reacts with two oxygen molecules spontaneously to regenerate the original compound [20]. This futile redox cycle consumes ~60 moles of NADPH to generate ~120 moles of ROS in ~2 min for β-lapachone, leading to the generation of permeable hydrogen peroxide (H_2O_2). This diffuses into the nucleus and causes massive oxidative stress and SSBs [16]. Initial DNA damage is mainly through the formation of altered bases, SSBs, and apurinic/apyrimidinic (AP) sites generated through incorporation of 8-oxo-deoxyguanine [21]. Ultimately, damage caused by H_2O_2 results in extensive SSBs and DSBs. These lesions lead to PARP hyperactivation that can be prevented by BAPTA-AM (chelates Ca^{2+}), PARP inhibitors, or the NQO1 inhibitor dicoumarol, in NQO1+ cells. In contrast, cells deficient in NQO1 due to NQO1 polymorphisms, *2[C609T] or *3[C465T], are unaffected by exposure to NQO1-bioactivatable compounds [14], lacking the enzyme activity for redox cycling Hyperactivation of PARP rapidly degrades the increased NAD+ pools generated as a result of the oxidation of NADH in the futile cycle [11, 20, 22]. NAD+ loss is not seen in cells treated with PARP1 inhibitors; instead, cells exposed to PARP inhibitors in combination with NQO1-bioactivatable drugs undergo a synergistic apoptotic cell death response [14].

4.3 Calcium release, DNA damage and μ-Calpain-dependent programmed necrosis

One of the key components in the cell death response by NQO1-bioactivatable drugs is the release of calcium from the core endoplasmic reticulum (ER) stores, which is otherwise inert [11, 23]. This results in specific programmed necrosis referred to as NAD+ -Keresis. Pre-treatment, with the calcium chelator, BAPTA-AM, suppresses PARP hyperactivation and results in specific inhibition of NQO1-dependent cell death by NQO1-bioactivatable drugs. Extensive DNA damage along with Ca^{2+} release from the ER results in the hyperactivation of PARP1 in NQO1+ cancer cells. PARP1 hyperactivation rapidly degrades the NAD+ and causes concomitant ATP losses within 30–40 min of drug treatment. μ-Calpain activation is observed upon treatment with NQO1-bioactivatable drugs within 8–24 h [16, 24]. The multitude of damage caused by treatment with these drugs overwhelms DNA repair machinery and depletes the cells of the energy resources, culminating in cell death [10, 11, 16, 20, 24–27].

4.4 NQO1-bioactivatable drugs lead to perturbations in metabolic pathways

Treatment with NQO1-bioactivatable drugs causes wide-scale metabolic changes in the cell, which can be attributed to cell death overwhelming the cellular machinery. Altering key enzymes in NAD metabolism results in synergy with NQO1-bioactivatable drugs. NAMPT is an important source of reducing equivalents for redox balance in cancer cells. Pretreatment with FK866, a NAMPT inhibitor, leads to accelerated cell death due to decrease in NAD+/NADH levels and reduced doses of NQO1-bioactivatable drugs [28]. NAMPT knockdown has also been shown to sensitize cancer cells to ROS induction through ionizing radiation [29, 30].

4.5 Exploiting NQO1-bioactivatable drugs as radiosensitizers

Cancer cells, tissues, and organs subjected to ionizing radiation experience a wide spectrum of DNA lesions including SSBs, DSBs, AP sites and DNA-protein cross-links. One unrepaired DSB is lethal to the cell [21, 31]. Hence, NQO1-bioactivatable drugs, when combined with IR (**Figure 1**), synergistically kill cancer cells due to the combined effect of DNA damage and PARP1 hyperactivation [21, 32]. Sublethal doses of NQO1 drugs and IR combine to release massive amounts of ROS due to

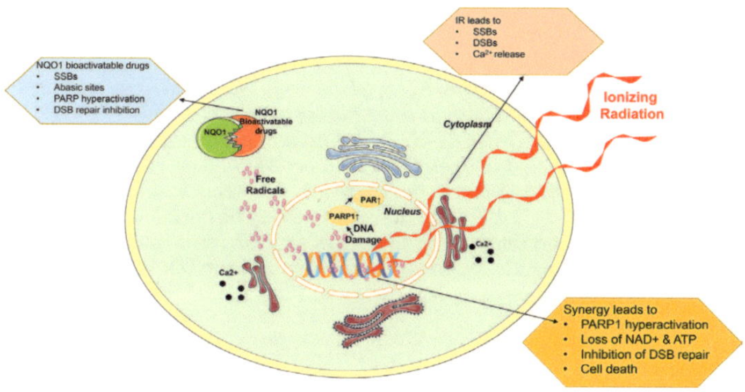

Figure 1.
Radiation sensitization by NQO1 bioactivatable drugs: sublethal doses of β-lapachone when bioactivated by NQO1 release massive amounts of ROS, resulting in synergy with IR and increased programmed necrosis. NQO1 bioactivatable drugs in combination with IR show tremendous synergy even at low doses. The combined effect of DNA damage and PARP hyperactivation provides more lethality to a cancer cell whereas NQO1 provides the specificity. This leads to increased ROS, gH2AX formation, hyperactivation of PARP, massive NAD and ATP losses, prevention of DSB repair, perturbations in the metabolic pathways, and μ-Calpain-mediated programmed necrosis known as NAD + -Keresis.

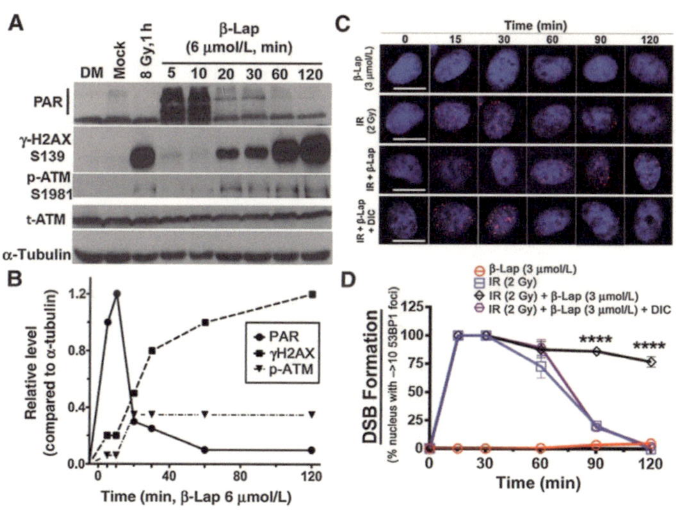

Figure 2.
*Sublethal doses of IR and β-lap in NQO1+ LNCaP cells cause PARP-1 hyper-activation and dramatic ATP loss: A, LNCaP cells expressing or lacking NQO1 were treated with IR + β-lap and monitored for PAR formation—UT, untreated control for IR; V, vehicle; DMSO only. B, Synergistic ATP loss was noted after IR + β-lap compared to single treatments alone. Results are means ± SE for experiments performed three times in duplicate. Student's t-tests compared single to combined treatments. ***p < 0.001, **p < 0.01.*

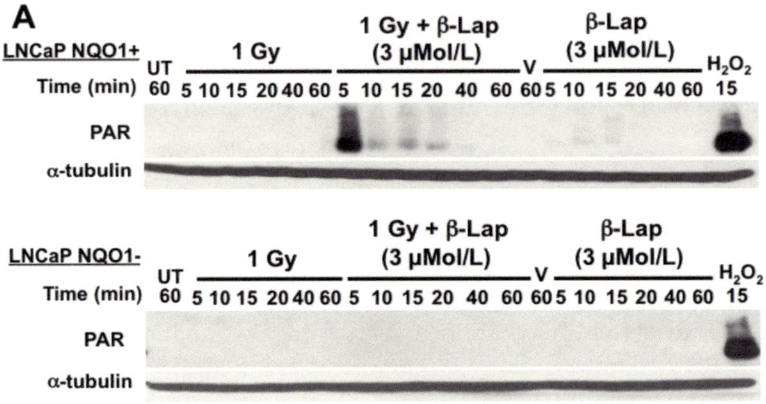

Figure 3.
*β-Lap inhibits DNA double strand break repair: A. log-phase A549 NSCLC cells were treated with or without β-lap (6 μM) and cell extracts prepared at various times during treatment to detect PAR-PARP formation, γ-H2AX (pS139), pS1981 ATM, total ATM (t-ATM) and α-tubulin steady-state levels by Western blot. A549 cells were also exposed or not to IR (8 Gy) and analyzed 1 h later. Mock, non-irradiated cells. DM, media alone. B. Graphical representation of data shown in **Figure 2A**. C. Representative images of A549 cells exposed or not to IR (2 Gy) alone, β-lap (3 μM, 2 h) alone, the combination [IR (2 Gy) + β-lap (3 μM, 2 h)], or the combination with DIC (50 μM, NQO1 inhibitor) and assessed for DSB breaks over time (0–120 min) using 53BP1 as the surrogate marker (in red). Cells were also stained for nuclear DNA using DAPI (in blue). Scale bar = 10 μm. D. Graphical representation of data presented in **Figure 2C**; ****p < 0.0001.*

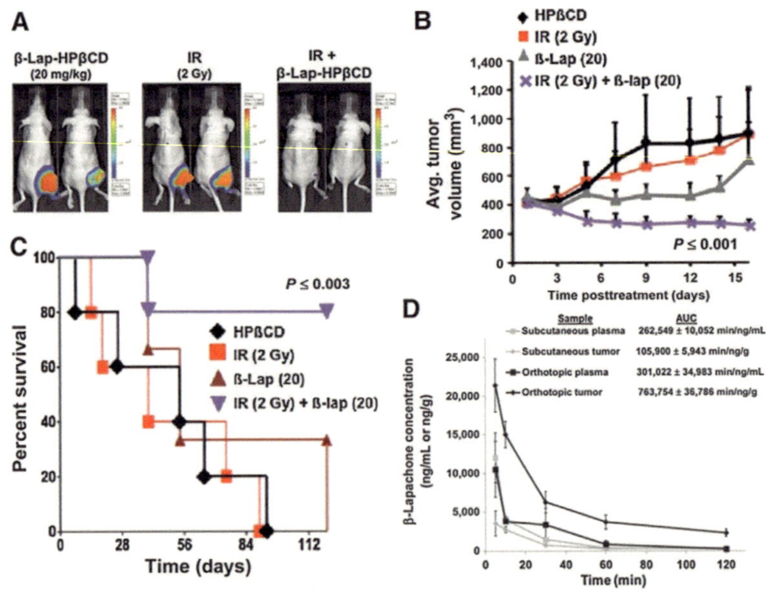

Figure 4.
*β-Lap radiosensitizes subcutaneous A549-luc xenografts in athymic nude mice: A. subcutaneous A549-luc xenografts (400 mm³) were generated in athymic nude mice and then treated with or without IR (2 Gy) then immediately with or without β-lap (20 mg/kg) for 5 treatments every other day. Representative antitumor responses (at day 20 post-treatment) are demonstrated for β-lap alone, IR alone, and the IR + β-lap combination. B. Antitumor responses (tumor volumes, mm³) over time are shown for the treatments described in **Figure 3A**. C. Overall survival of animals treated as described in **Figure 3A**. D. PK values for plasma and subcutaneous vs. orthotopic A549-luc tumors in athymic nude mice. Note the significantly high levels of β-lap in orthotopic vs. subcutaneous A549 tumor tissue, whereas plasma levels were identical in both sets of mice.*

their synergy, resulting in PARP hyperactivation, loss of nucleotides and increased programmed necrosis (**Figures 2** and **3**), beyond the capabilities of the single agents (IR or NQO1-bioactivatable drug) alone. Head and neck cancers, PDA and NSCLC have been shown to be sensitive to nontoxic doses of β-lapachone when combined with IR [21, 32]. Using NQO1-bioactivatable drugs as radiosensitizers leads to increases in ROS, γH2AX formation, hyperactivation of PARP1, massive NAD+ and ATP losses, inhibition of DSB repair, perturbation in carbon flux pathways and μ-Calpain mediated programmed necrosis known as NAD + -Keresis. The cell death responses observed are independent of any oncogenic drivers [21, 31–33]. This lethal combination between radiation therapy and NQO1-bioactivatable drugs prolongs long-term survival and promotes enhanced tumor shrinkage at non-toxic doses of each agent (IR and Drug, **Figure 4**). Thus, combining NQO1-bioactivatable drugs with radiation therapy, should be a long-standing treatment modality for tumors overexpressing NQO1.

5. Discussion

5.1 Advantages of NQO1-bioactivatable drugs vs. other radiosensitizers

The major advantage of using NQO1-bioactivatable drugs as radiosensitizers is the tumor selectivity afforded by the drugs themselves. Synergy is afforded by a number of tumor-selective responses to the drugs. First, the dependence of the drugs on NQO1 levels is perfect for the specific treatment of various difficult-to-treat human cancers, including non-small cell lung, pancreatic, breast, prostate, and head and neck cancers. Tumor selectivity requires approximately 100 units of enzyme activity, whereas lower levels of NQO1 results in mild metabolomic alterations used for the treatment of metabolic syndromes [34]. Second, the minimum time of exposure of 30–120 min fits the pharmacokinetics of the drug. It should be noted that all studies thus far indicate that the drugs have to be available immediately after or at the same time as exposure with IR. Pre-treatment prior to IR is ineffective. Third, synergy between NQO1-bioactivatable drugs and IR occurs due to PARP1 hyperactivation causing massive NAD+ and ATP loss, preventing repair of the DNA damage created by IR. NQO1-bioactivatable drugs are highly specific to tumors, causing little normal tissue toxicity, which is unaffected by IR treatment [14, 16, 20, 25, 31]. Preclinical in vivo data suggest that radiosensitization trials with NQO1-bioactivatable drugs are warranted for non-small cell lung, pancreatic, breast prostate, and head and neck cancers.

5.2 Future directions for NQO1-bioactivatable drugs

A clinical trial of radiation sensitization effects of the new drug, isobutyldeoxynyboquione (IB-DNQ), against non-small cell lung (NSCLC) and/or pancreatic adenocarcinomas (PDAC) is warranted. These cancers are almost uniformly NOQ1 over-expressive and they have routinely low levels of catalase [14]. We have developed CLIA assessments of NQO1 status and enzymatic levels for these studies. The pharmacokinetics of IB-DNQ in these cancers, particularly in NSCLC and PDAC cancers, is relatively short at about 6 h, but long enough for sensitization of tumors to the NQO1-bioactivatable drug + IR. Biomarker and DSB repair kinetics are ongoing in our laboratory in preparation for these radiosensitization studies.

Acknowledgements

This work was supported by NIH/NCI R01s - CA210489 and CA224493 to David A. Boothman.

Author details

Naveen Singh[1], Edward A. Motea[1], Xiumei Huang[2], Colton L. Starcher[1], Jayne Silver[1], I-Ju Yeh[1], S. Louise Pay[1], Xiaolin Su[1], Kristen A. Russ[3], David A. Boothman[1†] and Erik A. Bey[1*]

1 Department of Biochemistry and Molecular Biology, Indiana University School of Medicine, Indianapolis, Indiana, United States of America

2 Department of Radiation Oncology, Simon Cancer Center, Indiana University School of Medicine, Indianapolis, Indiana, United States of America

3 Translational Research Core, Simon Cancer Center, Indiana University School of Medicine, Indianapolis, Indiana, United States of America

*Address all correspondence to: beye@iu.edu

† Deceased

References

[1] Brady LW. The changing role of radiation oncology in cancer management. Cancer. 1983;**51**:2506-2514

[2] Lederman M. The early history of radiotherapy: 1895-1939. International Journal of Radiation Oncology, Biology, Physics. 1981;7:639-648

[3] Ahmad SS, Duke S, Jena R, Williams MV, Burnet NG. Advances in radiotherapy. BMJ. 2012;**345**:e7765

[4] Durand RE. Roles of thiols in cellular radiosensitivity. International Journal of Radiation Oncology, Biology, Physics. 1984;**10**:1235-1238

[5] Wardman P. Chemical radiosensitizers for use in radiotherapy. Clinical Oncology (Royal College of Radiologists). 2007;**19**:397-417

[6] Lee MW, Parker WB, Xu B. New insights into the synergism of nucleoside analogs with radiotherapy. Radiation Oncology. 2013;**8**:223

[7] Revesz L, Palcic B. Radiation dose dependence of the sensitization by oxygen and oxygen mimic sensitizers. Acta Radiologica. Oncology. 1985;**24**:209-217

[8] Raleigh DR, Haas-Kogan DA. Molecular targets and mechanisms of radiosensitization using DNA damage response pathways. Future Oncology. 2013;**9**:219-233

[9] Boothman DA, Greer S, Pardee AB. Potentiation of halogenated pyrimidine radiosensitizers in human carcinoma cells by beta-lapachone (3,4-dihydro-2,2-dimethyl-2H-naphtho[1,2-b]pyran-5,6-dione), a novel DNA repair inhibitor. Cancer Research. 1987;**47**:5361-5366

[10] Pink JJ, Planchon SM, Tagliarino C, Varnes ME, Siegel D, Boothman DA. NAD(P)H:Quinone oxidoreductase activity is the principal determinant of beta-lapachone cytotoxicity. The Journal of Biological Chemistry. 2000;**275**:5416-5424

[11] Bentle MS, Reinicke KE, Bey EA, Spitz DR, Boothman DA. Calcium-dependent modulation of poly(ADP-ribose) polymerase-1 alters cellular metabolism and DNA repair. The Journal of Biological Chemistry. 2006;**281**:33684-33696

[12] Boothman DA, Pardee AB. Inhibition of radiation-induced neoplastic transformation by beta-lapachone. Proceedings of the National Academy of Sciences of the United States of America. 1989;**86**:4963-4967

[13] Boothman DA, Meyers M, Fukunaga N, Lee SW. Isolation of x-ray-inducible transcripts from radioresistant human melanoma cells. Proceedings of the National Academy of Sciences of the United States of America. 1993;**90**:7200-7204

[14] Huang X, Motea EA, Moore ZR, et al. Leveraging an NQO1 bioactivatable drug for tumor-selective use of poly(ADP-ribose) polymerase inhibitors. Cancer Cell. 2016;**30**:940-952

[15] Oh ET, Kim JW, Kim JM, et al. NQO1 inhibits proteasome-mediated degradation of HIF-1alpha. Nature Communications. 2016;**7**:13593

[16] Huang X, Dong Y, Bey EA, et al. An NQO1 substrate with potent antitumor activity that selectively kills by PARP1-induced programmed necrosis. Cancer Research. 2012;**72**:3038-3047

[17] Froeling FEM, Mosur Swamynathan M, Deschenes A, et al. Bioactivation of napabucasin triggers reactive oxygen species-mediated cancer cell death. Clinical Cancer Research. 2019

[18] Siegel D, Yan C, Ross D. NAD(P)H:Quinone oxidoreductase 1 (NQO1) in the sensitivity and resistance to antitumor quinones. Biochemical Pharmacology. 2012;**83**:1033-1040

[19] Terai K, Dong GZ, Oh ET, et al. Cisplatin enhances the anticancer effect of beta-lapachone by upregulating NQO1. Anti-Cancer Drugs. 2009;**20**:901-909

[20] Bey EA, Bentle MS, Reinicke KE, et al. An NQO1- and PARP-1-mediated cell death pathway induced in non-small-cell lung cancer cells by beta-lapachone. Proceedings of the National Academy of Sciences of the United States of America. 2007;**104**:11832-11837

[21] Li LS, Reddy S, Lin ZH, et al. NQO1-mediated tumor-selective lethality and radiosensitization for head and neck Cancer. Molecular Cancer Therapeutics. 2016;**15**:1757-1767

[22] Bentle MS, Reinicke KE, Dong Y, Bey EA, Boothman DA. Nonhomologous end joining is essential for cellular resistance to the novel antitumor agent, beta-lapachone. Cancer Research. 2007;**67**:6936-6945

[23] Tagliarino C, Pink JJ, Dubyak GR, Nieminen AL, Boothman DA. Calcium is a key signaling molecule in beta-lapachone-mediated cell death. The Journal of Biological Chemistry. 2001;**276**:19150-19159

[24] Tagliarino C, Pink JJ, Reinicke KE, Simmers SM, Wuerzberger-Davis SM, Boothman DA. Mu-calpain activation in beta-lapachone-mediated apoptosis. Cancer Biology & Therapy. 2003;**2**:141-152

[25] Bey EA, Reinicke KE, Srougi MC, et al. Catalase abrogates beta-lapachone-induced PARP1 hyperactivation-directed programmed necrosis in NQO1-positive breast cancers. Molecular Cancer Therapeutics. 2013;**12**:2110-2120

[26] Chakrabarti G, Silvers MA, Ilcheva M, et al. Tumor-selective use of DNA base excision repair inhibition in pancreatic cancer using the NQO1 bioactivatable drug, beta-lapachone. Scientific Reports. 2015;**5**:17066

[27] Silvers MA, Deja S, Singh N, et al. The NQO1 bioactivatable drug, beta-lapachone, alters the redox state of NQO1+ pancreatic cancer cells, causing perturbation in central carbon metabolism. The Journal of Biological Chemistry. 2017;**292**:18203-18216

[28] Moore Z, Chakrabarti G, Luo X, et al. NAMPT inhibition sensitizes pancreatic adenocarcinoma cells to tumor-selective, PAR-independent metabolic catastrophe and cell death induced by beta-lapachone. Cell Death & Disease. 2015;**6**:e1599

[29] Chakrabarti G, Gerber DE, Boothman DA. Expanding antitumor therapeutic windows by targeting cancer-specific nicotinamide adenine dinucleotide phosphate-biogenesis pathways. Clinical pharmacology: Advances and Applications. 2015;**7**:57-68

[30] Chakrabarti G, Moore ZR, Luo X, et al. Targeting glutamine metabolism sensitizes pancreatic cancer to PARP-driven metabolic catastrophe induced by ss-lapachone. Cancer & Metabolism. 2015;**3**:12

[31] Dong Y, Bey EA, Li LS, et al. Prostate cancer radiosensitization through poly(ADP-ribose) polymerase-1 hyperactivation. Cancer Research. 2010;**70**:8088-8096

[32] Motea EA, Huang X, Singh N, et al. NQO1-dependent, tumor-selective radiosensitization of non-small cell lung cancers. Clinical Cancer Research. 2019;**25**:2601-2609

[33] Planchon SM, Pink JJ, Tagliarino C, Bornmann WG, Varnes ME, Boothman DA. Beta-lapachone-induced apoptosis in human prostate cancer cells: Involvement of NQO1/xip3. Experimental Cell Research. 2001;**267**:95-106

[34] Li LS, Bey EA, Dong Y, et al. Modulating endogenous NQO1 levels identifies key regulatory mechanisms of action of beta-lapachone for pancreatic cancer therapy. Clinical Cancer Research. 2011;**17**:275-285

Chapter 10

Brachytherapy in Endometrial Cancer

Mehmet Sait Bakir

Abstract

Endometrial cancer is the most common gynecologic cancer in developed countries with the cumulative risk rate of 1.71%. Endometrial cancer standard treatment is surgery. But adjuvant radiotherapy may be recommended for patients in advanced age who have high-grade disease, deep myometrial invasion, LVSI positivity, risk factors such as large tumor diameter, lymph node invasion, and advanced stage disease. Brachytherapy is applied in two ways, namely intra-cavitary or interstitial radiation therapy. Intra-cavitary brachytherapy is the presence of a therapeutic radioactive isotope within the body space, for example, vaginal and intra-uterine brachytherapy. Radioactive isotopes are directly inserted within the tissue in interstitial brachytherapy as in the treatment of cervical or endometrial cancers that have reached the lateral walls. The intra-cavitary brachytherapy technique is the most commonly used technique in gynecologic oncology. Standard treatment cannot be performed in a group of patients due to their medical disorders and clinical performances. In these patients, definitive radiotherapy is applied for clinical stage 1 patients, neo-adjuvant therapy is applied to patients with local advanced stage disease and brachytherapy alone or radiotherapy with addition of EBRT is applied as palliative treatment in patients who have complaints such as bleeding and pelvic pain.

Keywords: endometrial cancer, vaginal brachytherapy, high dose rate (HDR), medically inoperable, vaginal boost

1. Introduction

Endometrial cancer is the most common gynecologic cancer in developed countries with the cumulative risk rate of 1.71% [1]. The median age at the time of diagnosis is 63 years and about 90% of the patients are above 50 years of age. However, 4% of the patients are diagnosed under the age of 40 years [2]. The vast majority (80%) of endometrial cancer patients are diagnosed at early stages and while the 5-year survival rate is 95%, it significantly decreases in patients with local and distant metastases (68 and 17%, respectively) [3]. The standard treatment of endometrial cancer is total abdominal hysterectomy and bilateral salpingo-oophorectomy (TAH + BSO). Lymphadenectomy is performed in suitable patients when indicated [4, 5]. Adjuvant radiotherapy may be recommended for patients in advanced age who have high-grade disease, deep myometrial invasion, LVSI positivity, risk factors such as large tumor diameter, lymph node invasion and advanced stage disease (**Table 1**) [6–9].

	PORTEC-1	GOG 99
Age	>60	See below
Grad·	3	2–3
Myometrial invasion	>50% (outer 1/2)	>66.6%·(outer 1/3)
Lvmphvasctilar space invasion	N/A	Present
High-intermediate risk group	At least 2/3 of above	any age, all three of above risk factors age > 50, two of above risk factors age > 70, one of above risk factors

FIGO, International Federation of Gynecology and Obstetrics; PORTEC, postoperative radiation therapy in endometrial cancer; GOG, gynecologic oncology group.

Table 1.
High-intermediate risk groups in FIGO stage I endometrial cancer as defined by PORTEC-1 and GOG 99.

The risk groups had previously been addressed in many studies (PORTEC-1, GOG 99 studies) and finally a consensus was reached by the European Society For Medical Oncology (ESMO), European Society for Radiotherapy and Oncology (ESTRO) and the European Society Of Gynecological Oncology (ESGO) in 2014 (**Table 2**) [9].

In the randomized controlled studies of GOG (Gynecological Oncology Group) 99 and PORTEC-1 (Operative Radiation Therapy in Endometrial Cancer), the patients who had intermediate risk factors were divided to two groups and while one group received external beam radiotherapy (EBRT), the other group was followed-up without treatment. The groups in both studies have been presented in **Table 1** [6, 8].

No effect could be demonstrated on the overall survival in either of the two studies. However, the recurrence rate decreased to 3–6% from 12 to 15% in patients with intermediate risk factors who received EBRT. In the subgroup analyses, while the recurrence rate decreased to 5–6% from 18 to 26% in patients in the high-intermediate (H-I) risk group, it decreased to 2% from 5 to 6% in the low-intermediate risk group. Side effects of radiation therapy were seen at a high rate in both studies despite an excellent local control. While the toxic effect rate was 26% in the EBRT group in PORTEC 1, it was 4% in the untreated group ($p < 0.0001$) [10]. Hematological, genitor-urinary, gastro-intestinal and skin complications were also significantly higher in the GOG 99 study group compared

Risk group	Description
Low	Stage I endometrioid, erade 1–2, <50% myometrial invasion, LVSI negative
Intermediate	Stage I endometrioid, grade 1–2, ≥50% myometrial invasion, LVSI negative
High-intermediate	Stage I endometrioid, grade 3, <50% myometrial invasion, regardless of LVSI status Stage I endometrioid. 1–2, LVSI unequivocally positive, regardless of depth of invasion
High	Stage I endometrioid, grade 3, ≥50% myometrial invasion, regardless of LVSI status Stage II Stage III endometrioid. no residual disease Non-endometrioid (serous or clear cell or undifferentiated carcinoma, or carcinosarcoma)
Advanced	Stage III residual disease and stage IVA
Metastatic	Stage IVB

Table 2.
New risk groups to guide adjuvant therapy use.

to the untreated group [6]. In the long-term quality of life data of the PORTEC-1 study, urinary and intestinal functions were found to be poorer compared to the untreated group [11]. Local radiation therapies have come to the foreground due to the high incidence of the toxic effects of pelvic EBRT and their significance has gradually increased. Brachytherapy is applied in two ways, namely intra-cavitary or interstitial radiation therapy. Intra-cavitary brachytherapy is the presence of a therapeutic radioactive isotope within the body space, for example, vaginal and intra-uterine brachytherapy. Radioactive isotopes are directly inserted within the tissue in interstitial brachytherapy as in the treatment of cervical or endometrial cancers that have reached the lateral walls. The intra-cavitary brachytherapy technique is the most commonly used technique in gynecologic oncology.

2. Vaginal brachytherapy

2.1 Vaginal brachytherapy (VB) application

2.1.1 Vaginal applicators

Various vaginal applicators are available in gynecologic oncology depending on the location of the radiation source and whether it contains a cover or not. The Fletcher-Suit-Delclos system is among the most commonly used (**Figure 1**). Vaginal ring applicators are mostly used in HDR. Cylinder vaginal applicators, i.e., Delclos dome cylinder are used in patients undergoing hysterectomy (**Figure 2**).

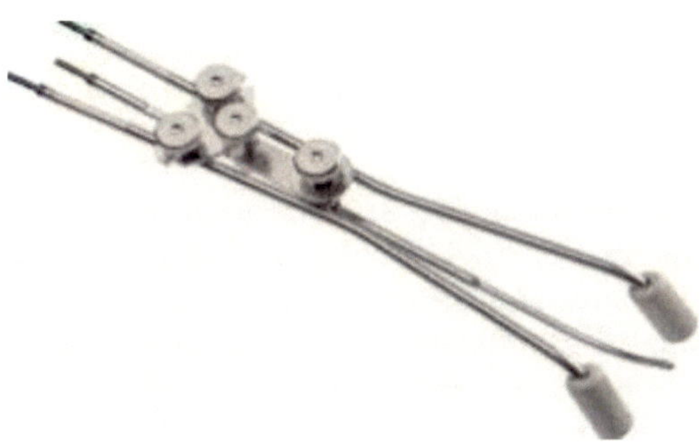

Figure 1.
Vaginal ring applicator.

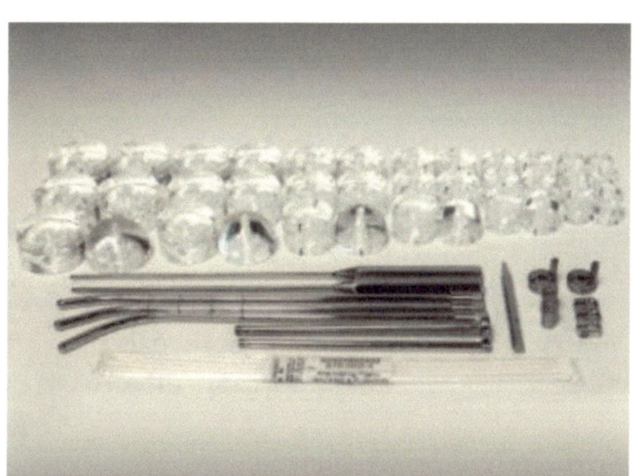

Figure 2.
Cylinder vaginal applicators (Delclos dome cylinder).

Single-channel cylinder applicator is among the most commonly used applicators; it minimizes the toxic effects as it is simple and since it covers the whole of the vaginal surface [12]. Multi-channel vaginal cylinder applicators are less harmful to neighboring tissues through providing asymmetrical dose radiation; however, they have a higher effect on the vaginal mucosa [13, 14].

Despite the presence of variable applicators, they have similar efficiency in the prevention of vaginal recurrence.

2.1.2 Dose depth

Despite the absence of a standard dose depth, vaginal lymphatics were reported to proceed 3 mm beneath the mucosa and treatment covering this depth was reported to be sufficient. Normally, a 1 cm depth is targeted. The most common monotherapy is a 0.5 cm depth and 7 Gy 3 fraction [12]. The doses effective in the vaginal surface when used as vaginal boost treatment have been reported by the Radiation Therapy Oncology Group [15].

2.1.3 Vaginal length

There is no consensus on the vaginal length to be treated. It has been reported that the proximal vagina can be treated between 1 and 10 cm [16]. The American Brachytherapy Society (ABS) has reported that the proximal vagina should be treated 3–5 cm or including 1/2–1/3 of the vagina [17]. Due to the possibility of high toxic doses causing vaginal stenosis and due to the decreasing frequency of distal vaginal recurrence, the treatment modalities that cover the whole vagina are gradually decreasing [12].

2.1.4 Dose rate

All vaginal brachytherapy applications had been carried out as LDR before the introduction of HDR [4]. Historically, low dose hourly 60 cGy had been used widespread in most brachytherapy regimens. This treatment modality given as LDR was taking long and it required hospitalization. About 96% of brachy therapists have switched to this method through the introduction of HDR applicators [17]. The advantages of HDR include less radiation exposure of the health staff and visitors as it enables remote control, thrombo-embolic events are less frequently encountered as the patients are treated in the outpatient setting and long-term immobilization is avoided. There is no difference between LDR and HDR with regard to recurrence and the overall survival [18].

2.1.5 Treatment plan

There are many ways for an accurate treatment plan in VB applications. When 2D and 3D CT-based treatment plans were compared, the 3D method was found to be superior as it reached the clinical target volume and produced less harm to neighboring tissues [19]. Many brachy therapists use the 3D treatment plan and its application at every session separately was not found to be superior to single session application, except for being expensive [20]. The CT-based treatment plan reveals the air between the vaginal cuff and the applicator effectively and enables a more effective treatment [21].

2.1.6 Dose and duration of vaginal brachytherapy

The toxic dose that emerges during VB is related to the amount of the total dose, dose velocity, total vaginal length, dose depth and the fraction time. In a study, the patients who received VB with HDR were allocated to four groups as 4 fractions of 9.0 Gy, 5 fractions of 6.0 Gy, 6 fractions of 5.0 Gy and 6 fractions of 4.5 Gy. A 1 cm depth from the vaginal surface was utilized. Vaginal, urinary bladder and rectal toxicity were found to increase as the amount of the dose increased along with the fraction [22]. In another study, no grade 2 or above vaginal, urinary bladder and rectal toxicity were encountered when 6 fractions of 4.0 Gy VB was applied targeted only to the vaginal surface [23]. The ABS recommends HDR VB as 24 treatment schemes as monotherapy and the 22 treatment scheme as boost dose [12]. In the PORTEC-4 study conducted for standardization of the dose and the fraction amount, the patients with H-I risk, early stage endometrial cancer were divided into treatment and observation groups; the treatment group was randomized as 3 fractions of 7.0 Gy or 3 fractions of 5.0 Gy. However, the study was terminated early as the patient collection and the untreated group were not proper. Therefore, further studies are required for standardization of the dose amount and the duration of fraction.

2.1.7 Protection from vaginal toxicity

Vaginal toxicity is a significant complication of VB and it impairs the quality of sexual life due to vaginal atrophy, shortness and narrowness. The sexual activity frequency and satisfaction are reduced in patients undergoing surgery and VB [24]. In a study, having sexual intercourse during the VB treatment was reported to prevent vaginal shortness and narrowness; however, atrophy-related dyspareunia was reported in 2/3 of the patients and furthermore, it was emphasized that the distal 2/3 of the vagina was more susceptible to toxic effects rather than the proximal 1/3 of the vagina [22]. Use of vaginal dilator for 6 months following radiotherapy was shown to decrease the vaginal stenosis [25]. In the Cochrane database, use of vaginal dilator during radiotherapy was not shown to have sufficient evidence. However, it accepts the observational studies suggesting that use of the regular vaginal dilator may improve the vaginal stenosis rates reported by the patients [26]. Estrogen cream is another option for protection of the vagina. Despite the absence of sufficient and strong evidence about the use of estrogen creams, they were shown to prevent vaginal atrophy in small studies [27]. A selection should be made after discussing the benefits and harms of this treatment option with the patient.

3. Adjuvant vaginal brachytherapy treatment

3.1 Adjuvant vaginal brachytherapy as monotherapy

As reported above, we know that pelvic EBRT reduces the recurrence; however, it leads to severe side effects compared to follow-up without treatment in endometrial cancer. Radiotherapy via the vaginal route was considered to be more proper as vaginal recurrences are seen most in post-operative endometrial cancer patients. Similarly, with pelvic EBRT, VB treatment was not shown to be effective on the overall survival. However, while the vaginal recurrence rate is 0–3.1% in VB, the pelvic recurrence rate is 0–4.1% [28–30]. These rates are similar with pelvic EBRT and related to the lower toxic effects.

In the randomized controlled PROTEC-2 study comparing the effectiveness of pelvic EBRT and VB treatment, all patients were H-I risk endometrial cancer patients who had undergone TAH + BSO, but not lymphadenectomy. The patients were allocated to three groups as the group that received 23 fractions 46 Gy as pelvic EBRT, the high dose rate (HDR) group that received 7 Gyx3 fractions and the low dose rate (LDR) group that received 30 Gy VB. While the 5-year vaginal recurrence was 1.8% with VB, it was 1.6% in the pelvic EBRT group (p = 0.74). The pelvic recurrence rate was higher in the VB group (3.8% vs. 0.5%, p = 0.02). However, the gastrointestinal side effects were significantly lower in the VB group compared to the EBRT group [30].

3.2 Adjuvant vaginal brachytherapy as boost

A better loco-regional control can be achieved by adding VB to pelvic EBRT and the rate of vaginal recurrence would be seen as 0–2.7% and the rate of pelvic recurrence as 0.3–4.0% [29, 31–33]. Despite the absence of EBRT+/-VB randomized controlled study, boost VB may be added in the treatment of high risk patients whose vaginal recurrence is high and who receive low dose EBRT (45 Gy at 1.8 Gy/fractions). There are randomized controlled studies comparing EBRT + boost VB and VB alone. In one of these studies, while the total pelvic recurrence rate was 0.4% in EBRT + boost VB group, it was 5.3% in the VB only group (p = 0.013). No difference was found between the groups with regard to vaginal recurrence and overall survival; however, the radiation toxicity was lower in the VB group [33]. In the studies of RTOG, applying 5–6 Gy VB boost only onto the vaginal surface as 45 Gy EBRTx3 fractions or 50.4 Gy EBRTx2 fractions is recommended [34, 35].

3.3 Vaginal brachytherapy and chemotherapy

The effect of adding chemotherapy (CT) to VB was investigated particularly in high risk endometrial cancer patients who had the likelihood of distant metastasis. In a study conducted by Landrum et al., the 2-year progression-free survival was 91% in 23 patients including H-I risk early stage endometrial cancer, uterine serous carcinoma (USC) and clear cell carcinoma (CCC). Vaginal recurrence occurred in one patient (4.2%); this patient also had distant metastasis [36]. The effect of VB + CT was investigated in the GOG 249 randomized controlled study. In that study, while one group received EBRT, another group received VB + CT (3 cycles of carboplatin and paclitaxel). The study included the GOG 99 H-I risk patients, patients with stromal invasion and stage 1–2 USC and CCC. While the overall survival was 92% in the EBRT group, it was 92% in the VB + CT group at the end of the 2-year follow-up (p = NS). There was no significant difference between the vaginal recurrence rates in the two groups. While hematologic toxicity, neuropathy and fatigue were more common in the VB + CT arm, grade 2 diarrhea was more common in the EBRT arm [37].

4. Vaginal brachytherapy treatment in high-risk histology

More aggressive treatments are used in uterine serous cancer (USC), clear cell carcinoma (CCC) and carcino-sarcoma (CS), which are the high risk histologies of endometrial cancer [38]. Most of the large studies including PORTEC-1, GOG 99 and PORTEC-2 [6, 8, 30] included early stage endometrial cancer patients and not high-risk patients. However, in the GOG 249 study, 20% of the patients were USC and CCC patients [37]. In a study conducted by Creasman et al., the outcomes of stage 1 high risk patients were found to be similar to those of grade 3 endometrioid type adeno-carcinoma patients [39]. Despite the presence of vaginal recurrence at a rate of 0–2.7% in stage 1–2 patients with high risk histology, the pelvic recurrence rate was found to be 0–9% [40–43]. In a study investigating USC patients, while the 5-year survival rate was 94% in patients who received VB + CT, it was 65% in patients who received LDR + EBRT but not CT [40]. In another study, USC patients received VB + CT (six cycles of carboplatin and paclitaxel) and the vaginal, pelvic and distant metastasis rates were found to be 0, 9, and 10%, respectively, and the 5-year survival rate was 90% [41]. The effectiveness of VB alone was investigated in endometrial cancer patients with high risk histology. Some authors reported that CT did not have a great contribution [42, 43].

4.1 Brachytherapy for treatment of medically inoperable endometrial cancer

As mentioned above, the standard treatment of endometrial cancer is TAH + BSO (total abdominal hysterectomy + bilateral salphingo-oopherectomy) and lymphadenectomy when indicated, however, this standard treatment cannot be performed in a group of patients due to their medical disorders and clinical performances. In these patients, definitive radiotherapy is applied for clinical stage 1 patients, neo-adjuvant therapy is applied to patients with local advanced stage disease and brachytherapy alone or radiotherapy with addition of EBRT is applied as palliative treatment in patients who have complaints such as bleeding and pelvic pain. While LDR VB+/−EBRT has been used recently in the treatment of these patients, HDR VB+/−EBRT is widely used today [44, 45]. The treatment of medically inoperable endometrial cancer patients is planned better and more effectively through advancements in radiology.

4.1.1 Patient characteristics

Medically inoperable endometrial cancer patients should be meticulously evaluated pre-operatively by a gynecologic oncologist. Most of these patients have cardiac diseases, pulmonary diseases, hypertension, diabetes mellitus, cerebro-vascular disease, renal disease, syndromes such as Marfan syndrome, advanced age and other malignancies. Morbid obesity is a relative contra-indication for the operation depending on the experience of the surgeon and the condition of the patient. Clinical performance of the patients is of vital importance as a pre-operative parameter. All of these patients should be evaluated pre-operatively for local or general anesthesia by experienced anesthetists. The hormone therapy (progestin, aromatase inhibitors) option is also available besides the radiotherapy option for clinical stage 1, grade 1 patients who are not eligible for surgery, for patients with endometrioid type endometrial cancer, for those below the age of 40 years and those willing to have a child [46]. Regression has been detected in 55% of the patients treated in this way [47].

Levonorgestrel-releasing intra-uterine devices (LNGIUDs) may be added to treatment of patients who have precancerous and stage 1, grade 1 endometrioid type endometrial cancer [48]. The patients are meticulously evaluated with CT or MRI with regard to tumor diameter, myometrial invasion depth, cervical involvement, ovarian involvement and pelvic para-aortic lymph node involvement if hormone therapy is planned, as oral regimens have the likelihood of recurrence at a rate of 25% despite the 50% or above success rates [49]. While endometrial cancer staging is done surgically according to the recent International Federation of Gynecology and Obstetrics (FIGO) 2009 classification, clinical staging is used in medically inoperable patients (**Table 3**) [50].

The patients should be meticulously evaluated for pelvic examination and distant metastasis if clinical staging would be used. Vagina, cervix and the uterus are evaluated, presence of a mass lesion is examined and the search for parametrium involvement is attempted through bimanual (rectal-vaginal) examination. Computed tomographies of the thorax, abdomen and the pelvis are performed for distant metastasis and MRI is used for assessment of the uterus and the pelvis as the negative predictive value is >85% for myometrial invasion in contrast-enhanced T2-weighted

IA-Uterine cavity sounds to <8 cm
IB-Uterine cavity sounds to >8 cm
Stage II-Involves the corpus and cervix
Stage III-Parametrium, adnexa, or vagina but confined to true pelvis
Stage IVA-Involving local structures (rectum/bladder)
Stage IVB-Metastatic

Table 3.
Clinical staging system for endometrial cancer.

Structure	Image data set	Definition
Gross tumor volume	T2-wcightcd MRI	Visible abnormality if present
clinical target volume	MRI or CT	Entire uterus, cervix, and upper 1–2 cm of the vagina
Organs at risk	MRI or CT	Sigmoid, rectum, bladder, bowel, and uninvolved lower third of the vagina

CT, computed tomography; MRI, magnetic resonance imaging.
Note. MRI is required if a gross tumor volume is to be contoured. The clinical target volume includes the entire uterus, cervix, and upper vagina. Organs at risk include bladder, rectum, and sigmoid.

Table 4.
Recommended structures for volume-based planning in medically inoperable endometrial cancer.

MRI and the positive predictive value is low [51]. 18-F-fluoro-deoxyglucose positron emission tomography (PET) is used for lymph node involvement [52, 53]. In a study conducted with PET-CT, the pelvic node involvement rate was 63% and the para-aortic lymph node involvement was 95% [54].

4.1.2 Dose standards and technical properties

The target volume has been defined as the whole uterus, cervix and the upper 3–5 cm of the vagina for inoperable endometrial cancer in the 2000 ABS guideline and mainly MRI, and if MRI is not available, CT was recommended for the treatment plan [55]. The risks for the neighboring organs should be considered when performing volume-based treatment through MRI or CT [56] (**Table 4**).

In a study of Gill et al., 38 inoperable endometrial cancer patients underwent volume-based treatment and the gross tumor volume (GTV) and the clinical target volume (CTV) were determined with MRI in 19 patients and with CT in the remaining 19. While 20 patients received a mean 37.5 Gy VB in 4–5 fractions, 20 patients received 45 Gy EBRT followed by 25 Gy boost VB treatment. While the local control rate was 90.6% for 2 years, the overall survival rate was 94.4%. Hemorrhage developed in only one patient during the applicator placement and she received blood transfusion. No patients had grade 3 or acute and late complications [57]. The patients should be referred to centers where MRI or CT is available or their treatment should be attempted by using ultrasonography and radiography.

4.1.3 Treatment

1. HDR VB may be used alone in patients who have clinical stage 1, grade 1–2 myometrial invasion of less than 50 [56]%. GTV is specified in the course of brachytherapy with MRI and the whole uterus and its serosa are irradiated (CTV). For minimal harm to the neighboring tissues (OAT), the limit is 70–75 Gy for the rectum and the sigmoid, and 80–100 Gy for the urinary bladder. The HDR dose schemas for these patients have been presented in **Table 5**.

2. Pelvic EBRT+HDR VB is recommended for clinical stage 1 patients with myometrial invasion >50%. EBRT is applied 45–50 Gy so as to include all pelvic lymph nodes, the whole uterus and 1–2 cm proximal of vagina. Dose schemas are presented in **Table 6** for these patients.

3. Patients with clinical stage 2 endometrial cancer are given pelvic EBRT + HDR VB. This treatment modality is also valid for clinics that do not have MRI. The doses presented in **Table 6** are used.

4. Higher doses of pelvic EBRT (including all lymphatic regions) up to 65 Gy + HDR VB are given to patients with clinical stage 3 endometrial cancer. The doses presented in **Table 6** are used.

4.1.4 Management of recurrent disease after definitive radiation

Radiotherapy options are quite limited in biopsy-proven recurrences after definitive radiation treatment. It may only be used for palliative purposes in vaginal hemorrhage and pelvic pain. Hormone therapy and chemotherapy options should be considered in patients with recurrence [58].

4.2 Treatment-related toxicity from the use of radiation therapy for endometrial cancer

In the literature, radiotherapy was shown to have been used in 60% of cervical cancers, 45% of endometrial cancers and 100% of vaginal cancers [59, 60]. Healthy cervical and uterine tissues are known to tolerate radiation therapy (RT) well. Although pregnancy is known to have occurred in women receiving 20–30 Gy RT for the uterus, an atrophic uterus improper for pregnancy develops in women

HDR total dose (Gy)	HDR dose fractionation	EQD_2 (Gy)
36	6 Gy × 6	48
38.4	6.4 Gy × 6	52.5
363	7.3 Gy × 5	52.6
34	8.5 Gy × 4	52.4
40–50	5 Gy × 9–10	50–62.5

Table 5.
HDR dose table.

EBRT (Gy)	HDR total dose (Gy)	HDR dose fractionation	EQD_2 (Gy)
45	19.5	6.5 Gy × 3	71.1
45	18.9	6.3 Gy × 3	69.9
45	20.8	5.2 Gy × 4	70.6
45	25	5 Gy × 5	75
45	17	8.5 Gy × 2	70.5
50.4	12	6.0 Gy × 2	65.6
50.4	22.5	3.75 Gy × 6	75.3

Table 6.
EBRT and HDR dose schemas.

receiving 40–50 Gy. The toxic effect of RT depends on the age for ovaries; exposure to 20 Gy usually results in ovarian insufficiency in an adult woman. The influence of RT on the vagina depends on the location (superior, medial, inferior, posterior or the anterior wall). While the proximal vagina seems to be resistant to high doses (>100 Gy), the distal and the posterior walls are susceptible to atrophy and stenosis. While the rectum and the urinary bladder can be treated with low risk with 45–50 Gy RT, the small intestine shows severe toxic effects against <30 Gy, depending on the treated volume. These toxic effects of RT are known to be related to the treated tissue amount, fraction number and dose, previous surgeries, concurrent chemotherapies, co-morbid conditions and the smoking status [61].

Acute toxicity is defined as conditions that develop in the course of RT.

Sub-acute toxicity is defined as conditions that develop between 4 and 12 weeks after termination of RT.

Late toxicity is defined as the irreversible reactions that develop 3 months after termination of the treatment.

4.2.1 Genito-urinary (GU) system toxicity

The patient is asked to come to the treatment with a full urinary bladder with the aim of moving away the bowels as the urinary bladder can tolerate RT relatively better than the bowels.

4.2.1.1 Acute radiation cystitis

This is among the most common RT-induced complications. The patients present with urinary symptoms (dysuria, frequency, urgency and nocturia). Infectious cystitis should be excluded. The symptoms usually recover spontaneously within 1–2 weeks. Genitor-urinary complaints were reported to be seen less frequently when adjuvant therapy was performed with intensity-modulated radiation therapy (IMRT) [62].

4.2.1.2 Late genito-urinary toxicity

This toxic effect of RT emerges as the urinary bladder epithelium and the micro-vascular circulation are affected. Fibrosis and collagen accumulate under the epithelium and the muscle layer, and the urinary bladder capacity decreases. This effect leads to over-activity and contraction of the urinary bladder resulting in urge incontinence. In the PORTEC-1 study, while grade 3–4 toxicity was not observed, the rate of grade 1–2 genito-urinary complication was 5% higher [11].

Hematuria and ulcer formation are the late GU findings. Recurrent urinary bladder stones may be formed. Ureto-vaginal or vesico-vaginal fistulae may also develop following brachytherapy [63].

4.2.2 Gastro-intestinal (GI) toxicity

Gastro-intestinal toxicity may develop during RT or later and impair the quality of life of the patients through leading to restrictions in the daily lives of the patients.

4.2.2.1 Acute RT toxicity

As the small intestine epithelium shows a rapid proliferation, it is affected to a higher extent by RT. While nausea and vomiting are seen at the beginning of the treatment, abdominal cramps and diarrhea are experienced during the following 2–3 weeks. This effect is considered to result from the disappearance of small intestine crypts and the inability to restore them in a short while [64]. The acute effects in the colon include fecal urgency and tenesmus. Acute colonic problems are seen in approximately 50% of the patients who receive 45–50 Gy as adjuvant; however, acute grade 3 toxicity is lower than 3% [10, 30]. There are randomized studies reporting that these acute effects may be significantly reduced by using IMRT [65].

4.2.2.2 Late GI toxicity

Late effects may develop between 6 months and several years in most patients. The pathophysiology includes chronic enteropathy with mucosal atrophy and loss of mucin-producing goblet cells. Fibrosis in the intestinal walls causes dysmotility and acute obstruction. There are no techniques that do not cause late intestinal complications, including IMRT. The late toxic intestinal effects include chronic diarrhea, malabsorption, recurrent ileus, mucosal ulcer, telangiectasias and rectal proctopathy.

4.2.3 Vaginal toxicity

Vaginal complications are commonly seen both during pelvic EBRT and VB. This toxic effect impairs the quality of life of the patients by leading to sexual dysfunction. Vaginal toxicity above grade 2 was not reported when the vaginal cuff was treated with HDR VB alone in a study [23].

4.2.3.1 Acute vaginal mucositis

Erythema and superficial ulcers develop as a result of vaginal surface epithelium injury in patients receiving brachytherapy. This leads to exudative vaginal discharge and may result in secondary infections.

4.2.3.2 Vaginal ulceration and necrosis

This complication is particularly seen when interstitial brachytherapy is used for treatment of full-thickness vaginal mucosa involvement [66].

4.2.3.3 Vaginal stenosis

This is a common late complication of both pelvic EBRT and VB. Dyspareunia is common due to reduced vaginal length. Vaginal stenosis and complete closure should be prevented to achieve a satisfactory follow-up. Stenosis usually develops 3–6 months after therapy. Vaginal dilators with proper thickness and length are used for the primary repair in these patients. While some authors propose that the use of vaginal dilators after RT reduces the stenosis, some others propose that it is not much effective [67].

Author details

Mehmet Sait Bakir
Division of Gyneacologic Oncology, Department of Gyneacology Obstetrics, Akdeniz University, Antalya, Turkey

*Address all correspondence to: sabakcil@gmail.com

References

[1] WHO. GLOBOCAN 2012: Estimated Cancer Incidence, Mortality and Prevalence Worldwide in 2012. 2012. Available from: http://globocan.iarc.fr/Pages/fact_sheets_population.aspx [Accessed: 03 April 2015]

[2] Lee NK, Cheung MK, Shin JY, et al. Prognostic factors for uterine cancer in reproductive-aged women. Obstetrics and Gynecology. 2007;**109**:655Y662

[3] National Cancer Institute. Endometrial Cancer Treatment. Physician Data Query (PDQ). 2015. Available from: http://www.cancer.gov/cancertopics/pdq/treatment/endometrial/healthprofessional [Accessed: 01 April 2015]

[4] Aalders J, Abeler V, Kolstad P, et al. Postoperative external irradiation and prognostic parameters in stage I endometrial carcinoma: Clinical and histopathologic study of 540 patients. Obstetrics and Gynecology. 1980;**56**:419-427. [PubMed: 6999399]

[5] Creasman WT, Morrow CP, Bundy BN, et al. Surgical pathologic spread patterns of endometrial cancer. A gynecologic oncology group study. Cancer. 1987;**60**:2035-2041. [PubMed: 3652025]

[6] Keys HM, Roberts JA, Brunetto VL, et al. A phase III trial of surgery with or without adjunctive external pelvic radiation therapy in intermediate risk endometrial adenocarcinoma: A gynecologic oncology group study. Gynecologic Oncology. 2004;**92**:744-751. [PubMed: 14984936]

[7] Canlorbe G, Bendifallah S, Laas E, et al. Tumor size, an additional prognostic factor to include in low-risk endometrial cancer: Results of a French multicenter study. Annals of Surgical Oncology. 2016;**23**(1):171-177

[8] Creutzberg CL, van Putten WL, Koper PC, et al. Surgery and postoperative radiotherapy versus surgery alone for patients with stage-1 endometrial carcinoma: Multicentre randomised trial. PORTEC study group. Post Operative Radiation Therapy in Endometrial Carcinoma. Lancet. 2000;**355**:1404-1411. [PubMed: 10791524]

[9] Colombo N, Creutzberg C, Amant F, Bosse T, González-Martín A, Ledermann J, et al. ESMO-ESGO-ESTRO endometrial consensus conference working group. International Journal of Gynecological Cancer. 2016;**26**(1):2-30. DOI: 10.1097/IGC.0000000000000609. PMID:26645990

[10] Creutzberg CL, van Putten WL, Koper PC, et al. The morbidity of treatment for patients with stage I endometrial cancer: Results from a randomized trial. International Journal of Radiation Oncology, Biology, Physics. 2001;**51**:1246-1255. [PubMed: 11728684]

[11] Nout RA, van de Poll-Franse LV, Lybeert ML, et al. Long-term outcome and quality of life of patients with endometrial carcinoma treated with or without pelvic radiotherapy in the post operative radiation therapy in endometrial carcinoma 1 (PORTEC-1) trial. Journal of Clinical Oncology. 2011;**29**:1692-1700. [PubMed: 21444867]

[12] Harkenrider MM, Grover S, Erickson BA, et al. Vaginal brachytherapy for postoperative endometrial cancer: 2014 survey of the American brachytherapy society. Brachytherapy. 2016;**15**(1):23-29

[13] Tanderup K, Lindegaard JC. Multi-channel intracavitary vaginal brachytherapy using three-dimensional optimization of source geometry.

Radiotherapy and Oncology. 2004;**70**:81-85. [PubMed: 15036856]

[14] Bahadur YA, Constantinescu C, Hassouna AH, et al. Single versus multichannel applicator in high-dose-rate vaginal brachytherapy optimized by inverse treatment planning. Journal of Contemporary Brachytherapy. 2015;**6**:362-370. [PubMed: 25834580]

[15] Jhingran A, Winter K, Portelance L, et al. A phase II study of intensity modulated radiation therapy (IMRT) to the pelvic for post-operative patients with endometrial carcinoma (RTOG 0418). International Journal of Radiation Oncology, Biology, Physics. 2008;**72**:S16-S17

[16] Owens K, Patel H, Yashar C, et al. Vaginal cuff brachytherapy for endometrial carcinoma: Results of limiting vaginal coverage to one centimeter length. Brachytherapy. 2007;**6**:98-99

[17] Small W Jr, Beriwal S, Demanes DJ, et al. American brachytherapy society consensus guidelines for adjuvant vaginal cuff brachytherapy after hysterectomy. Brachytherapy. 2012;**11**:58-67. [PubMed: 22265439]

[18] Fayed A, Mutch DG, Rader JS, et al. Comparison of high-dose-rate and low-dose-rate brachytherapy in the treatment of endometrial carcinoma. International Journal of Radiation Oncology, Biology, Physics. 2007;**67**:480-484. [PubMed: 17141980]

[19] Kim H, Kim H, Houser C, et al. Is there any advantage to three-dimensional planning for vaginal cuff brachytherapy? Brachytherapy. 2012;**11**:398-401. [PubMed: 22301073]

[20] Zhou J, Prisciandaro J, Lee C, et al. Single or multi-channel vaginal cuff high-dose-rate brachytherapy: Is replanning necessary prior to each fraction? Practical Radiation Oncology. 2014;**4**:20-26. [PubMed: 24621419]

[21] Humphrey P, Cornes P, Al-Booz H. Vaginal vault brachytherapy in endometrial cancer: Verifying target coverage with image-guided applicator placement. The British Journal of Radiology. 2013;**86**:20120428. [PubMed: 23407428]

[22] Sorbe BG, Smeds AC. Postoperative vaginal irradiation with high dose rate afterloading technique in endometrial carcinoma stage I. International Journal of Radiation Oncology, Biology, Physics. 1990;**18**:305-314. [PubMed: 2303363]

[23] Townamchai K, Lee L, Viswanathan AN. A novel low dose fractionation regimen for adjuvant vaginal brachytherapy in early stage endometrioid endometrial cancer. Gynecologic Oncology. 2012;**127**:351-355. [PubMed: 22850411]

[24] Bruner DW, Lanciano R, Keegan M, et al. Vaginal stenosis and sexual function following intracavitary radiation for the treatment of cervical and endometrial carcinoma. International Journal of Radiation Oncology, Biology, Physics. 1993;**27**:825-830. [PubMed: 8244811]

[25] Law E, Kelvin JF, Thom B, et al. Prospective study of vaginal dilator use adherence and efficacy following radiotherapy. Radiotherapy and Oncology. 2015;**116**:149-155. [PubMed: 26164775]

[26] Miles T, Johnson N. Vaginal dilator therapy for women receiving pelvic radiotherapy. Cochrane Database of Systematic Reviews. 2014;**9**:CD007291

[27] Pitkin RM, VanVoorhis LW. Postirradiation vaginitis. An evaluation of prophylaxis with topical estrogen. Radiology. 1971;**99**:417-421. [PubMed: 5553582]

[28] Eldredge-Hindy HB, Eastwick G, Anne PR, et al. Adjuvant vaginal cuff brachytherapy for high-risk, early stage endometrial cancer. Journal of Contemporary Brachytherapy. 2014;**6**:262-270. [PubMed: 25337127]

[29] Paydar I, DeWees T, Powell M, et al. Adjuvant radiotherapy in stage II endometrial carcinoma: Is brachytherapy alone sufficient for local control? Brachytherapy. 2015;**14**:427-432. [PubMed: 25911995]

[30] Nout RA, Smit VT, Putter H, et al. Vaginal brachytherapy versus pelvic external beam radiotherapy for patients with endometrial cancer of high639 intermediate risk (PORTEC-2): An open-label, non-inferiority, randomised trial. Lancet. 2010;**375**:816-823. [PubMed: 20206777]

[31] Nori D, Merimsky O, Batata M, et al. Postoperative high dose-rate intravaginal brachytherapy combined with external irradiation for early stage endometrial cancer: A long-term follow-up. International Journal of Radiation Oncology, Biology, Physics. 1994;**30**:831-837. [PubMed: 7960984]

[32] Cannon GM, Geye H, Terakedis BE, et al. Outcomes following surgery and adjuvant radiation in stage II endometrial adenocarcinoma. Gynecologic Oncology. 2009;**113**:176-180. [PubMed: 19217147]

[33] Sorbe BG, Horvath G, Andersson H, et al. External pelvic and vaginal irradiation versus vaginal irradiation alone as postoperative therapy in medium-risk endometrial carcinoma: A prospective, randomized study--quality-of-life analysis. International Journal of Gynecological Cancer. 2012;**22**:1281-1288. [PubMed: 22864336]

[34] Jhingran A, Winter K, Portelance L, et al. A phase II study of intensity modulated radiation therapy (IMRT) to the pelvic for post-operative patients with endometrial carcinoma (RTOG 0418). International Journal of Radiation Oncology, Biology, Physics. 2008;**72**:S16-S17

[35] Viswanathan AN, Moughan J, Miller BE, et al. NRG oncology/RTOG 0921: A phase 2 study of postoperative intensity-modulated radiotherapy with concurrent cisplatin and bevacizumab followed by carboplatin and paclitaxel for patients with endometrial cancer. Cancer. 2015;**121**(13): 2156-2163

[36] Landrum LM, Nugent EK, Zuna RE, et al. Phase II trial of vaginal cuff brachytherapy followed by chemotherapy in early stage endometrial cancer patients with high-intermediate risk factors. Gynecologic Oncology. 2014;**132**:50-54. [PubMed: 24219982]

[37] McMeekin D, Filiaci V, Aghajanian C, et al. A randomized phase III trial of pelvic radiation therapy (PXRT) versus vaginal cuff brachytherapy followed by paclitaxel/carboplatin chemotherapy (VCB/C) in patients with high risk (HR), early stage endometrial cancer (EC): A gynecologic oncology group trial. Gynecologic Oncology. 2014;**134**:438

[38] Greven K, Winter K, Underhill K, et al. Final analysis of RTOG 9708: Adjuvant postoperative irradiation combined with cisplatin/paclitaxel chemotherapy following surgery for patients with high-risk endometrial cancer. Gynecologic Oncology. 2006;**103**:155-159. [PubMed: 16545437]

[39] Creasman WT, Kohler MF, Odicino F, et al. Prognosis of papillary serous, clear cell, and grade 3 stage I carcinoma of the endometrium. Gynecologic Oncology. 2004;**95**:593-596. [PubMed: 15581969]

[40] Turner BC, Knisely JP, Kacinski BM, et al. Effective treatment of stage I

uterine papillary serous carcinoma with high dose-rate vaginal apex radiation (192Ir) and chemotherapy. International Journal of Radiation Oncology, Biology, Physics. 1998;**40**:77-84. [PubMed: 9422561]

[41] Kiess AP, Damast S, Makker V, et al. Five-year outcomes of adjuvant carboplatin/paclitaxel chemotherapy and intravaginal radiation for stage I-II papillary serous endometrial cancer. Gynecologic Oncology. 2012;**127**:321-325. [PubMed: 22850412]

[42] Barney BM, Petersen IA, Mariani A, et al. The role of vaginal brachytherapy in the treatment of surgical stage I papillary serous or clear cell endometrial cancer. International Journal of Radiation Oncology, Biology, Physics. 2013;**85**:109-115. [PubMed: 22543202]

[43] Townamchai K, Berkowitz R, Bhagwat M, et al. Vaginal brachytherapy for early stage uterine papillary serous and clear cell endometrial cancer. Gynecologic Oncology. 2013;**129**:18-21. [PubMed: 23262378]

[44] ACR-ASTRO Practice Parameter for the Performance of Low-Dose Rate Brachytherapy. Available from: http://www.acr.org [Accessed: 11 May 2015]

[45] American College of Radiology. ACR-ASTRO Parameter for the Performance of High-Dose-Rate Brachytherapy. Available from: http://www.acr.org [Accessed: 11 May 2015]

[46] Baker J, Obermair A, Gebski V, Janda M. Efficacy of oral or intrauterine device-delivered progestin in patients with complex endometrial hyperplasia with atypia or early endometrial adenocarcinoma: A meta-analysis and systematic review of the literature. Gynecologic Oncology. 2012;**125**:263-270

[47] Ushijima K, Yahata H, Yoshikawa H, et al. Multicenter phase II study of fertility-sparing treatment with medroxyprogesterone acetate for endometrial carcinoma and atypical hyperplasia in young women. Journal of Clinical Oncology. 2007;**25**:2798-2803

[48] Orbo A, Vereide A, Arnes M. Levonorgestrel-impregnated intrauterine device as treatment for endometrial hyperplasia: A national multicentre randomised trial. BJOG. 2014;**121**:477-486

[49] Gunderson CC, Fader AN, Carson KA, et al. Oncologic and reproductive outcomes with progestin therapy in women with endometrial hyperplasia and grade 1 adenocarcinoma: A systematic review. Gynecologic Oncology. 2012;**125**:477-482

[50] Mikuta JJ. International Federation of Gynecology and Obstetrics staging of endometrial cancer 1988. Cancer. 1993;**71**:1460-1463

[51] Wu LM, Xu JR, Gu HY, et al. Predictive value of T2-weighted imaging and contrast-enhanced MR imaging in assessing myometrial invasion in endometrial cancer: A pooled analysis of prospective studies. European Radiology. 2013;**23**:435-449

[52] Crivellaro C, Signorelli M, Guerra L. et al, Tailoring systematic lymphadenectomy in high-risk clinical early stage endometrial cancer: The role of 18F-FDG PET/CT. Gynecologic Oncology. 2013;**130**:306-311

[53] Antonsen SL, Jensen LN, Loft A, et al. MRI, PET/CT and ultrasound in the preoperative staging of endometrial cancerdA multicenter prospective comparative study. Gynecologic Oncology. 2013;**128**:300-308

[54] Chang MC, Chen JH, Liang JA, et al. 18F-FDG PET or PET/CT for detection of metastatic lymph nodes in patients with endometrial cancer: A systematic

review and meta-analysis. European Journal of Radiology. 2012;**81**:3511-3517

[55] Nag S, Erickson B, Parikh S, et al. TheAmericanBrachytherapy Society recommendations for high-dose-rate brachytherapy for carcinoma of the endometrium. International Journal of Radiation Oncology, Biology, Physics. 2000;**48**:779-790

[56] Consensus statement for brachytherapy for the treatment of medically inoperable endometrial cancer. Brachytherapy. 2015;**14**(5):587-599. DOI: 10.1016/j.brachy.2015.06.002. [Epub: 15 July 2015]

[57] Gill BS, Kim H, Houser C, et al. Image-based three-dimensional conformal brachytherapy for medically inoperable endometrial carcinoma. Brachytherapy. 2014;**13**:542-547

[58] Available from: http://www.nccn.org/professionals/physician_gls/pdf/uterine.pdf [Accessed: 20 January 2015]

[59] Delaney G, Jacob S, Barton M. Estimation of an optimal radiotherapy utilization rate for gynecologic carcinoma: Part II--carcinoma of the endometrium. Cancer. 2004;**101**:682

[60] Delaney G, Jacob S, Barton M. Estimation of an optimal radiotherapy utilization rate for gynecologic carcinoma: Part I--malignancies of the cervix, ovary, vagina and vulva. Cancer. 2004;**101**:671

[61] Eifel PJ, Jhingran A, Bodurka DC, et al. Correlation of smoking history and other patient characteristics with major complications of pelvic radiation therapy for cervical cancer. Journal of Clinical Oncology. 2002;**20**:3651

[62] Klopp AH, Yeung AR, Desmukh S, et al. Phase III randomized trial comparing patient-reported toxicity and quality of life during pelvic intensity modulated radiation therapy as compared to conventional radiation therapy. International Journal of Radiation Oncology, Biology, Physics. 2016;**96**(2S):S3

[63] Morris M, Eifel PJ, Lu J, et al. Pelvic radiation with concurrent chemotherapy compared with pelvic and Para-aortic radiation for high-risk cervical cancer. The New England Journal of Medicine. 1999;**340**:1137

[64] Carr KE. Effects of radiation damage on intestinal morphology. International Review of Cytology. 2001;**208**:1

[65] Barillot I, Tavernier E, Peignaux K, et al. Impact of post operative intensity modulated radiotherapy on acute gastro-intestinal toxicity for patients with endometrial cancer: Results of the phase II RTCMIENDOMETRE French multicentre trial. Radiotherapy and Oncology. 2014;**111**:138

[66] Eifel PJ, Levenback C, Wharton JT, Oswald MJ. Time course and incidence of late complications in patients treated with radiation therapy for FIGO stage IB carcinoma of the uterine cervix. International Journal of Radiation Oncology, Biology, Physics. 1995;**32**:1289

[67] Vaginal dilator therapy for women receiving pelvic radiotherapy. Cochrane Database of Systematic Reviews. Cochrane Systematic Review - Intervention Version published: 08 September 2010:pub22010:CD007291. DOI: 10.1002/14651858.CD007291

Chapter 11

Acquisition and Management of Data for Translational Science in Oncology

Thomas J. FitzGerald, Maryann Bishop-Jodoin, Fran Laurie, Richard Hanusik, Matthew Iandoli, Kathryn Karolczuk, Sandra Kessel, Fred Prior, Joel Saltz, Ashish Sharma, Michael Knopp, Mark Rosen, Ying Xiao, David Followill, Jeff Michalski, Ameer Elaimy, James Shen, Peter Lee, Maria Giulia Cicchetti and Janaki Moni

Abstract

Oncology clinical trials provide opportunity to advance care for patients with cancer. Bridging basic science with bedside care, cancer clinical trials have brought new and updated scientific knowledge at a rapid pace. Managing subject data in translation science requires a sophisticated informatics infrastructure that will enable harmonized datasets across all areas that could influence outcomes. Successful translational science requires that all relevant information be made readily available in a digital format that can be queried in a facile manner. Through a translational science prism, we look at past issues in cancer clinical trials and the new National Institutes of Health/National Cancer Institute initiative to address the need of database availability at an enterprise level.

Keywords: translational science, IROC, clinical trials, radiation oncology, NCTN, imaging, NCTN, TCIA

1. Introduction

Translational science provides the opportunity to apply advances in science directly to patient care. In oncology, new and important scientific information is moving forward at an enterprise level. Managing data for translational science requires a sophisticated informatics infrastructure that can harmonize multiple datasets on subjects in all areas that influence outcome. Medical history, stage of disease, disease location, surgery, pathology genomic/proteomics imaging, radiation therapy, and medical oncology are equally important in determining outcome both in tumor control and normal tissue function post-therapy. In this chapter, we describe opportunities moving forward to enhance our knowledge and application of science to patient care.

IntechOpen

2. Problems of the past

The primary mechanism for oncology clinical development over the past 50 years has been in the planning and execution of clinical trials. The oncology clinical trial program in the National Cancer Institute (NCI) began as small groups of clinical investigators driven by the common need to potentially improve the care of subjects undergoing cancer therapy. The groups quickly grew into larger organizations of adult and pediatric oncologists, which included representation from all oncology disciplines in surgery, medical oncology, and radiation therapy. By 1980, pediatrics was recognized as its own discipline and the Pediatric Oncology Group (POG) was established by the merger of the pediatric divisions of the former Cancer and Leukemia Group B (CALGB) and SWOG. In 1995, imaging was recognized as its own discipline and the American College of Radiology Imaging Network (ACRIN) was established to meet the growing need of imaging acquisition and imaging science in clinical trials. Although each of the established groups housed radiation oncology as a discipline committee, the Radiation Therapy Oncology Group (RTOG) was established to promote radiation oncology as a discipline with a pathway to evaluate radiation technology and comprehensive radiation therapy. In its halcyon moment, there were 10 cooperative groups each with its own statistical data center and tissue bank resource center. The cooperative groups have been responsible for generating many of the most important publications on oncology care over the past 60 years and have become the model for validating progress in oncology. Core services in imaging and radiation therapy were established to manage specified needs in cooperative group clinical trial management. These included the Radiological Physics Center (RPC) and the Quality Assurance Review Center (QARC) as well as the American College of Radiology (ACR). As radiation oncology matured into an image-directed discipline, the radiation oncology quality assurance centers assumed a greater responsibility into collecting images used to develop target volumes of choice for radiation therapy treatment planning. In pediatrics, the images were not siloed as segregate entities between radiology and radiation therapy but applied symbiotically to all investigators for target definition and assessment of response in a single data review system. This enhanced the synergism between radiologists and radiation oncologists in the care of children [1]. In 2007, a recommendation was made by a group designed to review and assess the cooperative group mechanism and functions. The recommendation was to decrease the number of the individual cooperative groups and consolidate core services including tissue banks, data management centers, and process review of quality assurance [2]. The pediatric groups had merged into the Children's Oncology Group (COG) and as the restructuring started to mature, COG was positioned to be one of the five funded groups. The transition was completed by 2014. SWOG (formerly South West Oncology Group) chose to remain a single entity. The National Surgical Adjuvant Breast and Bowel Project (NSABP), the Radiation Therapy Oncology Group (RTOG), and the Gynecologic Oncology Group (GOG) merged as an administrative entity now known as NRG Oncology. The Cancer and Leukemia Group B (CALGB), American College of Surgeons Oncology Group (ACOSOG), and the North Central Cancer Treatment Group (NCCTG) formed the Alliance for Clinical Trials in Oncology and the Eastern Cooperative Oncology Group (ECOG) merged with the American College of Radiology Imaging Network (ACRIN) to form the ECOG-ACRIN Cancer Research Group. Each of the groups maintains an operation center as well as a statistical and data management center with NRG having more than one center. Tissue banking overlaps between the groups. The image acquisition and management and radiation therapy quality assurance are managed by the Imaging and Radiation Oncology Core (IROC), which was constituted by the existing imaging and radiation therapy quality assurance centers. These centers include the Radiologic Physics Center (RPC), the Quality Assurance Review Center (QARC), the Wright Imaging Center at Ohio State, and the American College of Radiology (ACR) core quality assurance centers in imaging and radiation oncology [1, 3].

The integration of the cooperative groups established an economy of scale for the NCI clinical trials program. The five NCTN groups house a significant amount of data. These data include outcome data, tissue banks data, and IROC hosting invaluable information important for clinical trial outcome analysis. These data libraries house the largest volume of oncology-related information in the world. Because the data are acquired on clinical trials, the datasets and outcome information are the best in the world for consistency in data acquisition and management and completeness of the information. They are among the best resources in the world for performing outstanding translational science research and comparing institutional translational science against validated datasets. Currently, the data are fragmented and siloed within the multiple remaining statistical centers, tissue banks, and IROC. Moving salient trial information into a single or synergistic data system would be an important objective promoting translational science. Hundreds of thousands of complete datasets are readily available in these systems, which can be used to promote individual work and serve to validate work of translational scientists for the next generation of clinical trials. This is the goal of big data acquisition and data management of this information. Each subject on study has pathology, imaging, therapy, and data for outcome analysis. Validated datasets with consistent and uniform acquisition of information will permit accurate assessment of trial outcome and provide quantitative significance to the work. The potential for successful application of this effort is within our reach, the challenge is to define a pathway to achieve the goals of the work.

Problem solving in oncology is challenging. To move the field forward with strong translational science and apply balanced judgments for disease management, the information acquired for review must be robust to appropriately power the study question and have the quality needed to be certain that the conclusions are accurate and can be validated. Oncology data management can be challenging if the information under review is incomplete and unvalidated, resulting in inaccurate conclusions established in outcome analysis. The database must also undergo self-renewal as process improvements become standard for evaluating outcome imaging to validate patterns of failure and pathology to review change in biomarker status relative to disease progression. Tools for biomarker identification, imaging, radiation oncology, and applied medical oncology are under constant revision and databases for translational science need constant maintenance to insure accuracy and applicability. Future strategic translational science objectives are clear and unambiguous. The more complete and accurate the information acquired, the more successful science can be applied to the bedside. In the next section, we will describe challenges in clinical trial outcome interpretation when information is incomplete.

3. Problems in clinical trial interpretation

3.1 Hodgkin lymphoma

Hodgkin lymphoma is a unique disease than can affect children, adolescents, and adults of all ages. Chemotherapy has become the initial and primary therapy for this disease with choice of agents and duration of therapy based on stage at presentation, subject medical status, and response to induction therapy. The use of radiation therapy remains under continued refinement and influenced by both response to chemotherapy and volume of tumor at presentation. Pediatric Oncology Group protocol 8725 evaluated what would be today called intermediate and advanced stage subjects. In this study, subjects were treated with eight cycles of hybrid chemotherapy

(ABVD-MOPP). After completion of chemotherapy, subjects were randomized to observation or to receive radiation therapy to all sites of disease identified on imaging at presentation. In the original Journal of Clinical Oncology publication, there was no difference in outcome in subjects who received radiation therapy [4]. Retrospective analysis of the study required imaging at presentation and before radiation therapy. The results revealed that subjects who received study-compliant radiation therapy had a survival rate that was 10% superior to those who received chemotherapy only. For the subjects treated in a manner not compliant to study guidelines (deviation), the survival was identical to those who received chemotherapy alone. In other words, subject outcome with chemotherapy was not improved using consolidation radiotherapy in a non-study-compliant manner. Most study deviations were secondary to excluding original disease from the treatment field [4, 5].

Because of the study deviation rate, the next series of clinical trials in Hodgkin lymphoma required that the radiation therapy fields be reviewed pre-radiation therapy at the Quality Assurance Review Center (QARC/now IROC). The trials evaluated early stage subjects with therapy titration secondary to response after two cycles of chemotherapy and subjects with intermediate risk disease. With pretreatment review of radiation therapy objects, compliance to study was outstanding. However, the images at presentation and response were collected by QARC to (1) confirm response and (2) define radiation therapy treatment fields. The images were reviewed retrospectively for response confirmation and the central review agreed only 50% of the time with the site assessment, demonstrating the need to define response in a consistent manner if clinical trials were going to be designed to either titrate or augment therapy based on response to treatment [6].

COG AHOD0031 was the first clinical trial in the world to use central review of imaging objects to assess response to treatment and to review radiation therapy treatment objects in real time. The real time review of objects was imbedded into the trial design structure. The image review and the review of radiation therapy treatment objects were completed at QARC with immediate feedback to site and COG statistical center, which in turn triggered both secondary and tertiary points of randomization with therapy titration based on good to complete response and therapy augmentation if response was incomplete (**Figure 1**). The trial accrued more than 1700 subjects. The completeness of the database, including outcome images, have generated many secondary projects including response in bone with PET, radiomics of response to chemotherapy in pulmonary parenchyma and pleural effusions, and patterns of failure on protocol therapy [8–10]. The data management process involved in COG trials has established the infrastructure for translational science. Pathology objects are housed in tissue banks and outcome information is housed at the statistical center; nevertheless, this information could be made available as needed for secondary projects to be completed. One of the goals moving forward is to have all this information available in a single format. This will be discussed in greater length in The Cancer Imaging Archive (TCIA) section.

The advantage to the data management system housed at IROC for COG is the current ability to now manage clinical trials for many subsets of subjects with Hodgkin lymphoma in a nimble manner with international involvement. With digital data transfer tools, information can be reviewed in real time to effectively manage adaptive trials in a facile manner. Very young subjects, older subjects with medical co-morbidities, CD30 therapies, and immunotherapy are now under study with real-time review of response coupled with biomarker analysis [11]. Expanding this strategy to a global and quantitative function is how translational science can be applied on an enterprise basis. Creating a central resource of all cancer research information and objects for investigators would enhance next generation science.

DOI: http://dx.doi.org/10.5772/intechopen.89700

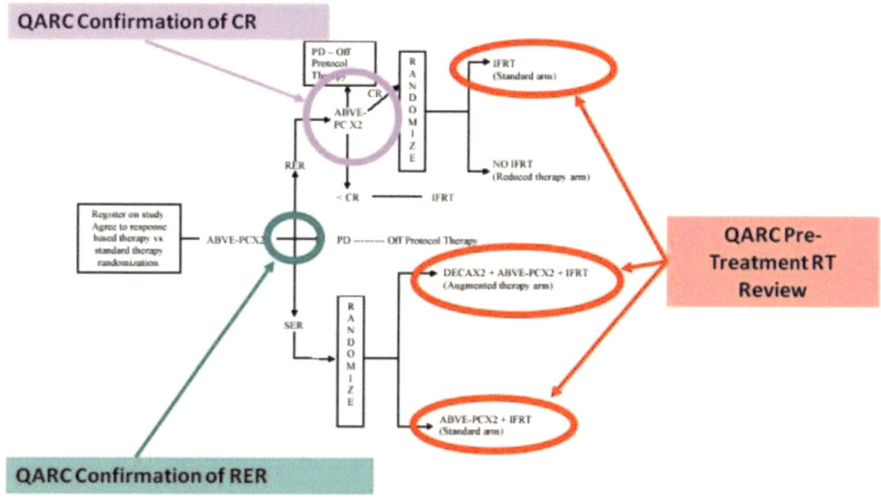

Figure 1.
Real-time imaging and radiation therapy object reviews on AHOD0031. This image is under the creative commons attribution license [7].

3.2 Breast

Clinical trials have been the infrastructure to process improvements in care for breast cancer patients. The NSABP (National Surgical Adjuvant Breast and Bowel Project) clinical trial B-06 confirmed the use of radiation therapy in the definitive management of breast cancer. Clinical trials have optimized chemotherapy in this disease, conformed the utility of hormonal therapy, and provided us the platform to titrate therapies including surgery. The advantages of clinical trials in breast cancer are self-evident [12, 13]. Likewise, clinical trials in breast cancer also reflect the problems associated with limited data acquisition and how unintentional omission of data acquisition negatively influences translational science.

The former CALGB conducted a series of well-designed clinical trials intended to evaluate the role of chemotherapy dose escalation with Adriamycin and Cytoxan with the sequential additional of Taxol in node positive subjects [13]. These trials performed in sequence predated the routine use of Her-2-Neu-directed therapy in this disease. Likewise, these trials in development predated the confirmation that radiation therapy provided a survival advantage for node positive breast cancer subjects treated with chemotherapy. The decision was made by the principal investigator not to either collect or inquire how local care to the breast and lymph nodes was applied and accomplished. The decision was made in this direction because there was no unambiguous information available at the time of trial development that local care or local control affected survival; therefore, the utility of data collection was not thought to be of consequence and did not merit the cost or effort. Evidence to the contrary was made public in 1997 when two separate clinical trials were published together, both demonstrating a survival advantage when node positive subjects were treated with radiation therapy on an adjuvant basis [14, 15]. This made clinical trial interpretation challenging because subject outcome relative to type, duration, and specific chemotherapy could not be solely assigned to the chemotherapy delivered. Many of the subjects on these series of studies also received radiation therapy to dose and volumes that were non-uniform and site/investigator specific.

To attempt and address this situation, Sartor and colleagues from QARC (now IROC Rhode Island) attempted to collect radiation therapy treatment information in a retrospective manner by contacting institutions about specific subjects. This was partially effective, however limited in execution because of several reasons. This effort was not the intention or part of the data management of the studies; therefore, site investigator enthusiasm to support the effect was non-uniform. The second issue was one that is now more visible in more modern clinical trials as to collect this information, institutional review boards (IRB) began to insist that subjects on study be re-consented for this effort. Accordingly, this became a significant barrier to project completion [16].

These trials accrued more than 3000 subjects and were well powered to achieve the objectives of the study. However, only less than one-third of the radiation therapy information could be collected and often the information received was incomplete. The information received clearly indicated that without protocol guidelines, dose and volumes treated were significantly heterogeneous and when treated, subjects received therapy that was non-uniform relative to dose and volume and conclusions would have been difficult to validate. There was a trend for subjects who received Taxol to also have received radiation therapy, imposing a question as to which therapy, or both, provided a care advantage.

A second issue foreshadowed a problem now seen in current breast cancer clinical trials. There were more than 300 local and or local regional failures in this study. If radiation therapy objects were collected and detailed information concerning the location and nature of the local failure, the application of the radiation oncology treatment fields, technique, and dose could be reviewed to better ascertain how radiation therapy can/should be applied along the chest wall and regional draining lymph nodes. The lack of information has led to a paralysis in our understanding of issues than remain today.

ACOSOG Z0011 (Z11) was a clinical trial designed to evaluate limited axillary surgery in subjects with breast cancer including those with limited nodal involvement. The objective was to validate that sentinel lymph node staging coupled with radiation therapy would be non-inferior to more comprehensive axillary surgery [17]. The trial asked for what is referred to as "tangential radiation therapy." This would imply that the axillary volume was treated to a partial volume. In studies evaluating this point using anatomical guidelines superimposed on radiation therapy treatment fields, approximately 60% of the axilla would be included in a traditional field that would not extend superiorly to the axillary vein nor posteriorly to the latissimus muscle [18]. The study proved to be positive relative to limited axillary surgery. However, radiation therapy treatment objects were not collected as part of the study, giving the impression that partial volume RT to the axilla could be considered a new standard of care. Jolie and colleagues decided to review this point and with several colleagues including support from QARC (IROC), attempts were made to gather specific information as to how radiation therapy was delivered to subjects on study. The investigators encountered similar barriers to data acquisition relative to site enthusiasm and IRB approval. However, the investigators were able to determine that a significant number of subjects were treated with more comprehensive radiation therapy to extended volumes including regional lymph nodes that were not study directed. Therefore, conclusions concerning the application of radiation therapy to limited volumes of the axilla are premature [19].

If radiation therapy digital datasets and radiation dose were collected as part of the study, it is possible that interventional review pre-therapy could have been performed and the data set could have been more uniform. In this situation, outcome images could be applied to patterns of failure analysis and define outcome relative to axillary therapy with more security. This issue continues to haunt even the most current breast cancer trial attempting to discern the appropriate radiation therapy target volume in subjects with limited and more extended axillary surgery. This has influence in normal tissue outcome and despite nearly 50 years of clinical trials, it remains unanswered. If the datasets were complete, it is possible we might be closer to understanding how to apply therapy for both tumor control and optimal normal tissue function. This is of increasing importance as radiation therapy is now being asked to treat nodal regions with more limited surgery. If information acquired on study was more complete, we may be further along in our understanding of field placement. This also limits our ability to perform translational science including pathology biomarkers for local failure and other potential areas of interest to the oncology community. These are problems of omission of data acquisition and limit our ability to use these datasets to review information in retrospect and apply knowledge to the next generation of clinical trials.

3.3 Head/neck

There is much to be learned as issues of head and neck management are influenced by biomarkers and relationship to viral origin of disease. To be accurate in data assessment, pathology and imaging objects need to be complete to intercompare both staging and therapy execution/outcome. Non-uniform treatment execution can limit study success and utility of the dataset for translational science.

Tirapazamine gained prominence as a hypoxic cell sensitizer to radiation therapy with favorable phase 2 results. In the HeadSTART clinical trial, Tirapazamine was randomized with traditional chemoradiotherapy for locally advanced squamous cell carcinoma of the head/neck. In this study, both imaging and radiation therapy quality assurance objects underwent on treatment review at QARC for study compliance. Pre-treatment review was not utilized because the trial included many international partners and most of the involved sites credentialed for participation had primitive digital transfer tools at the time of clinical trial participation. The trial management committee determined that pre-therapy review would potentially be a barrier to accrual. Nearly 25% of the cases required radiation field adjustments to ensure that full dose was received to gross tumor as seen on central review. Of the 211 requests for field alteration, 116 chose not to adjust the fields and 95 chose to make the adjustment. In all cases, the potential for deviation was due to potential exclusion of gross tumor from full dose and protocol-compliant radiation. If the adjustment was made on treatment, subjects had reasonable survival; however, their survival was less than those who had a compliant plan de novo. If adjustments were not made, except for two cases, the trial management committee agreed with the assessment of the on-treatment reviewer. The trial committee asked the primary on-treatment reviewer to score all study deviations into two categories, clinically meaningful or not. Clinically meaningful deviations excluded gross tumor from full-dose radiation therapy. Subjects with clinically meaningful deviations had a significant decrease in survival while those whose deviations were not considered significant had an outcome identical to those whose plans were adjusted for compliance on treatment. Both groups had survival less than the subjects who had a compliant plan upfront. The most unfortunate aspect of this study is the deviation rate on trial over rode the point of randomization on the study, rendering the experimental arm uncertain, secondary to quality of the radiation therapy. Therefore, the cases become less helpful for translational science endeavors including pattern of failure analysis as the outcome was influenced by the quality of the data [20, 21].

Current studies in head and neck cancer place emphasis on the role of immunotherapy in both comparing the traditional platinum-based therapy coupled with non-inferiority objectives to evaluate toxicity. In these trials, investigators have matured in the coverage of gross tumor. However, there is new disparity on coverage of targets deemed of intermediate and low risk as investigators are empirically titrating volume treated to ameliorate mucosal discomfort and late effects to multiple normal tissue volumes. Therapeutic titration will influence toxicity profiles. If investigators are titrating volumes, modern protocols may unfairly favor toxicity profiles generated by new regimens in comparison to historical standard. Complete datasets including outcome imaging with patterns of failure will be important to compare both tumor control and toxicity moving forward.

These are important datasets as strategies in artificial intelligence and machine learning in radiology and radiation oncology need to be developed from accurate and complete datasets, especially as the origin of disease becomes multifactorial in origin. If objects are not targeted correctly or per protocol, it will be impossible to develop accurate artificial intelligence (AI) machine tools that can be applied for translational science moving forward.

3.4 Lung

Treatment of patients with lung malignancy is challenging as metrics for normal tissue function extend beyond the anatomical constraints that can be defined in radiation oncology planning images. Both tumor control and normal tissue function are influenced by dose to target and radiation dose to normal tissue, including volumes of parenchyma receiving low, intermediate, and high doses. One of the challenges moving forward is to ensure that volumes are drawn accurately to assess tumor control and cardio-pulmonary function. RTOG 0617 study evaluated the role of targeted therapy coupled with both low- and high-dose radiation therapy to tumor target. Radiation therapy treatment objects were submitted for review without diagnostic images to validate that what was drawn for treatment reflected all the tumor anatomy. It was assumed, perhaps accurately, that the planning CT would be sufficient to confirm that all disease was included in the intended target. Although the study did not show a benefit to high-dose radiation, the paradox was that in the early phase of the trial, the higher dose arm had statistically worse local control. One explanation is that gross tumor may not have been fully contoured in selected cases and possibly influenced trial outcome. As such, without primary imaging and outcome imaging, it is difficult to confirm the pattern of failure, possibly rendering these datasets less useful for secondary analysis. Complete datasets would be helpful to validate trial outcome and increase the utility of the data for secondary analysis and translational science [22].

4. Analysis

Successful translational science requires that all relevant information be made readily available in an informatics format that can be queried in a facile manner. Incomplete datasets can lead to conclusions that may be inaccurate. Complete datasets will permit the facts to drive study outcome and investigators will feel the analysis is accurate. A senior clinical trial investigator once stated that the time to write your protocol is when you analyze your data as you finally begin to see the questions you should have both asked and anticipated in the design phase of the trial. This is why informatics platforms must have enterprise-level query function to help answer questions not anticipated in study design. Datasets from clinical trials potentially make the best tools for moving translational science forward as the (1) subjects are entered on trial for a specific purpose, (2) the stage and appropriateness for subject entry are confirmed with uniform standards, (3) information including pathology and imaging are collected and collated in a uniform manner, (4) subjects are treated in a uniform manner with treatment data available for review, and (5) outcome information is available including imaging to validate outcome as appropriate. These datasets permit evaluation of a potential new biomarker as (1) the information may be available in situ as a digital object and (2) additional tissue may be available as part of an exhaustible resource housed in a tissue bank. Nimble query function can permit intercomparison between subjects on the same trial or other subjects on different studies with similar demographics for analysis. This can potentially evaluate and compare those with similar biomarkers on different studies. The datasets become a rich resource for science. At the moment within both industry and the NCTN, the information is housed in disparate locations including statistical data centers that house subject demographics and outcome, IROC which houses images and radiation therapy treatment objects, and tissue banks which house both digital maps of known biomarkers and tissue help for additional studies when needed. As a result, efforts to perform secondary analysis on objects become challenging and often lost in process and sequential approvals for use. This can take considerable time and effort and often the scientific question is muted and defeated by processes designed for data protection.

To make science move forward at an enterprise level, this information needs to be housed in in a single platform designed to promote and support the modern scientist with nimble and comprehensive query function for robust data review. The next section will discuss how these objects are currently managed and present a strategy for modern science moving forward.

5. The cancer imaging archive (TCIA)

TCIA is an initiative of the National Institute of Health (NIH) and the National Cancer Institute (NCI) to address the need for enterprise database availability to promote translational science and to validate concepts and ideas against a strong database. The archive resides in the public domain and the objects are fully de-identified per government standards. The principal investigator of TCIA is Fred Prior, PhD, who is the chair of quantitative science at the University of Arkansas. Dr. Prior has long-standing expertise in database management and development of image datasets. He has applied his expertise to this effort coupled with co-investigators Joel Saltz, MD, PhD, and Ashish Sharma, PhD. Dr. Saltz is the chair of bioinformatics at Stony Brook University and an international expert in digital pathology and integrated database function. Dr. Sharma is at Emory University and is an informatics expert who helps move TCIA to enterprise function.

The digital archive houses imaging and outcome information that can be used for translational science. The current portfolio includes datasets from all cancer subtypes in adult oncology and will soon be updated with datasets from pediatric oncology. The information includes clinical information, imaging, radiation therapy datasets and treatment plans, pathology objects including genomics, and other supplemental information required for analysis. The current portfolio can be accessed through www.thecancerimagingarchive.net. TCIA is an important initiative as it makes information available to all interested scientists who can apply information directly to their projects of interest.

As TCIA moves forward, it will be essential to find mechanisms for enterprise-level data capture and uniform data formatting for all trials both within the NCTN and industry. Clinical trials within the NCTN will likely need to be designed in the future with data capture as part of the protocol and processes imbedded in the trial will need to be made uniform in the trial design to be uploaded to TCIA once the trial is complete and objects fully de-identified for the public archive. Investigators will want to be able to look at specific subjects' subsets in clinical trials and evaluate both image and biomarker expression for subsets both within individual trials and intercompare with other trials for outcome analysis. This will be true in all adult and pediatric oncology subtypes. We are learning more each day about response-directed therapies and the relationship of response and disease progression relative to biomarkers. The informatics tools will need to be robust to accommodate this element of data exchange and evaluation. Digital pathology will play an increasingly important role including capture of profiles that are identified to date in a manner similar to oncotype for breast cancer. Tissue will need to be stored for the biomarker not yet identified. Digital capture makes identified objects inexhaustible while tissue is exhaustible, hence the reason we need to store and protect this invaluable resource. Radiation therapy treatment plans will need to be fused with images that define targets and correlate to images that review the pattern of failure. It will be through these mechanisms we will all mature in our understanding of disease processes and the success/failure of our applied therapies [23, 24].

6. Conclusions

Enterprise-level function of comprehensive clinical trial datasets is closer to reality than it has been in the past. The quality of the dataset will significantly influence the quality of our understanding of the applied information and how we use clinical information moving forward. Efforts need to be made to optimize existing datasets in the NCTN and industry to help move knowledge forward in a manner we can validate and trust.

Acknowledgements

CA 180803.

Conflict of interest

The authors declare no conflict of interest.

Author details

Thomas J. FitzGerald[1*], Maryann Bishop-Jodoin[1], Fran Laurie[1], Richard Hanusik[1], Matthew Iandoli[1], Kathryn Karolczuk[1], Sandra Kessel[1], Fred Prior[2], Joel Saltz[3], Ashish Sharma[4], Michael Knopp[5], Mark Rosen[6], Ying Xiao[6], David Followill[7], Jeff Michalski[8], Ameer Elaimy[9], James Shen[9], Peter Lee[9], Maria Giulia Cicchetti[1] and Janaki Moni[1]

1 University of Massachusetts/IROC Rhode Island, Lincoln, RI, USA

2 University of Arkansas/TCIA, Little Rock, AR, USA

3 Stony Brook University/TCIA, Stony Brook, NY, USA

4 Emory University/TCIA, Atlanta, GA, USA

5 Ohio State University/IROC Ohio, Columbus, OH, USA

6 University of Pennsylvania/IROC Philadelphia, Philadelphia, PA, USA

7 MD Anderson/IROC Houston, Houston, TX, USA

8 Washington University of St. Louis/IROC St. Louis, St. Louis, MO, USA

9 University of Massachusetts Medical School, Worcester, MA, USA

*Address all correspondence to: tjfitzgerald@qarc.org

References

[1] FitzGerald TJ, Bishop-Jodoin M, Followill DS, Galvin J, Knopp MV, Michalski JM, et al. Imaging and data acquisition in clinical trials for radiation therapy. International Journal of Radiation Oncology, Biology, Physics. 2016;**94**(2):404-411

[2] FitzGerald TJ. A new model for imaging and radiation therapy quality assurance in the National Clinical Trials Network of the National Cancer Institute. International Journal of Radiation Oncology, Biology, Physics. 2014;**88**(2):272-273

[3] NCTN: NCI's National Clinical Trials Network: National Cancer Institute; 2019 [updated May 25, 2019]. Available from: https://www.cancer.gov/research/areas/clinical-trials/nctn

[4] Weiner MA, Leventhal B, Brecher ML, Marcus RB, Cantor A, Gieser PW, et al. Randomized study of intensive MOPP-ABVD with or without low-dose total-nodal radiation therapy in the treatment of stages IIB, IIIA2, IIIB, and IV Hodgkin's disease in pediatric patients: A pediatric oncology group study. Journal of Clinical Oncology. 1997;**15**(8):2769-2779

[5] FitzGerald TJ, Urie M, Ulin K, Laurie F, Yorty J, Hanusik R, et al. Processes for quality improvements in radiation oncology clinical trials. International Journal of Radiation Oncology, Biology, Physics. 2008; **71**(1 Suppl):S76-S79

[6] Mendenhall NP, Meyer J, Williams J, Tebbi C, Kessel S, Laurie F, et al. The impact of central quality assurance review prior to radiation therapy on protocol compliance: POG 9426, a trial in pediatric Hodgkin's disease. Blood Cells. 2005;**106**(11):753

[7] Fitzgerald TJ, Bishop-Jodoin M, Bosch WR, Curran WJ, Followill DS, Galvin JM, et al. Future vision for the quality assurance of oncology clinical trials. Frontiers in Oncology. 2013;**3**:31

[8] Friedman DL, Chen L, Wolden S, Buxton A, McCarten K, FitzGerald TJ, et al. Dose-intensive response-based chemotherapy and radiation therapy for children and adolescents with newly diagnosed intermediate-risk hodgkin lymphoma: A report from the children's oncology group study AHOD0031. Journal of Clinical Oncology. 2014;**32**(32):3651-3658

[9] Dharmarajan KV, Friedman DL, Schwartz CL, Chen L, FitzGerald TJ, McCarten KM, et al. Patterns of relapse from a phase 3 study of response-based therapy for intermediate-risk Hodgkin lymphoma (AHOD0031): A report from the Children's oncology group. International Journal of Radiation Oncology, Biology, Physics. 2015;**92**(1):60-66

[10] Dharmarajan KV, Friedman DL, FitzGerald TJ, McCarten KM, Constine LS, Chen L, et al. Radiotherapy quality assurance report from children's oncology group AHOD0031. International Journal of Radiation Oncology, Biology, Physics. 2015;**91**(5):1065-1071

[11] Fitzgerald TJ. Optimisation of adaptive therapy for advanced Hodgkin lymphoma. The Lancet Oncology. 2019;**20**(2):167-168

[12] Fisher B, Bauer M, Margolese R, Poisson R, Pilch Y, Redmond C, et al. Five-year results of a randomized clinical trial comparing total mastectomy and segmental mastectomy with or without radiation in the treatment of breast cancer. The New England Journal of Medicine. 1985;**312**(11):665-673

[13] Henderson IC, Berry DA, Demetri GD, Cirrincione CT,

Goldstein LJ, Martino S, et al. Improved outcomes from adding sequential paclitaxel but not from escalating doxorubicin dose in an adjuvant chemotherapy regimen for patients with node-positive primary breast cancer. Journal of Clinical Oncology. 2003;**21**(6):976-983

[14] Hayes DF, Thor AD, Dressler LG, Weaver D, Edgerton S, Cowan D, et al. HER2 and response to paclitaxel in node-positive breast cancer. The New England Journal of Medicine. 2007;**357**(15):1496-1506

[15] Moore A. Breast-cancer therapy–Looking back to the future. The New England Journal of Medicine. 2007;**357**(15):1547-1549

[16] Sartor CI, Peterson BL, Woolf S, Fitzgerald TJ, Laurie F, Turrisi AJ, et al. Effect of addition of adjuvant paclitaxel on radiotherapy delivery and locoregional control of node-positive breast cancer: Cancer and leukemia group B 9344. Journal of Clinical Oncology. 2005;**23**(1):30-40

[17] Giuliano AE, McCall LM, Beitsch PD, Whitworth PW, Morrow M, Blumencranz PW, et al. ACOSOG Z0011: A randomized trial of axillary node dissection in women with clinical T1-2 N0 M0 breast cancer who have a positive sentinel node. Journal of Clinical Oncology. 2010;**28**(18_suppl):CRA506-CRA

[18] Reznik J, Cicchetti MG, DeGaspe B, FitzGerald TJ. Analysis of axillary coverage during tangential radiation therapy to the breast. International Journal of Radiation Oncology Biology Physics. 2001;**51**(3):6-7

[19] Jagsi R, Chadha M, Moni J, Ballman K, Laurie F, Buchholz TA, et al. Radiation field design in the ACOSOG Z0011 (alliance) trial. Journal of Clinical Oncology. 2014;**32**(32):3600-3606

[20] Peters LJ, O'Sullivan B, Giralt J, Fitzgerald TJ, Trotti A, Bernier J, et al. Critical impact of radiotherapy protocol compliance and quality in the treatment of advanced head and neck cancer: Results from TROG 02.02. Journal of Clinical Oncology. 2010;**28**(18):2996-3001

[21] Rischin D, Peters LJ, O'Sullivan B, Giralt J, Fisher R, Yuen K, et al. Tirapazamine, cisplatin, and radiation versus cisplatin and radiation for advanced squamous cell carcinoma of the head and neck (TROG 02.02, HeadSTART): A phase III trial of the Trans-Tasman Radiation Oncology Group. Journal of Clinical Oncology. 2010;**28**(18):2989-2995

[22] Bradley JD, Paulus R, Komaki R, Masters G, Blumenschein G, Schild S, et al. Standard-dose versus high-dose conformal radiotherapy with concurrent and consolidation carboplatin plus paclitaxel with or without cetuximab for patients with stage IIIA or IIIB non-small-cell lung cancer (RTOG 0617): A randomised, two-by-two factorial phase 3 study. The Lancet Oncology. 2015;**16**(2):187-199

[23] Prior F, Smith K, Sharma A, Kirby J, Tarbox L, Clark K, et al. The public cancer radiology imaging collections of the cancer imaging archive. Scientific Data. 2017;**4**:170124

[24] Prior F, Almeida J, Kathiravelu P, Kurc T, Smith K, Fitzgerald TJ, et al. Open access image repositories: high-quality data to enable machine learning research. Clinical Radiology. 2019. pii: S0009-9260(19)30169-2. DOI: 10.1016/j.crad.2019.04.002. [Epub ahead of print]

Chapter 12

Implications of Radiosensitizer and Radioprotector Factors in Refining the Dose-Volume Constraints and Radiobiological Models

Camil Ciprian Mirestean, Călin Gheorghe Buzea, Roxana Irina Iancu and Dragoș Petru Teodor Iancu

Abstract

Radiotherapy is a cornerstone of the modern treatment of many types of cancer, having both curative and palliative roles. It is estimated that more than half of cancer patients will need radiation therapy in the course of evolution. The goal of radiotherapy is to maximize tumor control, reducing adverse effects on normal tissues in close proximity at the same time. Improving the therapeutic ratio is the main goal of the efforts made to improve the technique and accuracy of the radiotherapy by using the targeting of the tumor volume with the help of the imaging guide and the dose conformation around the target volume. The use of the multi-leaf collimator (MLC) allowed a better coverage of the target volume in the irradiation field, thus reducing the unnecessary irradiation of healthy tissues. The use of radioprotective agents and radiosensitizers is another strategy to maximize the effect of radiotherapy. Recently, interest has focused on the design of irradiation protocols that exploit the differences in biology in terms of the response to irradiation between tumor cells and normal tissues.

Keywords: radiotherapy, IMRT, VMAT, SIB, dosimetry

1. Introduction

The transition in the 1990s from conformal 3D radiotherapy to intensity-modulated intensity radiotherapy (IMRT) allowed the high-dose irradiation of volumes with irregular shapes [1, 2]. The use of radioprotective agents and radiosensitizers is another strategy to maximize the effect of radiotherapy. Recently, interest has focused on the design of irradiation protocols that exploit the differences in biology in terms of the response to irradiation between tumor cells and normal tissues [2, 3].

From the clinical point of view, tissue radiosensitivity is reported as the difference in the degree of response at the same dose of irradiation or at different doses required to produce the same response to different subjects. The radiosensitivity and radioresistance of the different types of tissues is determined by the mitotic rate and the cellular repopulation, being proven that the cells with low rates of

IntechOpen

repopulation are more radioresistant. Especially for cells with long post-mitotic life, for which the main mechanism of radiation induced hypoplasia and atrophy, is death in interphase, the response is obtained only at high doses of radiation [1, 2, 4].

2. Dose-volume-toxicity correlations - from radiobiology to guidelines and clinical practice

With all the technical and ballistic advances in the planning and delivery of radiation therapy that has occurred in over 100 years since the use of radiation in anticancer treatments, it has not been possible to obtain a perfect therapeutic ratio for which the irradiation of healthy tissues tends to zero. Historically, the first initiative to guide doctor radiation oncologists was the publication of Rubin and Cassarett, a collection of reports on toxicities and doses to which they were reported. The 1980s were a significant evolution in the field of radiation oncology, the radiotherapy being transformed from a two-dimensional (2D), based on the approximate evaluation of the position of the radiosensitive organs based on the anatomical landmarks and subsequently of the 2D simulator with conventional radiographs, to a three-dimensional (3D/volumetric) process. This evolution has shown that previous knowledge about tumoricidal doses and tolerance of radiosensitive organs to irradiation does not present accuracy and new information is needed regarding partial organ volumes and toxicities [2, 5].

In this context, a scientific committee has carried out an extensive review on the dose data received from different organs and toxicities, reaching the consensus to evaluate the data using a volumetric division of organs in one-third, two-thirds, and the whole organ. The consensus of eight experts from reference centers in the United States was published under the name “Emami Paper.” The paper was a reference for assessing the risk of toxicity associated with doses, but being a literature review until 1991, it contained data from the previous 3D-CRT technology. Another limitation of the study was the evaluation of toxicities after conventional irradiation (2 Gy/fraction), and at that time neither the dose-volume histograms were routinely used in dosimetry. From the clinical point of view, only the most severe toxicity was evaluated, without any grading system for these adverse effects [1, 2, 6, 7].

The next decades have brought a revolution in terms of oncological treatments. A multidisciplinary approach has become a standard in oncology, and sequential and increasingly concomitant therapeutic associations are increasingly used. In terms of technology, most cobalt units have been replaced with linear accelerators, and radiotherapy planning based on CT simulation has become standard. 3D-CRT and IMRT techniques based on IGRT have been widely implemented, and delineation of tumor target volumes using CT, MRI, and PET-CT imaging has become a standard. The complexity and the large number of factors that influence the response to the irradiation of the tumors and the probability of the complications of the normal tissues have made it necessary to develop predictive models for the clinical complications associated with the radiation therapy. The large number of data reported in relation to the different toxicities and conditions of registration make analysis difficult to identify value parameters. A group of clinicians and researchers performed a retrospective analysis called “Quantitative Analysis of Normal Tissue Effects in the Clinic (QUANTEC).” The aim of this approach was to review the available literature on the correlation of dose-volume parameters with the complications of normal tissues, the study being the analysis of the literature of the last 18 years. The paper QUANTEC, resulting from the collective effort of 57 experts, appears with the support of the American Association of Radiation Therapy (ASTRO) and American Association of Medical Physics (AAPM) and is published in the supplement of the journal "International Journal of Radiation Oncology, Biology, Physics" (the Red Journal) [2, 5–8].

The QUANTEC group aimed to provide a reliable prediction at the time of radiotherapy planning of the risk of occurrence of toxicity depending on the volume parameters extracted from the dose-volume histograms.

Although these publications contain a comprehensive review of scientific papers of the information published in order to be a guide for clinicians, the use of this guide cannot substitute for the judgment of the radiation oncologist clinician, considering the large number of intrinsic and extrinsic factors on which the radiosensitivity of each organ depends [7, 8].

There is no model that accurately predicts normal tissue responses to irradiation for routine clinical use, most models being more descriptive than predictive. The use of the multi-leaf collimator (MLC) allowed a better dosimetric coverage of the target volumes also offering a significant reduction in the irradiation of the healthy tissue from the proximity of tumors.

$$(BED) = n \cdot d\left(1 + \frac{d}{\alpha/\beta}\right) \tag{1}$$

The isoeffect formula for conversion to standard fractionation is commonly used in cases where another fractionation scheme (hypofractionation or hyperfractionation) is used to assess the toxicity risk according to the "QUANTEC" data:

$$(\mathrm{EQD2}) = \mathrm{D}\frac{\mathrm{d} + (\alpha/\beta)}{2 + (\alpha/\beta)} \tag{2}$$

The α/β index is calculated based on information from cell survival curves on in vitro cell cultures, assigning values for the α/β ratio, and using these values to calculate a normal dose of tissue tolerance may be risky in estimating clinical complications [2, 7, 9].

Organs at risk (OAR) are those organs that if irradiated can be structurally and functionally affected. The structures that are in the proximity of the irradiated volume or by their anatomical function are defined as OAR, receive a certain dose during the treatment. These OAR's have been divided from the radiobiological/functional point of view into serial organs and parallel organs. The spinal cord is the most relevant example of OAR with serial architecture. Each subunit of the spinal cord is vital to the functioning of the entire organ. The parallel structural organization is based on the functional independence of the subunits. The impairment of a limited number of structures does not compromise the function of the whole organ; the dysfunction occurs if a large number of subunits have been affected, because the remaining functional ones do not have sufficient compensatory capacity. An example of an organ with parallel architecture would be that of the parotid glands. In these cases the average dose absorbed throughout the organ is the most significant predictor of toxicity [5, 7, 8].

Using a Lyman mathematical model and the algorithm proposed by Kutcher and collaborators, a radiobiological model was proposed based on extrapolation of Emami guides to any dosimetric distribution, using dose-volume histograms (DVH). The Lyman-Kutcher-Burman (LKB) model was and is one of the most used radiobiological mathematical models, but the multitude of factors involved in producing toxicities made this model an ideal one, without being implemented in clinical practice as a standard. The QUANTEC is one of the most valuable analyzes on dose-volume parameters based on numerous retrospective studies. However, the therapeutic and technical diagnostic advances in the multimodal treatment of the pathological pathology make it necessary to update and validate new recommendations regarding the dose-volume parameters correlated with toxicities [7–10].

With the implementation of inverse planning techniques (IMRT and volumetric intensity-modulated volumetric arc therapy (VMAT)), it became necessary to define a risk-exposed volume (RVR) in order to obtain an optimal dose distribution using the planning software, trying to limit the risk of developing high-dose regions outside the target volume. ICRU83 defines RVR as the difference between the volume included in the external contour and the volumes CTV and OAR. With the implementation of IMRT, the dose received by RVR can be a predictor of the risk of radioinduced carcinogenesis, and a reduction of large volumes receiving low doses is necessary. In fact, there are numerous intrinsic and extrinsic factors that influence the radiosensitivity of each tissue/organ, related to the patient (age, comorbidities, Karnofsky score/ECOG performance status) and dependent on the radiosensitivity of each organ (serial dose-effect organization, the most eloquent case being of the spinal cord, parallel radiobiological organization volume-effect structure as in the case of liver and lungs, mixed serial and parallel organization described in the literature in the case of kidneys), but it is also influenced by the previous treatments applied. Radiotherapy treatment influences the response of radiosensitive organs by parameters as the maximum dose, average, minimum, dose rate, general treatment time, irradiation beam energy, and irradiated volume. Systemic treatments (radiosensitizing and radioprotective agents, chemotherapy, biological and immunotherapy) influence the tissue radiosensitivity and determine the variability of the different responses at the same irradiation dose. The most recent studies show the involvement of molecular and genetic profiles in radiosensitivity. According to Emami and QUANTEC studies, cerebral radionecrosis usually occurs late from 3 months up to a few years after radiotherapy with initially a 5% risk at 5 years after treatment at a dose of 60 Gy received by one-third of the brain by standard fractionation. Using the ratio $\alpha/\beta = 3$ in formulas derived from the quadratic linear model, radiation necrosis was estimated at <3% for a dose <60 Gy, increasing to 5% if the brain tissue received dose is 72 Gy. The toxicity caused by the irradiation of the brainstem can be potentially lethal. The Emami study considered TD 5/5 of 50 Gy for the entire brainstem and 60 Gy in one-third of the brainstem as the tolerance limit, but reviewing the study literature evaluates a brain stem tolerance up to 54 Gy with <5% risk of brainstem necrosis or neurological toxicity. It is also recommended to limit doses up to 59 Gy per volume (1–10 cc). In exceptional situations the brainstem can tolerate up to 59 Gy (<< 1 cc) and can receive up to 64 Gy [2, 8, 11].

Toxicity by spinal cord irradiation is also severe, and myelopathy is often disabling. For a ratio $\alpha/\beta = 0.87$, the risk of myelopathy is 0.2% at 50 Gy and 5% at 59.3 Gy, using the quadratic linear model. The values used in the literature for the α/β ratio are usually higher and make necessary to convert the dose of treatment per fractions to 2 Gy [8, 9, 12].

Radiation-induced optic neuropathy (RION) is severe toxicity leading to a rapid assessed blindness. Emami's recommendations are TD 5/5 of 50 Gy for the entire organ.

Based on the QUANTEC review, a dose of 50 Gy received by the whole organ is associated with <1% risk of toxicity, and the risk increases from 3–7% for doses between 55 and 60 Gy, the increase in toxicity rate being significant for doses greater than 60 Gy [2, 7, 8].

For the radiotherapy of thoracic tumors, radiation-induced pneumonitis is one of the most common toxicities in patients treated with radiation for cancers of the lung, breast, and other mediastinal tumors, often being the dose-limiting toxicity. Parameter V20 was identified as the most significant predictor of pneumonitis.

Radiation-induced pericarditis is associated with increased levels of mortality, the most relevant cardiac toxicity of irradiation. It was considered that the pericarditis risk is less than 15% when the mean pericardial dose was <26Gy, another dosimetric constraint considered predictive for pericarditis being V30 (pericardium) <46% in the case of breast cancers irradiation [2, 7].

Radiation-induced liver disease (RILD) usually occurs between 2 weeks and 3 months after radiation therapy. Emami guideline estimates an associated risk of <5% toxicity for an average dose of ≤30 Gy received by the liver, with a reduction to a maximum of 28 Gy required in patients with pre-existing liver disease.

Radiation-induced renal dysfunction is manifested in a variety of ways, from clinical symptoms to biochemical or imaging changes, most commonly with decreased creatinine clearance or even renal failure. An average dose of 18 Gy is considered to be associated with a 5% risk of toxicity at 5 years, with limitation to an average dose of 20 Gy being considered a feasible option in clinical practice [2, 5, 7].

Treatment toxicity for pelvine tumors includes femoral neck and head necrosis, associated with possible fracture. Factors such as osteoporosis and androgen treatment in the background increase the risk of irradiation toxicity. A 52 Gy dose for the entire femoral head was considered the recommended limit according to Emami publication, limiting the dose below 50 Gy and reducing the risk of neck/femoral neck necrosis to <5%. However, there are studies that report toxicities for large doses delivered on smaller volumes [7, 9, 13].

Without proposing to present all the recommendations of these guides, we have exemplified some recommendations and their predictive value on the toxicities for radiotherapy of tumors of the cervical, thoracic, abdominal, and pelvic regions.

The development of mathematical models in cancer biology and radiotherapy treatment is a step motivated by the desire to evaluate the probability of tumor control and the probability of healthy tissue complications. The technical evolution of radiotherapy and the complexity of the treatment plans have led to the emergence of increasingly complex treatment plans, with unpredictable difficulty to evaluate dose distributions. The desire to obtain an optimal plan and to increase the tumor control, limiting the risk of complications at the lowest possible level, has oriented the research toward the development of radiobiological models with a predictive value of the tumor response and the toxicity rate. The development of radiobiological models originated three decades ago, but in recent years efforts have been intensified to introduce these models into clinical practice. The inability to consider variables as clinical data and histological type of tumor made it difficult to introduce these models as standard in the process of evaluating treatment plans. However, some producers have included radiobiological models in commercial TPS that use DVH curves in the treatment plan and biological parameters such as histologic type and characteristics of nearby healthy tissues to calculate tumor control probability (TCP) and normal tissue complication probability (NTCP). The radiobiological models included in the TPS software are based on the Poisson TCP model and the LKB model for the calculation of NTCP [9, 14].

Although not yet implemented as a standard of assessment in clinical routine, TCP and NTCP models offered the radiation oncologist and medical physicist a useful tool in evaluating treatment plans and selecting the best treatment plan but also in evaluating geometrical errors and in comparison of the most modern radiotherapy techniques.

Dosimetric comparisons between treatment plans have been used extensively in validating treatment plans generated by the inverse planning techniques IMRT and VMAT, determining according to EMAMI/QUANTEC recommendations and the latest RTOG recommendations the possibility of reducing the risk of toxicities associated with irradiation. The use of radiobiological models has shown a small benefit in TCP and a significant reduction of NTCP when using the IMRT technique in prostate cancer radiotherapy. TCP/NTCP models were also used to compare sequential IMRT plans with SIB-IMRT plans. The use of the boost integrated in the

VMAT technique demonstrated the ability to reduce the average dose received by the rectum and bladder by 13 and 17% [2, 7, 15].

Also the use of radiobiological models can highlight the percentage with which the TCP value increases by increasing the dose to a certain value. In the case of comparative VMAT single-arc vs. VMAT double-arc treatment plans, the use of NTCP radiobiological models revealed similar values regarding the risk of radionecrosis of the femoral heads, on irradiation plans for prostate cancer although the dosimetric distribution is significantly different between the two plans. However, some authors report lower mean NTCP values for VMAT double-arc plans.

Biological optimization based on NTCP of treatment plans has become a feasible alternative, based on dose-volume optimization, demonstrating the possibility to reduce up to 3 times the doses received by the parotid glands in the case of locally advanced nasopharynx cancers treated by IMRT technique [16, 17].

Patient repositioning based on imaging guidance is routinely performed in most radiotherapy centers using modern radiotherapy techniques using daily setup and four-dimensional computer tomography (CBCT) images performed with onboard imaging (OBI) systems which are increasingly used to compare planned and treated target volumes. TCP and NTCP radiobiological models can be used to evaluate the effect of systematic and random errors on the probability of tumor control and on the risk of toxicity, using information from the DVH curves. Some authors have used EPID portal dosimetry to check the dose received by critical organs as heart for the purpose of evaluating NTCP [2, 16–18].

Another direction of interest was the evaluation with the help of the NTCP of the advantage of the new four-dimensional computer tomography (4D-CT) technology in radiotherapy planning. The radiobiology studies proved a minor benefit in TCP in many situations. This evaluation has the role to give a suggestive image of the situations in which the 4D-CT technique offers a clear advantage over 3D image-based planning. Reposition during treatment is made according to the geometric variations of the target volumes and to the changes in the anatomical conformation of the body. The adjustments in treatment position using CBCT imaging is often used without being able to accurately estimate the consequences from the point of view of toxicities and tumor control [2, 18–20].

Currently, replanning of treatment using weekly CBCT imaging for radiotherapy patients can be done during the course of treatment, to provide a more accurate dose and to avoid erroneous treatment due to daily movement of organs. Adaptive radiation therapy is defined as changing the radiological treatment plan delivered to a patient during a course of radiation therapy to take into account temporal changes in anatomy, such as tumor contraction, weight loss, or internal movement, etc. However, the biological consequences of this intervention during the course of treatment may remain unclear to some practitioners. The clinical impact of adaptive radiotherapy has been evaluated using biological modeling of bladder cancer. In the Wright et al. study, various adaptive planning target volumes (PTV) were generated from the inter-fractional variation of the bladder observed in the first four CBCT sessions. In addition to IMRT plans that deliver 60 Gy to a given PTV, simultaneous integrated impulse (SIB) plans have been generated. For uniform clonogenic cell density throughout the bladder, TCP ranged from 53–58% for 60 Gy planes, while it was between 51 and 64% for SIB planes. They showed that dose tracking and TCP calculation can provide additional information on standard criteria, such as geometric coverage for selected cases [20–23].

It is assumed that the use of IGRT can lead to an improvement in TCP by increasing the PTV dose coverage in daily treatment while decreasing NTCP by using low uncertainty CTV-PTV margins in the case of prostate cancer radiotherapy, demonstrating the ability to improve therapeutic for both IMRT and 3D-CRT plans.

With all the efforts made to develop radiobiological models, they remain ideal models. Including the individual biological parameters of the patients in the treatment decision will contribute to the understanding of differentiated response of tumors to radiotherapy and will be able to transform these models into feasible models applicable in clinical practice. The number of malignant stem cells and their intrinsic cell radiosensitivity, cell repopulation, tumor and tissue hypoxia, and the ability of tumor cells to reoxygenate and repair DNA damage are factors whose introduction into the radiobiological mathematical models will increase the accuracy of each case of tumor control and toxicity predictions. Thus, a step forward will be taken in the use of these models in clinical practice within the concept of personalized medicine, modulating the treatment for each patient in order to obtain the best therapeutic ratio.

Identifying new biomarkers to guide radiotherapy tailored to each case depending on the radiosensitivity of tumor cells and healthy tissue requires the identification of a large number of pre-therapeutic factors with predictive value on tumor toxicity and control. If the data obtained from the tumor histology and the patient performance status and comorbidities are taken into account in the evaluation and pre-therapeutic optimization of the plans, the biological parameters of the tumor are rarely considered in the modulation of the treatment. Also, early response to imaging-evaluated therapy may be a predictive factor of tumor control [2, 23–25].

The development, validation, and integration of imaging biomarkers using CT, PET-CT, and MRI to improve the response to radiotherapy are part of the areas of interest of clinical and preclinical studies, this research directive being integrated under the name of "radiomics." There are two directions for using predictive biomarkers for individualized treatment, to choose the treatment offered to a patient (e.g., intensifying and choosing a multimodal therapy for a hypoxic tumor with radiation and chemotherapy resistance factors or de-escalating treatment for tumors with radiosensitivity-associated factors such as HPV viral etiology for head and neck cancers). The modulation of the treatment by altered therapeutic and fractional associations (hypo- and hyperfractionation) aims to obtain a higher TCP with the limitation of NTCP of the tissues from the vicinity of target volumes, avoiding the risk of toxicity [2, 24, 26, 27].

Biomarkers can also be used for early evaluation of therapeutic outcomes to decide whether to discontinue or continue a therapeutic procedure or modify the initial treatment, but validating some biomarkers and including them in radiobiological models that are part of the clinical decision algorithm is still a strategy used only in preclinical and clinical studies. Regarding systemic therapy significant progress has been made, by discovering new therapeutic targets that have changed the clinical oncological practice, making it necessary to identify biomarkers to guide the therapeutic decision. HER-2 and hormone receptor status evaluated at breast cancer patient biopsy is currently used for therapeutic protocol decision, EGFR mutation targets treatment for targeted molecular therapy in lung cancer, KRAS mutational status is integrated into colorectal cancer treatment to allocate patients for anti-EGFR therapies for KRAS wild-type tumors, PD-L1 expression becomes a marker of response to immunotherapy in more and more nonplastic locations, and even though we have presented only a few suggestive examples, there is an increasing number of biomarkers with potential predictive for response to radiotherapy [2, 5, 27, 28].

Radiation oncology has a long history of research into understanding the implications of genetics in the variation of the response to treatment for each patient in order to personalize the therapy. The identification of new biological signaling pathways will explain the variation in the individual response of some tumors to irradiation. The use of elements from the genetic signature of each patient could constitute biomarkers of the clinical response to irradiation by modifying radiosensitivity of the tumor and healthy tissue. Since 1936 the different effects for subjects of irradiation with an identical radiation dose have been demonstrated by the occurrence of early skin toxicity, the near-Gaussian frequency distribution of individual sensitivity being highlighted. Subsequent research has shown the involvement of genetic syndromes in the early onset of toxicities, with the subtraction of cell hypersensitivity to irradiation, caused by affecting the DNA chain repair mechanisms. In addition to the ATM gene associated with ataxia-telangiectasia syndrome, other genes such as NBS1, LIG4, and MRE11 have been linked with syndromes associated with high radiosensitivity, caused by impaired DNA chain repair mechanisms [29, 30].

Modern radiobiology research has highlighted the applicability of genomics in predicting the adverse effects of radiotherapy, based on the application of genomics in radio-oncology. Advances in high-throughput approaches will support increased understanding of radiosensitivity and the development of future predictive analyses for clinical application. There is an established contribution of genetic risk factor to adverse radiotherapy reactions. The radiosensitivity of an individual is an inherited polygenic feature, and in order to elucidate the genomic involvement in radiosensitivity, the Radiogenomics Consortium was set up to allow large data cohorts for research development, and the REQUITE project would collect standardized and genotyped data for~5000 patients [31]. Linking their information with the dosimetric data will lead to the generation of multivariable models that can be used in the clinic, identifying new genes that have an impact on the radiosensitivity of the toxicity pathogenesis and the tests that will be incorporated into the clinical decision-making process [30, 32].

The development in the last decades of imagistic techniques and their non-invasive or minimally invasive character allowed the dynamic evaluation of the changes of the biological characteristics of the tumor. Molecular imaging brings pre-treatment information but also has the ability to evaluate the changes produced by the treatment since the first irradiation fractions. CT and MRI imaging already has a significant role in radiotherapy planning, CT simulation becoming a standard, and MRI imaging contributes to a more precise delineation of tumor invasion into adjacent organelles. The increasing use and availability of PET-CT imaging and its inclusion in treatment planning make it possible to use different tracers as a biomarker of tumor radiosensitivity in click practice [33]. *18F*-Fluorodeoxyglucose (18F-FDG) is one of the most used biomarkers in experimental and clinical investigations, the SUV values before and during the treatment being investigated as possible biomarkers of the treatment by chemotherapy and radiotherapy. The concept of "biological dose painting" is based on the delimitation of target volumes on functional criteria; the irradiation of a tumor with different doses and the escalation of the doses in areas with high uptake of 18F-FDG were discussed with the introduction of IMRT and VMAT techniques that allow the irradiation with different doses of some subvolumes from the target volume. 18F-FDG can identify tumor regions with high cell density and radioresistant regions due to hypoxia. Identifying the most common relapses after radiotherapy in the areas with higher uptake of 18F-FDG is a new argument for dose escalation in these regions.

The observation that in several cases of locally advanced cancers the tumor control after irradiation was not satisfactory made necessary a careful analysis of the areas where recurrence occurs. The analysis of the characteristics of the tumors with recurrence risk revealed an increased risk for the hypoxic regions or with an increased number of clonogens with proliferation capacity. One of the strategies used to control the tumor response is to use the boost on subvolumes with radioresistance pattern, considering the results of the studies that prove the survival rates associated with better locoregional control [34, 35].

The use of routine boost for all patients is a controversial topic. For head and neck cancers and for prostate cancer, there was a benefit in escalating doses by 10–20% in the topographic regions of the tumor with an increased risk of recurrence. An EORTC trial shows a minor benefit of breast boost but with a significant increase in toxicity rate.

Using radiobiological models, an increase of up to 20% of the TCP was observed in the case of a 10–30% dose escalation on a sub-volume of 60–80% of the primary tumor target volume. The introduction of IGRT and PET-CT hybrid imaging opens the horizons of a new challenge, the topographic identification of the region where the boost will be made, based on the clinical rationale balancing the benefit and the toxicities.

Adaptive risk optimization uses a biological objective function instead of an objective function based on dose-volume constraints, maximizing TCP for different regions of the tumor with recurrent risk while also minimizing NTCP for risk organs [2, 26, 36].

The tendency to include biological information in radiotherapy will lead to the use of cellular, molecular, and physiological characteristics in the treatment planning. PET-CT radiotracers 18F-FMISO-PET,^{60}Cu-ATSM-PET, and blood oxygen diffusion (BOLD)-MRI are frequently investigated in translational research related to tumor hypoxia. Investigation of tumor proliferation proved benefits from 18F-labeled fluorotime (FLT) as a biomarker.

The development of multivariable radiobiological models and dose prescription protocol based on functional data obtained from hybrid imaging is part of the tendency to include modern radiotherapy in the precision medicine trend, exploiting variations in tumor radiosensitivity and healthy tissues in clinical practice [2, 21, 37, 38].

Author details

Camil Ciprian Mirestean[1,2], Călin Gheorghe Buzea[3], Roxana Irina Iancu[4,5] and Dragoș Petru Teodor Iancu[3,5]*

1 Euroclinic Oncological Center, Iasi, România

2 University of Medicine and Pharmacy Craiova, România

3 Regional Institute of Oncology, Iasi, Romania

4 Universitary Emergency "St. Spiridon" Hospital, Iasi, Romania

5 University of Medicine and Pharmacy "Gr. T. Popa", Iasi, Romania

*Address all correspondence to: dt_iancu@yahoo.com

References

[1] Rubin P, Constine LS, Marks LB. ALERT Adverse Late Effects of Cancer Treatment: Volume 1: General Concepts and Specific Precepts, Volume 2: Normal Tissue Specific Sites and Systems. New York: Springer; 2014

[2] Bortfeld T, Schmidt-Ullrich R, De Neve W, Wazer DE. Image-Guided IMRT.Berlin Heidelberg: Springer; 2006

[3] Pacelli R, Caroprese M, Palma G, Oliviero C, Clemente S, Cella L, et al. Technological evolution of radiation treatment: Implications for clinical applications. Seminars in Oncology. 2019;**30**: pii: S0093-7754(19)30098-3

[4] Choi EJ, Ryu YK, Kim SY, Wu HG, Kim JS, Kim IH, et al. Targeting epidermal growth factor receptor-associated signaling pathways in non-small cell lung cancer cells: Implication in radiation response. Molecular Cancer Research. 2010;**8**(7):1027-1036

[5] Dobbs JE, Barrett A, Roques T. Practical Radiotherapy Planning. 4th ed. Boca Raton, Florida: CRC Press; 2009

[6] Emami B, Lyman J, Brown A, et al. Tolerance of normal tissue to therapeutic irradiation. International Journal of Radiation Oncology, Biology, Physics. 1991;**21**(1):109-122

[7] Emami B. Tolerance of normal tissue to therapeutic radiation. Reports of Radiotherapy and Oncology. 2013;**1**(1):36-48

[8] Bentzen SM, Constine LS, Deasy JO. Quantitative analyses of normal tissue effects in the clinic (QUANTEC): An introduction to the scientific issues. International Journal of Radiation Oncology, Biology, Physics. 2010;**76** (3 Suppl):S3-S9

[9] Van der Kogel A, Joiner M. Basic Clinical Radiobiology. 4th ed. London: Hodder Arnold Publication; 2009

[10] Warkentin B, Stavrev P, Stavreva N, Field C, Fallone BG. A TCP-NTCP estimation module using DVHs and known radiobiological models and parameter sets. Journal of Applied Clinical Medical Physics. 2004;**5**(1):50-63

[11] Mayo C, Yorke E, Merchant TE. Radiation associated brainstem injury. International Journal of Radiation Oncology, Biology, Physics. 2010;**76**(3 Suppl):S36-S41

[12] Kirkpatrick JP, van der Kogel AJ, Schultheiss TE. Radiation dose-volume effects in the spinal cord. International Journal of Radiation Oncology, Biology, Physics. 2010;**76**(3 Suppl):S42-S49. DOI: 10.1016/j.ijrobp.2009.04.095

[13] Jensen I, Carl J, Lund B, et al. Radiobiological impact of reduced margins and treatment technique for prostate cancer in terms of tumor control probability (TCP) and normal tissue complication probability (NTCP). Medical Dosimetry. 2011;**36**(2):130-137

[14] Mesbahi A, Rasouli N, Mohammadzadeh M, Motlagh BN, Tekin HO. Comparison of radiobiological models for radiation therapy plans of prostate cancer: Three-dimensional conformal versus intensity modulated radiation therapy. Journal of Biomedical Physics and Engineering. 2019;**9**(3):267-278

[15] Luxton G, Hancock SL, Boyer AL. Dosimetry and radiobiologic model comparison of IMRT and 3D conformal radiotherapy in treatment of carcinoma of the prostate. International Journal of Radiation Oncology, Biology, Physics. 2004;**59**(1):267-284

[16] Gago-Arias A, Sánchez-Nieto B, Espinoza I, Karger C, Pardo-Montero J. Impact of different biologically-adapted radiotherapy strategies on tumor control evaluated with a tumor response model. PLoS One. 2018;**13**(4):e0196310

[17] Rana S, Greco K, Samuel E, Bennouna J. Radiobiological and dosimetric impact of RayStation pencil beam and Monte Carlo algorithms on intensity-modulated proton therapy breast cancer plans. Journal of Applied Clinical Medical Physics. 2019;**20**(8):36-46

[18] Battista JJ, Johnson C, Turnbull D, Kempe J, Bzdusek K, Van Dyk J, et al. Dosimetric and radiobiological consequences of computed tomography-guided adaptive strategies for intensity modulated radiation therapy of the prostate. International Journal of Radiation Oncology, Biology, Physics. 2013;**87**(5):874-880

[19] Liu Q, Liang J, Zhou D, Krauss DJ, Chen PY, Yan D. Dosimetric evaluation of incorporating patient geometric variations into adaptive plan optimization through probabilistic treatment planning in head and neck cancers. International Journal of Radiation Oncology, Biology, Physics. 2018;**101**(4):985-997

[20] Roland T, Mavroidis P, Gutierrez A, et al. A radiobiological analysis of the effect of 3D versus 4D image-based planning in lung cancer radiotherapy. Physics in Medicine and Biology. 2009;**54**(18):5509-5523

[21] Nahum AE, Uzan J. (Radio) biological optimization of external-beam radiotherapy. Computational and Mathematical Methods in Medicine. 2012;**2012**:329214

[22] Wright P, Muren LP, Hoyer M, et al. Evaluation of adaptive radiotherapy of bladder cancer by image-based tumour control probability modelling. Acta Oncologica. 2010;**49**(7):1045-1051

[23] Siochi RA, Kim Y, Bhatia S. Tumor control probability reduction in gated radiotherapy of non-small cell lung cancers: A feasibility study. Journal of Applied Clinical Medical Physics. 2014;**16**(1):4444

[24] Bansal A, Kapoor R, Singh SK, et al. Dosimetric comparison of standard three-dimensional conformal radiotherapy followed by intensity-modulated radiotherapy boost schedule (sequential IMRT plan) with simultaneous integrated boost-IMRT (SIB IMRT) treatment plan in patients with localized carcinoma prostate. Indian Journal of Urology. 2012;**s28**(3):300-306

[25] López Alfonso JC, Parsai S, Joshi N, Godley A, Shah C, Koyfman SA, et al. Temporally feathered intensity-modulated radiation therapy: A planning technique to reduce normal tissue toxicity. Medical Physics. 2018;**45**(7):3466-3474

[26] Fonti R, Conson M, Del Vecchio S. PET/CT in radiation oncology. Seminars in Oncology. 26 July 2019. pii: S0093-7754(19)30079-X

[27] Gurtner K, Kryzmien Z, Koi L, Wang M, Benes CH, Hering S, et al. Radioresistance of KRAS/TP53-mutated lung cancer can be overcome by radiation dose escalation or EGFR tyrosine kinase inhibition in vivo. International Journal of Cancer. 29 July 2019

[28] Anakura M, Nachankar A, Kobayashi D, Amornwichet N, Hirota Y, Shibata A, et al. Radiosensitivity differences between EGFR mutant and wild-type lung cancer cells are larger at lower doses. International Journal of Molecular Sciences. 2019;**20**(15):E3635

[29] Williams JR, Zhang Y, Zhou H, Gridley DS, Koch CJ, Slater JM, et al.

Overview of radiosensitivity of human tumor cells to low-dose-rate irradiation. International Journal of Radiation Biology. 1996;**69**(3):279-290

[30] Kerns SL, Chuang KH, Hall W, Werner Z, Chen Y, Ostrer H, et al. Radiation biology and oncology in the genomic era. International Journal of Radiation Oncology, Biology, Physics. 2008;**72**(3):909-917

[31] van Lin EN, Futterer JJ, Heijmink SW, et al. IMRT boost dose planning on dominant intraprostatic lesions: Gold marker-based three-dimensional fusion of CT with dynamic contrast-enhanced and 1H-spectroscopic MRI. International Journal of Radiation Oncology, Biology, Physics. 2006;**65**(1):291-303

[32] West C, Azria D, Chang-Claude J, Davidson S, Lambin P, Rosenstein B, et al. The REQUITE project: Validating predictive models and biomarkers of radiotherapy toxicity to reduce side-effects and improve quality of life in cancer survivors. Clinical Oncology. 2014;**26**(12):739-742

[33] Sanchez-Nieto B, Nahum AE, Dearnaley DP. Individualization of dose prescription based on normal-tissue dose-volume and radiosensitivity data. International Journal of Radiation Oncology, Biology, Physics. 2001;**49**(2):487-499

[34] Bradley J, Thorstad WL, Mutic S, Miller TR, Dehdashti F, Siegel BA, et al. Impact of FDG-PET on radiation therapy volume delineation in non-small-cell lung cancer. International Journal of Radiation Oncology, Biology, Physics. 2004;**59**(1):78-86

[35] Kairemo K. PET/CT in External Beam Radiation therapy dose planning. Current Radiopharmaceuticals 2015;8(1):1

[36] Briens A, Castelli J, Barateau A, Jaksic N, Gnep K, Simon A, et al. [Adaptive radiotherapy: Strategies and benefits depending on tumor localization]. [Article in French]. Cancer Radiothérapie. 2019. pii: S1278-3218(19)30311-7

[37] Reynaert N. PET and MRI based RT treatment planning: Handling uncertainties. Cancer Radiothérapie. Ṅ2019. 2019;**23**(6-7):753-760

[38] Mackay RI, Hendry JH. The modelled benefits of individualizing radiotherapy patients' dose using cellular radiosensitivity assays with inherent variability. Radiotherapy and Oncology. 1999;**50**(1):67-75